VOID

Library of
Davidson College

the people's handbook of medical care

Random House / New York

the people's handbook of medical care

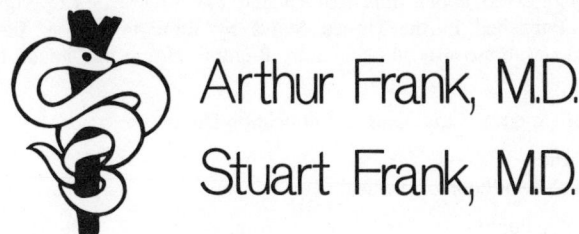

Arthur Frank, M.D.
Stuart Frank, M.D.

Copyright © 1972 by Arthur Frank, M.D. and Stuart Frank, M.D.

All rights reserved under International and Pan-American Copyright Conventions. Published in the United States by Random House, Inc., New York, and simultaneously in Canada by Random House of Canada Limited, Toronto.

Library of Congress Cataloging in Publication Data

Frank, Arthur.
The people's handbook of medical care.

1. Medicine, Popular. I. Frank, Stuart, joint author. II. Title. [DNLM: 1. Medicine—Popular works. WB 120 F827p 1972]
RC81.F82   1972   616   72–4593
ISBN 0-394-47925-4

Manufactured in the United States of America by American Book–Stratford Press, New York, N.Y.

98765432

to Barbara
to Suzanne
to our parents
and to the people, our patients, who teach us

Contents

Introduction	xi
1: The Business of Medicine and How to Deal with It	3
Doctors	4
Hospitals	6
Medical Costs	8
How to Identify Good Sources of Medical Care	13
What to Do in an Emergency	17
2: Your Medical Rights and Privileges	20
Obtaining Medical Care	20
Emergency Rooms	22
Treatment of Minors	25
First Aid	26
Fees	27
Liability	27
Privacy and Confidentiality	28
Reportable Diseases	29
Mental Patients	30
Medical Care in Jails	31
3: Recognizing Disease	34
Pain	34
Fever	42
Breathing Irregularities and Coughing	47
Bleeding and Anemia	55
Functions of the Brain	58
Functions of the Heart	70

Intestinal Functions	83
Skin and Hair	97

4: Medical Emergencies — 106

Shock	106
Head Injuries	108
Eye Injuries	115
Chest Injuries	120
Abdominal Injuries	128
Fractures, Strains, and Sprains	132
Cuts and Bruises	141
Burns	151
Bullet and Stab Wounds	156
Cardiac Arrest and Cardiac Massage	159
Tetanus	170

5: Common Ailments — 174

The Common Cold	174
Hepatitis and Jaundice	179
Infectious Mononucleosis	186
Urinary Tract Infections	188
Hemorrhoids	192
Traveler's Diarrhea	195
Vaginitis	199
Menstrual Problems	203
Hiccups	205
Nosebleed	207
Earaches	210
Toothaches and Dental Problems	214
Acne	217
Bad Breath	222
Thrombophlebitis	224
Motion and Sea Sickness	227
Insects, Rabies, and Snakebites	230
Sunstroke and Frostbite	241

6: Social and Political Medicine 246

Psychotropic Drugs 246
Medical Draft Counseling 272
Tear Gas and Chemical Warfare 278
Venereal Disease 291
Sex and Pre-Marital Counseling 300
Birth Control 303
Pregnancy 312
Abortion 324
Rape 326
Psychiatric Problems 329

7: Food, Nutrition and Obesity 347

8: Medical Supplies and Equipment 371

What to Get 371
Where to Get It 384

Appendices

I. Chapters of the Medical Committee for Human Rights 393
II. Free Clinic Directory 399
III. Medical Fitness Standards for Appointment, Enlistment, and Induction 410
IV. 4-F Memo 449
V. Summary of State Abortion Laws 471

Index 475

Introduction

This handbook has evolved out of our experiences as doctors providing general medical care, working in neighborhood free clinics, and organizing medical care for political and civil rights demonstrations. It was suggested by our recognition of the failure of the American medical care system to provide anything like the "right to health" for millions of people, who for reasons of income, skin color, language, age, or life style, have no access to adequate or dignified treatment.

This material reflects four simple but quite strongly held convictions: First, people can learn to be responsible for a substantial part of their own medical care, for such care is increasingly expensive, inadequate, or administered under such degrading conditions as to be of little value. Second, much information about medicine is couched in needlessly obscure terms. In order for the public to learn to take care of itself, medical information must be made accessible; it should be presented in informal language free of "mystery" and awe. Third, the inadequacy of existing medical books for the general public and the failure of medical training programs to recognize the social perspective of some medical problems is astonishing. Little, for example, has been written about the treatment of tear gas injuries; much of what is written about the treatment of drug problems is naïve, puritanical, and punitive. No book explains how to take care of a friend with hepatitis, how to tell if you have gonorrhea, how to get rid of crabs, what to do if you get raped, how to manage with a cast, how to deal with emergency-room medical care, or what to do if you are hit with a billy club. And finally, we believe that the persistent American fantasy about the beneficence, ubiquity and omniscience of the medical profession needs to be discussed in a more realistic perspective. People can obtain better medical care if they understand how medical care is provided.

The People's Handbook of Medical Care, therefore, differs from the standard medical handbook in several ways:

It describes the medical industry and how it works.

It contains information on the manifestations of disease to provide the reader with a practical concept of illness and a means by which to interpret symptoms.

It discusses the patient's medical rights and privileges.

It emphasizes the measures which should be taken if adequate professional care cannot be anticipated; if there is no ambulance available; if there is no hospital nearby, or none that will readily accept you. Suggestions on secondary treatment as well as first aid are included.

It indicates the serious nature of certain injuries and distinguishes between life-threatening situations and common problems which do not require a doctor or hospital. It emphasizes how you can take care of yourself with a minimum of expensive, sometimes dangerous, and often unnecessary medications.

It includes information about certain types of diseases which are made more serious simply because so much misinformation about them is available.

It describes precautionary measures to be taken by those who anticipate exposure to violence.

It identifies the medical supplies that might be needed, tells how to get them, and how to equip a medical aid station.

The People's Handbook of Medical Care is not an encyclopedia. Reading it will not make you an expert or enable you to practice expert medicine on yourself or anyone else. It does not answer all questions, or deal with all situations. It does not discuss, except indirectly, the medical problems of an aging population (heart disease, cancer, etc.) or the unique problems of infants and children.

Since we are obliged to generalize and to discuss the usual course of events, we must qualify our recommendations, relying heavily upon the reader's judgment to recognize when his circumstances require modification. There is very little in this book that is sacred, and nothing that is applicable to every situation. We trust that our readers will vindicate the faith we have in their judgment and will not take as gospel everything we say.

No book like this is ever exclusively the product of one or two individuals. Ours is no exception. We are indebted to our professional and lay colleagues from whose experiences we have learned a great deal. We have never worked alone at a demonstration or in a clinic. Our friends in the Medical Committee for Human Rights have long been leading the fight for the concept of health care as a human right, and we have profited greatly by our discussions with MCHR people and others from all over the country. We hope to continue to profit from those who will be kind enough to call our attention to the errors or omissions which may have appeared in this book.

We are grateful also for the help of a number of individuals: in particular, Steve Walsh, who assisted with the organization of the section on Psychiatric Problems; Aaron Altschul, who carefully reviewed the chapter on Food, Nutrition and Obesity; Fran Freeman, Denise Bechtel and Ralph Bernheimer for typing and editorial assistance; Jerry Schwartz for the list of Free Clinics; and Frank Goldsmith for the list of chapters of the Medical Committee for Human Rights. We are also indebted to the National Center for Family Planning Services of the Department of Health, Education and Welfare, and Jan Liebman of Planned Parenthood for some of the information from which the updated list of state abortion laws was prepared;

and to the Central Committee for Conscientious Objectors (CCCO) for the 4-F Memo which is reproduced in part in the Appendix.

A. F.
S. F.

the people's handbook of medical care

1 The Business of Medicine and How to Deal with It

Medicine is a business as well as a science and an art. Anyone who regards it simply as a sacred calling beyond the greed and avarice of twentieth-century America is putting himself at a substantial disadvantage in negotiating for the purchase of the very specialized services that doctors and hospitals are selling.

The average person regards the medical profession with awe and fear. He hopes to avoid it for as long as possible, but when he is forced to deal with it he usually regresses to the behavior of an anxious nine-year-old and allows himself to be led passively through a maze of out-patient and in-patient care, referrals, consultations, x-rays, operations, enemas, and sleeping pills. This mindless cooperation is seldom resented by the patient and is particularly agreeable to the health professionals. Consequently, the system, with its public relations and its shiny, complicated equipment, creates the illusion of working tolerably well—at least for middle America. It obviously collapses under the weight of such problems as the care of 30 million American poor, the elderly, the family that doesn't speak English, the radical, or the individual with unusual appearance or life style.

The medical care business thrives on the passivity of the patient and reinforces the mysticism of medicine. It should be recognized that this atmosphere of benevolence is used primarily for business purposes. The patient should not be distracted from using his critical faculties in dealing with the medical industry. He should try to understand the financial aspects of medical care and then evaluate the quality of the service he has arranged to purchase. At the very least, choosing medical care should be given the same consideration that applies to the process of selecting the man who works on the inside of one's car.

When the patient buys medical care he is at a disadvantage by virtue of the illness or injury which forces him to obtain the service under stress. It is therefore worthwhile to get some background information about how the system works, how it is constructed, who feeds it and who oils it.

Doctors

The medical care system depends upon doctors. It depends also on many other health professionals but, in the U.S., health care and doctors are synonymous. New ways to provide some types of health care by less expensive non-doctor personnel are already being used, and will ultimately reduce the medical mystique. In the meantime, however, your care, unless you do it yourself, depends largely on a doctor. The medical profession polices itself very poorly. The incompetent doctors, the alcoholics, the psychotics are rarely weeded out, and then only with great soul searching and self-righteous deliberation. Nevertheless, most doctors are not charlatans; and you can often obtain adequate, even superior medical care from many doctors.

After finishing college, the doctor spends an additional four years in medical school. His education is fairly intensive but it is universally acknowledged that medical school alone does not provide enough training for a graduate to take care of all the varieties of very sick people that he will encounter in his practice. When he graduates, the doctor will spend more time working and studying in a hospital that may or may not be affiliated with a medical school. This training consists of fewer lectures, labs, and libraries, and more patients, hospital wards, and operating rooms.

Virtually every medical school graduate will spend a year as an intern.* Interns are doctors. In most states they can be licensed to practice medicine, although their license may limit

---

* An internist is not the same as an intern. The former is a specialist in internal medicine, a highly developed specialty concerned with adult medical diseases excluding surgery, dermatology, psychiatry, etc.

their activities to the hospital in which they receive their training, and even then they can practice only under supervision. Most interns, particularly those who plan to specialize, continue their training as a resident. A residency is a program of hospital training in a medical specialty, for example, pediatrics, psychiatry, surgery, and takes from two to five additional years, depending on the specialty, after completing an internship. Residents are fully licensed to practice medicine. It is these interns and residents who make up the "house staff," those doctors who take care of hospitalized patients and who staff the hospital's clinics and emergency room.

Specialty training for the doctor is entirely optional. Once he has a license, a physician can practice medicine. The nature of his practice, whether he specializes or not, what he specializes in—none of these is determined by license or law, but rather by an informal balance of his training and interests, his experience, the regulations of the hospital to which he admits his patients, and his own integrity. Most medical specialties set forth procedures by which a doctor can be recognized as competent. This recognition, however, or "board certification," as it is called, is only a highly respected formality. It frequently is a measure of access to hospital privileges. It is not a legal certification to practice as a specialist and no legal certification is required for a doctor to practice whatever he wants. Medical organizations such as the American College of Surgeons or the American Board of Internal Medicine have very high certification standards, requiring specific training and the completion of detailed examinations. This certification is an excellent way to be reassured of a doctor's basic skills in that specialty.

Lack of certification does not mean, however, that your doctor doesn't know what he is doing. Many capable doctors practice in a particular specialty without having been certified in it. Specialty skills are helpful in the treatment of complex or rare illnesses, but they are not always necessary. Most medical problems are simple and can be handled by a capable general practitioner. The dilemma for the general practitioner, and for the patient, is the rapid expansion of knowledge. It is extraordinarily difficult for a busy doctor to maintain his skills in a number of medical areas simultaneously. It is hard enough for a doctor to keep current in one special area and almost impossible to do it in many. The honest general practitioner finds that he must refer a steadily expanding fraction of his patients for specialty care, and you will have to trust his judgment on when your problem exceeds his skills. Since most doctors have too many patients anyway, money will seldom be a factor in his decision about whether to send you to another doctor.

There is a rapidly developing trend for doctors to join together and practice in a group. The solo practitioner, the doctor who practices in an office by himself, is going the way of the general practitioner. Not only is it too impractical for a doctor to be available twenty-four hours a day every day, but modern medicine is far too complex for him to be comfortable and honest about treating all the medical problems which he might encounter. Doctors join together in groups to consult with each other, to provide day and night care, to save expenses, and to make more money. The size, type, and financial arrangements of medical groups are extremely varied. The benefits to the patient under the care of a medical group are obvious: although he may see a different doctor sometimes, it is reassuring to know that one of them is always available and that consultations among them are accessible.

Most, but not all, doctors have a hospital affiliation. Those who do not, refer patients who need hospitalization to more experienced doctors and some (a dermatologist, for example) only rarely have occasion to hospitalize anyone.

Hospitals

Administratively and financially there are three types of hospitals: private, public, and voluntary or non-profit.

7 † The Business of Medicine and How to Deal with It

Private hospitals, operated for a profit, are not charitable, have very few benevolent feelings, seldom have a capable house staff and rarely provide high-quality care. In a large city they may offer opulent facilities (at a price), peace and quiet and, if you desire, anonymity. In many rural areas they may be the only hospital around and may be owned and operated by the only doctor around. In these latter cases it takes an individual doctor with iron integrity and incredible honesty to avoid a real or apparent conflict of interest. Larger private hospitals may have a number of physicians on their staff, each caring for his own patients with a minimum of interference or control by his colleagues or by the hospital administration. Private hospitals may not be accredited (a procedure which requires that they conform to certain reasonable standards regarding facilities, staff, and functioning), even though they may be fully licensed in a community. The quality of the care you get at a private hospital depends mostly on the doctor, but you can assume that, except for rare circumstances, the hospital itself will be of marginal assistance and marginal quality. Private hospitals should be avoided if you have an option.

Public hospitals are run by a governmental agency: the city, the county, the state, or the federal government. Originally these hospitals were designed to care for the poor. Recently built public hospitals may care for patients other than the medically indigent and may operate much like voluntary hospitals. Traditionally, public hospitals hire doctors to take care of patients who cannot afford private medical care. The salvation of this unlikely and impractical system has been the hospitals' affiliation with the medical schools. Most of the large public hospitals enjoy an affiliation in which the patients and facilities of the hospital are used to augment the medical school's teaching program. In return, the medical school provides the hospital with qualified and motivated house staff and supervising senior attending staff to care for the patients. The big public hospitals are highly respected for the training they provide for doctors, and for the exhaustive care given the patients, but are much criticized for the quality of the hospital services.* Often, the care is of high quality, although the surroundings may be outrageously primitive, the ancillary services may be inadequate or entirely absent, and the comfortable amenities may be totally neglected (for example, thirty to forty sick people lined up in beds in one large room). A public hospital which is not affiliated with a medical school should be avoided if possible.

Voluntary or non-profit hospitals operate somewhere between the public and the private hospitals. The sources of their financial support may include public funds (a bond issue, for example), private contributions, church support or patient fees. Depending on the local circumstances, these hospitals may or may not care for indigent patients and may do so by various complicated arrangements with government agencies, private physicians, or through their own clinics. They may have a house staff; if they do, this should be marked as a plus. They may have a medical school affiliation; if they do, this is another big plus. They may have a sense of responsibility to their community and a sense of social conscience, but such commitments from voluntary hospitals are not common. They are usually governed by a quasi-public board of trustees with the details of their organization dependent on their sources of money. Apart from a house staff, their doctors are usually local physicians who have an arrangement with the hospitals which permits them to admit their private patients.

Medical Costs

It is unfortunate that money should be even a remote consideration in obtaining or providing medical care. When you are sick, even with a minor discomfort, and much more with a serious illness, good treatment should be available to you and

---

* Cook County Hospital in Chicago, Bellevue Hospital in New York, Boston City Hospital, and some others have excellent reputations which far exceed their geographical jurisdiction responsibilities.

9 † The Business of Medicine and How to Deal with It

its cost or how it will be paid for should be irrelevant. But this just isn't so. Someone has to pay for the doctors' time, the x-rays and the medications. And with very little outside help, that someone is you.

It is very expensive to get sick. If there were no assistance with medical bills, the costs of medical care would be prohibitive for 99 per cent of the American population. Most doctors in America still use a system called "fee for service" in their practice, which means simply that you pay for each office visit, hospital visit, or house call. Sometimes a blanket fee can be arranged to pay for an illness requiring an operation or for pregnancy and delivery. (Prepayment plans discussed later are a form of medical insurance.) If you are hospitalized, room charges, laboratory charges, operating room charges are all in addition to the fee you pay the doctor. The average daily cost of a hospital bed is about $75. And that is precisely what you are paying for—the bed. Everything else (except, but not always, the meals) is extra. It is a rare patient who gets out of the hospital for less than $100 per day. It's a very expensive and not too pleasant hotel room for someone who wants to rest up or dry out for a few days.

In America there are three categories of medical care: 1) an unreasonably expensive system for the rich; 2) an increasingly deteriorating system for the middle class; and 3) an unconscionably bad system for the poor. Although the medical industry and the AMA will loudly deny it, the quality of medical care often depends on one's ability to pay, and the three categories pay in four different ways:

Class A for the rich who pay directly;
Class B for those who have medical insurance;
Class C for those on some form of public assistance or welfare, and
Class D for those with no financial resources.

The Class A rich can count on getting much attention for their money; but they cannot count on the best medical care, especially if they choose their doctor on the basis of reputation and personality, or what is known as "bedside manner." Those who pay directly have immediate access to a physician and to hospitalization, even if neither is required. You qualify for this arrangement if you have substantial resources or if you are willing to go into debt.

Most of middle America falls into Class B, those covered by medical insurance. The medical industry and the AMA have continued to condemn any form of "socialized medicine" by pointing with pride to the fact that 75 per cent of Americans are covered by voluntary medical insurance. They carefully neglect to mention the fact that the average medical insurance does not include out-patient charges (those medical charges which are incurred outside a hospital), includes only a variable part of the hospital charges, and covers only about one-third of medicine bills. You may be covered by your own medical insurance either through your place of employment or school or by your parents' insurance, depending on your age and the fine print on the policy. Medical insurance is an unfortunate necessity, but you should get it if you can afford it and if it is available to you.

Medicare is, in effect, a form of medical insurance. Your payments to the social security system during your working years enable you to purchase this inexpensive insurance when you are over sixty-five and when the cost of this insurance would normally be too high for most older people.

Under the present system of medical insurance, the doctor bills the insurance company for whatever services he provides. Other than through the overstrained mechanism of the doctor's integrity, there is no satisfactory way to avoid extra, often unneeded services since the doctor's fees are directly related to the amount of service he provides. Because the doctor controls the amount of medical care you receive, there tends to be some overutilization. One way to eliminate this built-in inefficiency involves financing medical care by prepayment: you pay a fixed charge every month to receive preventive care or care during an illness. In prepayment there is a clear incentive for the doctor to function efficiently, to avoid unnecessary operations or treatment and to try to keep you well by the few techniques that exist for effective preventive health. Experience suggests that, in general, these systems provide high-quality health care at a lower cost than the fee-for-service system. While it eliminates incentives for overutilization by the doctor, it does not exclude the reverse, underutilization, or unavailability. Particular attention must be taken by doctors and patients to assure that quality is maintained in a prepaid system. Since some prepaid systems are actually patient-owned cooperatives the opportunity for consumer assurance of quality and consumer control exists here as it does in no other form of medical practice. If you live in an area where prepayment plans exist, it may be to your advantage to see if they are suitable for your needs.

If you are entitled to some sort of public assistance or welfare, particularly for medical bills, then you fall into Class C. It is worth your while to apply for such assistance even though this process invariably involves much paper work and getting tangled up in the government's guilt-ridden system of making you feel less than human for not being rich. Medicaid (Title XIX as it is sometimes called) will pay for most of your medical bills if you are eligible. The benefits and eligibility requirements vary widely and you should find out what they are in your area. Even if you are not eligible for Medicaid you may still be able to get some other kind of financial assistance. The resources and benevolence of the states, communities, or counties are remarkably different. In some cases, you can apply retroactively after you have been hospitalized or have received medical care.

If you fall into Class C you may find that your doctor gives you less attention than he does to his private patients, the erroneous implication being that you aren't free to choose your doctor, or dismiss him if you are dissatisfied. Don't give up this right. If you have Medicaid you are entitled to private medical care despite the fact that some government agency is paying the bill. Your doctor or the hospital may need an occasional reminder of this.

People in Class D, those with no financial resources, are in trouble. This group is generally not selected from among the very poor, since the very poor can often get some kind of public assistance. Rather, it is chosen from those who can't qualify for public assistance; those who don't want any or don't know of its availability; people who don't settle anywhere long enough to receive it; and, most commonly, the working poor who earn slightly more than the sum that would enable them to qualify for Medicaid but have no resources, no insurance, and no continuing income when they are sick. If they are sick long enough they will become eligible for Medicaid, but that seems to contradict the principle of good early care. The availability of treatment for people in Class D depends mostly on the good will of an individual doctor, on the resources in the community, and on the nature of the illness or injury. Some doctors will attend a patient for nothing or for a token amount, but usually only if the patient is worthy, respectful, and properly deferential. In large cities most voluntary hospitals will take care of a patient if they have to, regardless of his ability to pay, or if the illness or injury is so serious or life-threatening that they can't avoid it. They don't like to. They will bill the patient for services, be very unpleasant about collecting their bill, very ungracious about providing the services, and will release the patient or get him to a government hospital as soon as they can. In rural areas, tales of seriously sick and injured people being turned away from a voluntary or private hospital for lack of a cash deposit are unfortunately more common. Hospitals are usually not reimbursed by anyone or any agency for an unpaid bill. If they don't get some kind of outside funds, a non-paying patient represents a budget loss which they often cannot afford to sustain.

How to Identify Good Sources of Medical Care

Let us assume that you are not desperately ill or injured, that it is not three A.M., a weekend or a holiday, and that you simply want to find a doctor.

We will take the liberty here of making some very rough generalizations to serve as guidelines.

• Younger doctors are a new breed. The salvation of the medical profession probably lies in the new physicians. Many have rejected the traditional conservative approach of their older colleagues. This is particularly true in many of the large cities.

• Any hospital which has a house staff will be a better source of medical care than one without.

• Any hospital affiliated with a medical school will be better than one without such an affiliation. This assessment must be tempered by judgment, however, since many such hospitals are city hospitals with antiquated facilities and outrageous shortages of staff and equipment.

• Medical school hospitals may place you in contact with medical students who are functioning in association with the house staff. This opportunity should be welcomed, partly because you have a responsibility to contribute to their education and partly because they frequently have the responsibility to give you a very detailed and thorough evaluation. You may find them taking more time and more than a passive interest in your health as part of their training.

• If time permits, contact the local chapter of the Medical Committee for Human Rights (MCHR: see Appendix 1 for a list of Chapters), a group of doctors, nurses, and medical personnel who are interested in a humanistic approach to medical care. They will sometimes be able to refer you to a physician or to help establish facilities for the provisions of first aid at the scene of a demonstration. They may be able to assist with hospitalization or providing medical care if someone is arrested (see Chapter 2 on legal considerations).

- Remember that some hospital emergency rooms will be used as police staging areas during a crisis, and you might find yourself in the middle of hostile forces when you present yourself for medical care. If you can be selective, try to choose a hospital distant from the action. Remember that hospital policy is established by hospital trustees; these men are generally selected by the same criteria that college trustees are selected, not because of their unusual competence in medical (or educational) problems, but in consideration of their age, politics, and financial contributions. Needless to say, they are interested in preserving the status quo. The individual practitioner may or may not reflect hospital policy.

If you are not likely to need hospitalization but you want a doctor, your access to medical care is through:
1. a private doctor in his private office;
2. a hospital clinic or emergency room;
3. a student health clinic; or
4. a community or "people's" clinic.

There are major advantages and disadvantages to each of these. A prime factor, unfortunately, which you must never lose sight of, is your ability to pay. If you can't or won't pay, then skip 1. If you don't qualify as a student, skip 3. If you have serious hangups about dealing with the system, then try 4, but recognize that the resources of the community or people's clinic are frequently very limited.

It is extremely difficult for you to measure the qualifications and competence of the doctor you choose if you decide to go through route 1. The luxury of his address or quality of his furniture means little. The diplomas tell you that he is a graduate of a medical school and has had training at a hospital, but not how carefully he has kept up to date since then. If you call the local medical society for the name of a recommended doctor, you will get a name from their list of members. If you know what kind of specialist you want, they will give you a name from their list of members in that specialty. Any doctor can join the local medical society in most communities, and incompetence is rarely a deterrent to membership. If you call a hospital and ask for the name of a doctor, they will do the same, but their list is from their own staff. Your friends may give you the name of a doctor they know and like, but they too have no way to judge his competence, and they often like him because he's a nice guy or they feel comfortable with him. Personality and rapport should not be ignored, but you are not voting for class president—you are looking for a doctor, and competence should be your prime consideration. If you know a doctor socially and ask him to recommend someone, you will get as good advice as is available. He probably will be able to refer you to one of his colleagues, a process which should eliminate the obvious incompetents and frauds in the profession. He might also refer you to the most capable doctor around, since most doctors know who the best doctors in their community are.

If route 1, private medical care, is what you want, you must still be careful. Private group practice can be excellent but some aspects of care by the solo practitioner bear caution. The single practitioner has been described as "the last of America's pushcart industries." If you want a private physician you should obtain the services of someone who at least has rapid access to consultation, x-rays, and laboratory facilities. These services are not commonly found in the office of most solo practitioners.

Route 2, the hospital clinic or emergency room, is often the physician of the poor. There are frequent and long delays and the care can be very abrupt and impersonal. In spite of the uncomfortable surroundings, the quality of the care is sometimes better than in a randomly selected private office. Diagnostic facilities and the availability of consultation are variable; good in some cases, but haphazard, inconvenient, or absent in others. The impersonal nature of the hospital emergency room tends to be synonymous with anonymity, which depresses some people but may be preferable for others.

The decision to seek medical care at a hospital or emergency room during or after a political demonstration is often very difficult. The primary consideration should be based on the nature of your injury, rather than the jeopardy in which you may place yourself by presenting yourself to this type of facility. Obviously, if your injury is threatening to life or limb, the latter consideration becomes secondary. You may not be in any condition to make this decision and you may have to abide by the choice made by friends you know and trust.

Most emergency rooms are equipped to handle all types of problems, from a sore throat to a heart attack. Although the primary function of an emergency room is to provide emergency care, some hospitals have come to realize that the patient makes the initial decision about what represents a true emergency to him and what can wait until morning, so emergency rooms generally take care of all types of problems. In some hospitals, and usually during normal working hours, the emergency room staff will refer some non-emergency patients to one of their clinics for evaluation and treatment. Aside from the additional waiting time and inconvenience, the medical treatment is the same.

Emergency room or hospital clinic treatment is not free, except in public hospitals established to provide care for indigent patients. Even in public hospitals you will be charged if your income is above a minimum level, and your insurance company will be billed if you have medical insurance or Medicaid. Standard and substantial fees are charged for the services provided in emergency rooms.

Route 3, the student health clinic, is useful, usually free (or costs very little) and in some cases provides high quality and sympathetic assistance. Be wary of it though, even if you have legitimate access to its facilities, if you are sensitive about faculty access to your medical records. Although this surely must vary from campus to campus, there may be reason to doubt the sanctity of medical records in some cases when the school has control of the clinic. Regardless of other technical or legal considerations about what is privileged or private information, the school could interpret its role *in loco parentis* (in the place of the parents) as giving it authority to examine your medical records if necessary.

17 † The Business of Medicine and How to Deal with It

Route 4, the community or people's clinic, is an excellent choice for people with few or no financial resources. The very existence of free community clinics is strong indictment of the deficiencies of public medicine in America today. If your problem does not require hospitalization or is likely to be unsympathetically received in regular clinics (e.g., drugs, abortions), or if you reject the formidable hospital atmosphere and would prefer to deal with a more understanding and sympathetic staff in less starched surroundings, then you should consider the free clinic.

The free clinic movement is expanding rapidly. Some clinics provide limited services, such as counseling or drug treatment; others are equipped to provide complete free health services. Some serve only as referral centers or switchboards. A few are established to provide medical care for particular groups, such as Spanish-speaking or American Indian patients.

All of the free clinics have inadequate budgets and are chronically pressed for money. They are able to function only because they are staffed by volunteers and accept donations of equipment and supplies. But since the phone bill and the rent have to be paid, they will be happy to accept a small donation as token payment for the medical care or advice you have received.

What to Do in an Emergency

Despite our traditional belief that medical care should be available on a twenty-four-hour-a-day basis, everyone, including a doctor, has to sleep; everyone wants to take some time off. Medical care can usually be obtained somewhere and somehow around the clock, but you should recognize that the medical care system functions much less efficiently and often more expensively during the off-hours.

You are in the best position to determine what is an emergency. Don't be afraid to make that judgment, since no one else will make it for you. It should be based on the questions: Can it wait until tomorrow (or Monday)? Will the delay make things worse, more difficult, or even impossible to treat later? Are you so uncomfortable that treatment is needed simply to relieve the problem between now and the initiation of more definitive therapy? We suggest that you answer these questions liberally and always in your own favor. If there is any doubt at all, err on the side of caution and get help.

Remember that the decision of whether or not you will need hospitalization is not yours to make. In every case, this is a decision that will have to be made by a physician. Many emergency problems will clearly not need a hospital bed (e.g., a severe toothache needing pain medication or a lacerated hand needing sutures).

If you need emergency care we suggest the following:

- If you have a personal physician, contact his office. If he is not available, someone will probably be taking his calls for him and should be able to tell you what to do.

- If you are part of a system where arrangements for emergency medical care are already established (e.g., student health, prepayment health plans), follow their instructions or call for instructions.

- Do not ask for or expect a house call except under unusual circumstances. House calls are old-fashioned medicine. Unless you really cannot move or be moved, or you have no one at all to look after the kids, you should remember that much better medical care, with access to laboratory tests and x-rays, can be given in a doctor's office or hospital emergency room than can be given out of a doctor's bag in your bedroom. There is no increased risk in going out in the cold or rain if you have a cold or the flu. House calls are also much more expensive. You will have to pay for the doctor's traveling time, since the only things he is selling are his time and his wisdom, and he is the most expensive part of the system. If you really can't move, you may well need hospitalization, and the house call may delay everything since you have to get to the hospital anyway. House calls may, in fact, be useful only for non-emergency chronic care problems, particularly for old people

19 † The Business of Medicine and How to Deal with It

or invalids where routine care is given and needs can be anticipated. This is often better handled routinely by a visiting nurse or physician's assistant.

- If you don't have any previous arrangements, don't waste your time randomly shopping for a doctor in the Yellow Pages. You should go to the best hospital emergency room you know of in your community. Try to remember to take your health insurance details or Medicaid card with you. As we have noted, emergency rooms may not solve your problem, since some communities don't have a hospital or an emergency room, or the emergency room is not open twenty-four hours a day, or it is not staffed twenty-four hours a day, or it requires a cash deposit or a health insurance policy before anyone will see you. If this is the case, there are no useful generalizations. What you do will depend entirely on the local circumstances and resources and what other sources of care you might be able to identify. In communities such as these, it might be wise to think about some possible alternatives in advance.

2 Your Medical Rights and Privileges

For some segments of the population the right to medical care is not automatic. If you are old, poor or young; if your clothes are unusual or your hair is long; if you are black or chicano; if you are involved in a demonstration or protest; if you make your doctor feel uncomfortable or anxious or old or inadequate, your chances of getting optimum medical care are markedly reduced. The previous chapter describes how the system works. When it doesn't work you are relatively powerless medically and legally.

This chapter deals with various legal considerations which determine how you obtain medical care, how you pay for it, what your obligations are and which are your physician's, what rights and privileges you have and what to do if they are abused or neglected.

Since you need services of a doctor when excitement, confusion, or emergency impair your good judgment, your chances for success can be improved if you understand certain legal principles around which medical care is arranged.

Obtaining Medical Care

No doctor can be forced to treat you. Even if he is the only doctor available and you are obviously very sick or seriously injured, he can refuse to assist you and face no penalties more severe than those of his conscience and perhaps the ethics committee of his local medical society (not, traditionally, a very serious threat). This may seem cruel, but it is based on the contractual relationship between two parties. The relationship between yourself and your doctor may appear to you to be a personal one, but in the eyes of the law it is a contract—

written, verbal, or even implied. The implied contract is established when you seek treatment and the doctor administers care. Seeking treatment does not necessarily mean that you have requested his services; if you are confused or delirious or unconscious, the law assumes that you are seeking medical care. If a friend or passing stranger solicits care on your behalf and it is delivered, a contract is made.

One of the main reasons some doctors refuse to provide care in an emergency is that once the process is started the doctor is required to provide proper treatment until his services are no longer needed, that is, until he is discharged by the patient or he properly withdraws from the case. To do otherwise constitutes a breach of the contract and abandonment. The doctor may withdraw from the case only if he gives reasonable notice of his intention to do so and allows the patient ample opportunity to obtain the services of another physician, neither of which is likely in a serious emergency until the doctor and the patient get to the hospital. Laws modifying this obligation have been passed in a number of states, but it is still reasonable to assume that many doctors will continue to be reluctant to stop at the side of the road when they see an accident.

The contractual obligation is further complicated by the fact that the doctor must provide not only continuous but proper care. It matters very little that he is a psychiatrist who hasn't seen anyone with a bullet wound in twenty years, or a pediatrician who hasn't treated a heart attack since he left medical school. He is liable for his errors in judgment for proper diagnosis and treatment, in a delicate and difficult situation, usually distracted by emotion and almost always without adequate facilities.

Once the contract exists, you have a substantial amount of power over your contractual servant, the doctor. He knows, even if you don't, that you can require him to provide proper care.

Emergency Rooms

A hospital, like a doctor, does not have to accept any patient. Any time for any reason it can refuse to make its services available.* Nor is a hospital required to have an emergency room, but once it does, it has an obligation to accept any emergency patient. The doctor's half of the contract is, in effect, already implied by the offering of services through an emergency room. If it is determined that there is an unmistakable emergency, whether illness or injury, the emergency room must treat you. It cannot refuse because of your inability to pay, but it can assert that your problem is not an emergency. If you feel, nevertheless, that emergency treatment is necessary, your firm insistence should convince them, particularly if it is coupled with suggestions of your contemplation of litigation. Your persistence, however, will not create good will or endear you to the staff.

Although it deals primarily with emergencies rather than routine care, the emergency room is not under any conditions released from its obligation to provide adequate and proper care. If you are likely to be using an emergency room, you should be familiar with how it works and some of the subtleties in your relationship with it.

If you have to document your injuries for any reason, it is wise to use your proper name when you register. The medical record of John Doe will not be useful to you if they are needed in court. But you are under no obligation to tell the doctor how your injury was sustained. He should not conduct a legal inquiry into the nature of your injury. He should care only

---

* This broad concept is being challenged in a number of cases where hospitals have refused to provide services to certain individuals despite the fact that the hospitals had received public funds. It is thought by some that, in accepting public funds to operate, the hospitals have also accepted a responsibility to treat all individuals and have relinquished their option of selecting their patients. An emergency room, however, does not have the privilege of selectivity.

that you have a bullet wound, not who shot you. It should make no medical difference to him whether you were beaten up by the police, your boyfriend or a gang of roving kids. Be careful, though, of exaggerated secrecy which might work to your own medical disadvantage. The doctor will have to know whether you were cut with a knife or by a piece of shattered glass, since in the latter case he'll need to probe the wound to remove possible fragments. If the laceration on your finger was caused as you smashed it into someone's front tooth, or as you flew through the front window of your car, he might want to take x-rays to check for a fracture; if it occurred when your knife slipped, x-rays are probably unnecessary.

The hospital must legally report certain kinds of medical problems to the police. The principle of the confidential doctor/patient relationship is not always sacred. If you are reluctant to discuss your problem with the police, try to avoid the emergency room. Use caution and judgment in requesting a public ambulance. Use it by all means, if you need it, but remember that in some cities the ambulance may be accompanied or operated by the police. The staff of the emergency room may be hostile or sympathetic, but the likelihood that they will fail to notify the police should be counted as close to zero. If you don't want to deal with the police you will have to measure this reluctance against the severity of your injury and the alternatives available to you. (It should be noted, however, that all physicians, not only those in a hospital emergency room, must notify the police of reportable incidents.)

Sometimes the police are present in the emergency room. They may be in and out when there is "trouble" or when hospital facilities are being used as a police staging area. Regardless of the presence or activities of the police in the emergency room, they should not interfere with your proper medical treatment. They should not be permitted to delay treatment, remove you from the emergency room prematurely, interfere with your right to privacy or harass you. If they want to question you, you have a right to the normal procedures of police interrogation and/or arrest, and you have a right not to answer their questions until you have advice from a lawyer.

State laws differ as to the right of various officials to obtain, with or without your permission, blood or urine samples for measuring the concentration of alcohol or drugs. In an increasing number of states owning a driver's license implies consent to have blood drawn for the determination of alcohol content. If you are in command of your senses, it is worthwhile to remember that the person who draws the blood should not use alcohol or iodine to clean your arm. The alcohol, even the small amount present in the iodine solution, can contaminate the blood drawn and give the erroneous impression of a high alcohol content in your blood. As of the time of the preparation of this book, there were no satisfactory laboratory tests available to detect marijuana or LSD in blood or urine, but there are relatively simple tests to detect most other drugs.

In an emergency room, as in any medical treatment, you have a right to know what the doctor thinks is wrong and what he plans to do about it. You have a right to know the results of any laboratory tests or x-rays, what medications you are receiving, and the name of the doctor treating you. If you are contemplating civil litigation or bringing charges against an assailant, it would be wise to tell this to the doctor so that his records will reflect those aspects of the case that bear on these specifics.

It isn't fair to assume that the doctor will necessarily be hostile or antagonistic to you, but if he is, you are in a very insecure bargaining position, since he has "all the marbles." Acknowledge the situation but be firm and civil. You can probably achieve more personal benefits if you avoid verbal combat. If you are mistreated you should consider the possibility of bringing a malpractice suit, but unless the situation is desperate and deteriorating, you would probably do well to avoid an outright threat, since it will merely elicit hostility.

The emergency room can be a frightening and depressing place. Blood, noise, ambulances, police and excitement, the presence of desperately sick and seriously injured patients, as well as the dying. Don't be intimidated. Generally you will be seen in your proper turn, but the seriously ill will usually be moved ahead of you. You have to make the distinction between appropriate staff manipulation of sequence and subtle abuse of your rights. Avoid commenting on how rapidly someone else has been seen and focus on the fact that you can't breathe, are bleeding to death, or are in agonizing pain. You will probably accomplish very little by demanding your proper turn, and you will risk antagonizing the staff, which is usually already overworked.

Treatment of Minors

No physician can treat a patient who is under twenty-one or eighteen in some states unless he has the consent of the patient's parents or guardian. There are important exceptions to this rule, but the doctor who determines that an exception exists is exposing himself to risk. If he delivers unauthorized treatment and the parents disapprove, the doctor can be charged with assault, held liable for damages, and subjected to criminal prosecution. The consent of an adult relative isn't good enough, it has to be the parent or guardian.

In a bona fide emergency, if obtaining consent is impossible or unreasonable, or if delay will add unnecessary risk or danger, the doctor can treat without authorization. In other cases when a problem is serious but not life threatening, when consent is difficult to obtain, or when a minor is old enough to understand the implications of the treatment, some doctors will use their judgment and go ahead. If a minor is "emancipated" he can legally contract for treatment of non-serious or non-emergency problems. A minor is considered to be emancipated if he is responsible for his own livelihood and debts, if he has left his parents' home, and if he functions independently of his parents. Simply being married is not enough, the other conditions must be met as well. Some states are liberalizing their rules about the treatment of minors for certain problems like venereal diseases, pregnancy, and the provision of contraceptive devices. You'll have to find out what the local rules are, but, in general, if you are under age you will have a difficult time. The final determinant, of course, is what you tell the person at the front desk when you register.

First Aid

First aid can range from helping to pick up a stranger who has tripped on the sidewalk to applying tourniquets, giving artificial respiration, and cardiac massage, as long as it is administered by someone who does not normally practice medicine. The administration of medical treatment in this sense does not constitute the practice of medicine.

If you are not a physician and are doing your sincere best to help, the fact that you haven't the remotest thought of receiving any compensation does not get you off the hook. You are liable for damages if you do something wrong. When you help you can only perform to the limit of your skill. You cannot be expected to have the same degree of skill as a professional, but you are expected to use good judgment, common sense, and to do no harm. The same rules of liability apply to you as well as to a physician.

These words of caution are not intended to alarm or dissuade you from helping people who are in trouble. When people are sick or injured, the passers-by "don't want to get involved" and the overemphasis on potential liability has made it increasingly difficult to get help. In addition to the common sense, good judgment, and even wisdom that you may summon for an emergency, don't forget compassion. On the other hand, if someone helps you and makes an error, don't be so quick to call a lawyer.

Two examples where bad judgment complicated the best

intentions may serve to illustrate this point. In one, a confused, dazed and "glassy-eyed" man was left standing alone by a friend who went to get help. The patient collapsed, and the friend was judged liable for his failure to use good judgment in allowing the sick man to remain standing unattended. In the other case, a man suspected that his co-worker was having a heart attack, helped him briefly and then urged him to walk to a nearby hospital, about a mile away. That he suspected a heart attack and then counseled a long walk appeared to be inconsistent with what a reasonable man would have done in similar circumstances.

Fees

The doctor is entitled to be paid for his services even if you have not specifically consented to treatment. If you were drunk or unconscious when he started his treatment, you are still obliged to pay. However, the doctor cannot discontinue his services if you don't pay your bill promptly, or even at all. He can withdraw from the case for any reason, only if he gives you ample advance notice and adequate time to obtain the services of another physician. It should be added that the legality of his fee does not depend on the success of his treatment, or upon your satisfaction with his services.

Liability

A physician must treat his patients properly. If he doesn't and the patient is injured or his illness is made worse as a result, the physician is liable for those damages, and the patient may sue and recover money to compensate him. The situation has become a touchy subject with doctors in recent years because of the rising number of malpractice suits which have accompanied a great increase in public sophistication about medicine and the increasing complexities of practicing medicine.

Malpractice doesn't mean that your doctor can make no mistake. This is clearly impossible. It does mean that what he does has to be consistent with the prevailing standards of good practice, and that he must exercise skill and care comparable to that of his colleagues. A bad result, a wrong diagnosis or bad judgment does not necessarily constitute malpractice. If, however, the bad result was because of negligence, or the wrong diagnosis occurred because the doctor did not exercise due skill, care and diligence, or the bad judgment exceeded the limit that is expected of prudent men, then he may be liable. If the weight of evidence consistently establishes that reasonable men would have acted otherwise, the courts may consider that he acted improperly. The same conditions apply to non-physicians administering first aid.

You should be reminded that if you do not cooperate or complete the treatment as outlined by the doctor, he is absolved of responsibility for what goes wrong.

Privacy and Confidentiality

You have a right to be treated privately. Technically, you should not be exposed to shame, humiliation or mortification. The traditional view that your discussions with your doctor are as confidential as a priest's hearing of confession may or may not be true. There is much variation from state to state about the conditions of confidentiality in the doctor/patient relationship. What you tell your doctor is confidential, but what the law allows him or can require him to reveal varies. Some, but not all, confidential communications to your doctor are privileged. Privileged information is that information which cannot be disclosed in a legal proceeding without the specific consent of the patient. In general, ordinary information communicated to your doctor must be held in the strictest confidence. The law, however, tends to protect society and limits the confidentiality in two general ways. One is when the patient expressly wishes otherwise (as in his legal proceedings, or when he requests that his doctor fill out a form, etc.). The other is when the law requires otherwise. About two-thirds of the states have enacted specific laws which forbid the physician to disclose any information acquired in his medical role.* The remaining one-third generally adhere to traditional common law which does not recognize the legal status of the medical confidentiality. The states that do have privilege laws frequently qualify them in such a way that the doctor can be compelled to testify in some cases, or the judge can use his discretion to determine what answers would best serve the interests of justice.

There appear to be some kinds of information which are not considered confidential or privileged. The physician can be required to testify that he treated a patient and to provide details about the place, the duration of the treatment and the number of visits. This may seem trivial, but it has played a major role in the establishment of medical care facilities at times of demonstrations or civil disorders. In August, 1968, for example, the Medical Committee for Human Rights (MCHR) established medical units for people injured during the police riot that accompanied the Democratic National Convention. The names of those receiving treatment were, unfortunately, not privileged and were subpoenaed in various investigations. Since that time all MCHR facilities have abandoned the use of patients' names and now use numbered records. The patient keeps a copy of his number for future reference.

Reportable Diseases

Sometimes your doctor has no choice about what he must report to various police and/or public health authorities. In general, he must report births, deaths, acts of violence (even if

---

* The states that have some kind of protection of confidence include Alaska, Arizona, Arkansas, California, Colorado, District of Columbia, Georgia, Hawaii, Idaho, Illinois, Indiana, Iowa, Kansas, Kentucky, Louisiana, Michigan, Minnesota, Mississippi, Missouri, Montana, Nebraska, Nevada, New Mexico, New York, North Carolina, North Dakota, Ohio, Oklahoma, Ore-

self-inflicted) and many, but not all, types of contagious diseases, including hepatitis and venereal disease. In many states he must report cases of epilepsy to be computerized into the mechanism for the issuance of driver's licenses.

Mental Patients

There are two ways an individual may be placed in a mental hospital.

Voluntary commitment: Anyone can sign himself into a mental hospital. If you are dealing with a friend or relative who is having serious psychiatric problems, getting him to commit himself voluntarily is the best way to handle the problem of hospitalization. Getting in, however, is easier than getting out. The rules vary from state to state but, in general, hospital officials can delay your release for a time while they initiate what amounts to involuntary commitment proceedings. Don't assume that they will always try to hold you against your will, but remember that they can if they want to.

Involuntary commitment: Most states have definite procedures for involuntary detention of mentally ill people, but the laws determining who can initiate the process and the degree to which the courts are involved differ from state to state. Sometimes any citizen can sign commitment papers; sometimes it takes a physician or a psychiatrist or a law enforcement or health officer. There is also much variation in how this is initiated. The duration of an involuntary commitment in an emergency situation ranges from about three to seven days, and there are books of rules about follow-up, release proceedings, mechanism for prolonged commitment, and the relationship of it all to prisons and hospitals. Special

---

gon, Pennsylvania, South Dakota, Utah, Washington, West Virginia, Wisconsin, and Wyoming. For further information consult *Privileged Communication between Physician and Patient* by C. DeWitt, published by C. C. Thomas, Springfield, Ill., 1958.

provisions are made for commitment for alcoholism, drug addiction, and sex crimes.

All of the proceedings tend to be irrational and to protect the state rather than the individual. This probably reflects our society's cultural fear of strange people and our simplistic solution of locking them up and throwing away the key.

The entire commitment process is complicated enormously by what happens once a patient is admitted. Although a few mental hospitals are very good, many are ineffective. A number of cases have recently been brought to court to require the state to administer treatment to an individual while he is in a mental hospital. The effectiveness of hospitalization is further compromised by what amounts to incarceration and deprivation of the rights of mental patients, as if they were criminals rather than sick people. For example, in less than one-fourth of the states is a patient's right to communicate with the outside world protected by law; in less than half is his right to receive visitors protected by law; in less than a tenth is he guaranteed the right to correspond with his attorney; the use of physical restraints is restricted in less than one-fourth of the states; and less than one-fourth of the states assure that he will receive a periodic examination for consideration for discharge.

Medical Care in Jails

This is another of those muddled areas which seem chronically and conveniently to escape the attention of most legislative authorities. You can assume that once you get arrested you are a ward of the state, which is then theoretically responsible for your welfare, including specifically your medical care.

The most difficult time to obtain medical care in jails occurs around the time of the arrest. The difficulty is compounded many times if you are part of a mass arrest and the facilities for holding and processing prisoners are limited or strained. What happens depends on how obvious your injury or illness is, how accessible medical care facilities may be, how busy the police are, whether or not there was any police mistreatment of you or how much they worked you over while bringing you in, how much the police dislike you for your appearance, color, or for the nature of the circumstances in which you were arrested, and how long a delay there is before they can get you processed. Particularly troublesome are long delays in temporary facilities for people who have illnesses or injuries unrelated to their arrest when they get busted, or those who are taking regular medications which are not available in jail. People in the latter category who anticipate trouble should carry some medical certification attesting to their need for medication, which they can present to the police as soon as possible.

Under normal circumstances, an arrested person is taken to a temporary facility, usually the nearest precinct lockup. Within a few hours, he is arraigned and either released on bail or transferred to a long-term detention center. If at the time of the arrest the prisoner presents a medical problem, as judged by the arresting officer, he may be taken to a hospital emergency room for evaluation and treatment under guard. Upon release by the hospital physician he is returned to the precinct lockup. Once arrested, a prisoner may request medical attention, but the recognition and primary evaluation of his medical complaints, as well as the decision to do something about them or ignore them, rest with the police officer and not with a medical person. Although making this decision may distress some policemen, who usually don't like to be put in a position that forces them to diagnose their inmates, it apparently has not upset the system enough to induce it to change. The net effect is that many arrested persons, particularly those arrested for drunkenness, are denied access to medical care even under normal circumstances.

If you are in need of medical attention and are not able to obtain it promptly, there is relatively little that you can do. It may be useful to note the name and badge number of the uncooperative policeman, but there's always the cruel recognition that once you have the number there isn't much you can do with it. Making a scene may either help or make things a lot worse.

A critical issue concerns your right to have your own doctor (or one sympathetic to your interests) attend you while you are in jail. To exercise that right you must identify your own doctor, either privately, through your lawyer, or through an organization like the Medical Committee for Human Rights. It is pointless to go shopping through the Yellow Pages while you are in jail.

It may be worthwhile to get a private physician if you are very sick and feel that you are not getting proper treatment, if you want to document fully any injuries or illnesses in case of pending litigation, or if you are fearful of police brutality and want the police to recognize that your state of health is under surveillance.

In the view of many you should be as free to select your physician as you are to select your attorney and he should be able to see you while you are in jail. Unfortunately this view is not shared by virtually any jail or prison official, and it usually takes a court order and very unusual circumstances to get your own doctor into jail to see you. To our knowledge there has never been a definitive test of the issue in a broad sense. It is likely to be tested soon, probably in the context of some mass arrest and incarceration of demonstrators.

3 Recognizing Disease

The human body has an uncanny ability to recognize that something is wrong with it. A collection of signs and symptoms, discomforts and abnormalities, and pains and pressures signal the onset of illness or injury. Sometimes the abnormality is obvious; more often it is not. When you have a knife wound or a tear gas burn there is nothing elusive about the diagnosis and the cause and effect relationship is clear enough. When you are dealing with a cough or confusion or abdominal pain, you may know that something is wrong, but a clear understanding of what is responsible for the symptoms is more obscure.

This chapter categorizes and discusses, not the diseases, but the manifestations of the diseases. It is useful to understand symptoms; know why they exist, what they mean, and what might be done about them. You will be better able to decide what is serious and what is trivial if you have some perspective on the normal and abnormal functioning and physiology of the human animal. Some of the discussion in this chapter overlaps discussions in later ones (for example, headache as one type of pain is described here and as a manifestation of head injury elsewhere).

Pain

Pain is probably the single most definitive suggestion that something is wrong. It is often the earliest manifestation of disease, frequently the most prominent, generally the most disabling, usually the most frightening, and probably the most common. Fortunately it is not always serious. The problem is to determine when it is serious and when it is not.

Too many medical textbooks and most physicians separate pain into two categories: organic (or physical) and emotional. They accept the former as a diagnostic and therapeutic challenge, and dismiss the latter as a phenomenon of a disturbed mind to be placated, tranquilized, and tolerated. This is particularly unfortunate since pain hurts in either case, regardless of its cause, and the patient is uncomfortable.

The problem is complicated still further by marked individual variability in reaction to pain. Although most people have about the same threshold levels of perception of pain (in a standardized laboratory sense), their interpretation of it is modified by fear, emotional state, cultural patterns, the possibility (conscious or unconscious) of secondary gain or respite from responsibilities, and the coexistence of depression, excitement, hysteria, or other factors. Seemingly trivial pain may elicit intense agony in one person and severe pain may produce casual indifference in a more stoic individual. The danger is in imparting one's own values to the patient. It is his pain and his interpretation and his reaction to it. If you are assisting someone you can (and should) get some information by gauging the intensity of the pain, but you must use your judgment and err on the side of caution.

In addition to the intensity of the pain, a number of other factors are useful to determine what is wrong and how to deal with it. The constancy of the pain (steady or intermittent), the duration (minutes or days), the mode of onset (sudden or gradual), the quality (burning, sharp, pressure, knifelike), the location (diffuse, localized, superficial, or deep), and the factors which relieve or intensify the pain are the basis upon which an effort is made to establish its cause and cure.

However, even without specific information about the cause of specific kinds of pain, a moment or two of careful consideration should tell you a great deal. For example, you would probably be more concerned about the onset of explosive pain (headache or abdominal pain) than slowly developing pain. You would probably worry more about pain that lasted for two to three days than pain lasting twenty minutes. Pain related to a specific incident (head injury or toothache) would probably be of more concern if it grew more intense with the passage of a few days rather than less, as could be expected if the problem were spontaneously resolving.

Your good judgment, of course, is assisted by one other factor. Serious pain *usually* does not occur as an isolated symptom. Be careful, however, because this is a potentially dangerous generalization and is *usually, but not always,* true. Some examples are:

—a headache with dizziness, somnolence, and confusion is not just an ordinary headache.

—a stomach ache is usually neglected until there's a little fever or some diarrhea.

—you might think that some chest pain is the beginning of a chest cold until you start coughing up blood, and then it's time to worry.

Be careful. Isolated pain may mean serious disease as well. Some kinds of chest pain may be the beginning of a heart attack. Use your common sense and good judgment. If you are twenty years old you are not likely to be having a heart attack. If you are sixty, then your concern might be more valid.

Some kinds of abdominal pain may be the only sign of an ulcer, but the chances are that you'll soon find that the pain is relieved by food or antacids and this will modify your judgment of its severity.

The decision about when to seek medical help is a difficult one, and much as we'd like to simplify the understanding of pain and lay down some rules, there are too many exceptions to make rules of any value. Perhaps one generalization is worthwhile, however. Don't be a hero. When, in your considered judgment, and in the judgment of your friends or family, the pain gets to be more than you can handle and it interferes significantly with your normal activities, then you would be wise to seek medical advice. Obviously, the circumstances will temper your judgment, but, insofar as possible, try to make rational and unemotional decisions.

HEADACHES

There are dozens of kinds of headaches. Some are more serious than others, but obviously the headache that signifies a serious abnormality is far less common than the ordinary, garden-variety headache. As with all types of pain, there are features of some headaches which suggest that you are dealing with something serious. As with other types of pain also, the generalizations are not foolproof. Below are some rough guidelines. Your judgment, your perspective, and your familiarity with your normal patterns or those of the patient should be added to these rough rules.

• Sudden onset of pain (without a specific cause, such as a toothache) is more likely to be serious than the slow nonspecific onset of most headaches. If you can tell just when it started, and what you were doing at that time, then the onset is sudden.

• As a corollary to this, if the pain awakens you from a sound sleep, it should not be neglected. Be careful to note if you weren't awakened by something else and happened to notice that, incidentally, you had a headache. Don't neglect a headache which is present when you wake up in the morning either; it probably is not a tension headache or eyestrain and is often due to something like congested sinuses (which can be treated) or high blood pressure (which should be treated).

• If the pain is associated with an alteration in consciousness or confusion or dizziness or somnolence, you should get some help. If the pain follows a head injury (see Chapter 5), particularly if there has been any loss of consciousness, these symptoms of confusion are extremely common. If there has been no trauma, the headache associated with confusion represents an emergency. If there has been a head injury, the patient requires careful and dedicated observation. The symptoms should improve with time. If they don't, or if they get worse, or if new symptoms appear (such as weakness or fever), then you need professional attention. Make sure that someone checks the patient, talks to him, and watches regularly and frequently for slurred speech or lack of coordination (this means at intervals all night, and he should be awakened to do it). Check the size of the pupils, the black part in the center of the eye. They should be equal to each other in size; if they are not, there may be serious trouble.

• Fever tends to be associated with serious headaches. Consider what comes first. Fever itself, from whatever cause, can produce a headache. If fever appears to be primarily related to the headache and no other obvious cause is apparent for the fever, the headache has a more ominous significance.

• Watch out for a stiff neck. Most stiff necks are of no consequence. The abrupt onset of a stiff neck, along with a headache, fever, and other general symptoms, should alert your concern. You should be able to bend your neck down, with your mouth shut, to touch, or almost touch, your chest without causing pain. Neck movements should not elicit pain. A stiff neck, together with a headache and/or fever, may be associated with inflammation of the meninges, the thin tissue covering the brain, and this is one of the early signs of meningitis (an infection of the meninges).

THE TREATMENT OF PAIN

The problem of treatment of pain deserves brief comment because:

- —it shouldn't be as complicated as it seems; simple and inexpensive therapy is available;
- —there is too much deception (and even outright fraud) in advertisements about pain remedies;
- —the wrong drugs get used for the wrong reasons, the pills are wasted, and nothing useful is accomplished.

First, it is important to differentiate among categories of drugs. Medicines usually have a single most useful function and they should be used for that function only.

Analgesics (pain medication)—drugs used primarily to relieve pain (e.g., aspirin, morphine).
Sedatives—drugs used primarily to induce sleep (e.g., phenobarbital, chloral hydrate).
Tranquilizers—drugs used primarily to modify (up or down) emotional or psychic states (e.g., Thorazine, Librium, Miltown).

There is an overlap in each class and all medications have some variable degree of side effects. Thus, morphine, an analgesic, elicits some euphoria, and a tranquilizer or sedative will often relieve pain by putting you to sleep. An ideal analgesic drug will relieve severe pain without putting you to sleep.

For the treatment of pain, whatever its cause, there is a surprisingly small selection of measures at our disposal:

—the non-drug treatment.
—the drugs which you can get without a prescription:
  the simple, useful, inexpensive medications; and the complex, more expensive, more colorful and over-advertised medications.
—the more potent and more dangerous drugs which require a doctor's prescription.

The non-drug therapy is simple and cheap, but unfortunately only sometimes effective. Basically, these remedies fall into three groups:

Heat: A heating pad, hot-water bottle, hot towel or even a hot bath are wonderful for painful muscles, joints and some skin problems. It's usually worth a try if the affected part can be submerged or heated. Remember that heat itself may be painful and it shouldn't be so hot as to burn the skin. In general, a swollen area (ankle, wrist, jaw) should not be heated.

Cold: A few ice cubes in a towel or a wet towel which has been stored in the refrigerator will often provide relief for pain related to swelling (e.g., a sprained ankle or a black eye) or for many skin problems (cold is better for itching). Be careful not to freeze the skin.

Counter-irritants: Grandma's mustard plaster and the old horse liniment produce a mild, but not unpleasant, irritation of the skin. Since the brain can be easily fooled when it comes to perception of discomfort, it *may* ignore the underlying deep pain for the more extensive sensation on the skin. It is still possible to find liniments on the druggist's shelves ranging from oil of wintergreen and Sloane's liniment to Vick's Vap-O-Rub, and some of the preparations which may be advertised to produce heat are sometimes worth a try.

The non-prescription drugs: Your best bet here is unquestionably aspirin. It is an excellent drug with relatively few side effects. Most adults can use two tablets every four hours. Buy the cheapest reliable aspirin you can get. When you buy the more expensive varieties you have an opportunity to pay for the advertising and you get nothing extra in return. Aspirin is aspirin and all brands are the same except for trivial differences in compounding. Don't waste your money on the expensive bottles.

Since aspirin is the backbone of all simple therapy, it is also the basic ingredient in almost all the combination kinds of drugs sold for seemingly special purposes. The medications which are extensively advertised contain aspirin (read the label: aspirin is acetyl salicylic acid but it may be in some form like sodium salicylate) and frequently something like phenacetin and/or caffeine (a mild stimulant with no analgesic properties). The standard APC tablets contain just that, aspirin, phenacetin, and caffeine. Some people find that these work better than aspirin alone. That's fine. But again, don't waste your money on the expensive advertised varieties when the inexpensive brands are identical.

Some of the pharmaceutical companies have deleted the

phenacetin from their products because of reported cases of kidney problems in individuals who consumed enormous doses for many years. Phenacetin is not a problem for the occasional user. The phenacetin may or may not be in the product, and many companies have changed their product without appearing to change their basic label or their advertising. The fact that no one appears to miss it testifies to its questionable usefulness.

In a fair number of people aspirin causes stomach irritation. A "buffered" variety (watch the advertising again) frequently prevents the stomach irritation, but if buffered aspirin isn't available, a glass of milk or a few crackers taken with any aspirin will do just as well.

Except for aspirin there isn't much that's available over the counter that is very useful. There are all kinds of elaborate products, extensively advertised on television, promising special kinds of relief for special kinds of pain. They are usually made up of the same old stuff or some minor variation thereon. None is significantly better than aspirin or APC; all are substantially more expensive. If aspirin and time don't alleviate the pain, there are stronger drugs available, but these will need a prescription.

The prescription drugs: As a rule of thumb, the more effective a drug is in relieving the pain, the more likely it is to have potentially serious side effects. The two most troublesome side effects are sedation (problems with driving, keeping alert, etc.) and potential addiction (morphine will get anyone hooked, eventually), but there are a number of other peripheral problems as well. Some of the prescription drugs (like Darvon) are relatively free of risk, but although these require a prescription, they appear to be no more effective than aspirin if that good.

If aspirin doesn't relieve the pain, or at least take the edge off it, you will need to get a prescription for a stronger medication and you will need medical advice.

The spectrum of prescription pain killers ranges from Darvon and codeine to Demerol and morphine. It's foolish to take morphine for a toothache when codeine (safer and less addicting) will do. Generally we recommend codeine (or a codeine combination) if aspirin is ineffective, as a safe, inexpensive, effective pain medication, but recent studies suggest that codeine too may not be significantly better than aspirin.

Fever

When you are ill and must deal so often with subjective and vague symptoms, it is comforting to know that the measurement of temperature is simple, quantifiable, and precise. Either you have a fever or you don't. It is the single most precise diagnostic tool in the hands of the layman.

Before we discuss the utility of its measurement or its meaning, it is worth pausing for a brief discussion of physiology. A little bit about what creates and controls body temperature will help in understanding what makes a normal temperature into a fever and knowing what to do about it.

PHYSIOLOGICAL CONSIDERATIONS

Despite wide variations and even markedly abrupt changes in air temperature, humans comfortably and easily maintain body temperature within a normal range of about $1.0°-1.5°$ F. Even minor changes in body temperature indicate that something is wrong, and it is remarkable how accurately an individual can sense the minor changes of a few degrees that signify the presence of a fever.

Body temperature is almost always higher than air temperature. The maintenance of such a high temperature depends primarily upon the normal metabolic processes of the body (i.e., the utilization or "burning" of food in order to produce the energy to operate the chemical mechanisms of the body). Obviously, as the body's processes are accelerated, as in vigorous exercise, the metabolic rate, energy production, and heat production are increased. Shivering is a familiar regulatory mechanism for the body to rapidly increase the small muscle activity and to generate heat.

The regulation of temperature depends on complex control devices in the brain which slow or accelerate the production of heat and turn the controls for the loss of heat up or down. As heat is produced the excess is lost through radiation, convection or conduction away from the body (i.e., you lose heat to the surrounding environment). Temperature control is achieved primarily through the selection of clothing and by the automatic dilatation or constriction of blood vessels which carry warm blood to the skin and limbs where heat is lost. This latter mechanism is particularly striking in the large surface of a rabbit's ears, which are an extremely efficient temperature-regulating device in that animal. A more obvious mechanism in humans is sweating; the cooling effect is achieved by the evaporation of water from the skin. Dogs and other animals use this same procedure in panting: water evaporates from the surface of the tongue.

MEASURING TEMPERATURE

These physiological considerations lead to some generalizations about the measurement of temperature. It will be slightly higher after vigorous activity and it will be slightly lower after one comes inside on a very cold day. "Normal" values vary slightly from one person to another. Body temperatures are usually lowest in the early morning and rise steadily during the day, generally reaching a peak in the early evening. (This, by the way, is not reversed in people who reverse the day-night/work-sleep schedule.) It probably accounts also for why patients with a fever are most comfortable when they awaken.

Rectal temperatures are about $0.5°-1.0°$ higher than oral temperatures. (They are not more accurate, just higher because the tip of the thermometer is closer to the body's warmer central core.) Oral temperatures, taken with a closed mouth, are quite adequate but are difficult to obtain accurately in little children or in an adult who has to breathe through his mouth.

General observations:
- A thermometer is cheap and every household should have one.
- There is nothing sacred about 98.6° F. and many people have a normal temperature somewhere between 97° and 100°.
- People with a fever generally feel as if they have a fever.
- Shake the thermometer down below 98° F. before you use it. Hold tight.
- Don't wash the thermometer in hot water. It may break.
- Don't worry about a temperature of less than 100° (unless it gets down to less than about 96° F.). If it is very low, take it again, carefully, two to three full minutes, with your mouth closed. If you are feeling well and the temperature still reads less than 96° F., check to see if the thermometer is not broken, and while you are checking you might ask yourself why you took your temperature in the first place.

CLINICAL CONSIDERATIONS

The uncomfortable symptoms (such as headache and shaking chills) which are associated with a fever usually fluctuate in intensity. Rarely, and mostly with long-standing chronic disease, is the fever sustained at a constant high level. Usually, it moves up and down. This temperature instability is responsible for, or at least associated with, the uncomfortable symptoms. Chills accompany the rising temperature and are followed by a flushing sensation. As the temperature starts to drop, profuse sweating occurs. This pattern is typical but not always present. Stable fevers may be uncomfortable but are usually not associated with this disabling triad of chills, flush, and sweating. Perception of the fever varies. You may be distracted from the fever by the intensity of associated symptoms and the nature of the underlying disease. Some of these associated symptoms are almost universally present with a fever and may not, in themselves, be cause for alarm. Others may be quite serious.

A headache is common and usually is of no consequence. Some confusion may occur, and its presence should be viewed with serious concern. It is not uncommon in old people. Convulsions may be seen in children. These should be treated vigorously by efforts to lower the temperature with aspirin and/or sponging (see treatment of fever) and to maintain it below 103° F. The high temperature of some illnesses appears to activate a latent herpes virus which is always present in the skin of some people. These susceptible people get fever blisters or cold sores, which are annoying but not serious.

The familiar and almost classic pattern of abrupt onset of high temperature, headache, respiratory symptoms and/or gastrointestinal symptoms, malaise and muscle and joint pains is usually a response to a viral infection. Unfortunately, we can never be sure.

CAUSES OF FEVER

Almost any illness can cause a fever. The listing of possibilities is not useful. Generally any kind of injury to body tissues will produce a fever. Most commonly, fevers are associated with infectious diseases, bacterial or viral. It may also be associated with extensive soft tissue destruction, particularly if there has been some kind of maceration of tissues.

Other than its presence, which indicates that something is wrong, a fever is not a particularly useful diagnostic sign.

TREATMENT

Obviously, treatment of the fever is best accomplished through treatment of the underlying disease. The challenge is to identify the underlying disease and initiate therapy, if any is available. We assume, however, that you have done that, and that you have proceeded in a rational manner. You still have a fever and are awaiting the achievement of the imminent therapeutic miracle. What can you do to obtain some comfort? Generally speaking, aspirin will be the drug of first choice. It is the most effective simple pain relieving drug and is the most effective drug for its simple action to lower body temperature.

The dilemma is the choice between lowering the temperature with aspirin or leaving the temperature alone. If you use aspirin you will get temporary relief of the associated symptoms but you will also get the discomfort and symptoms of a rapidly changing temperature, as the aspirin pushes the temperature down and it slowly climbs back up again. Two aspirins are worth a try, however, and you will probably find yourself more comfortable if you keep the temperature down by taking them on a fairly regular schedule, every three to four hours.

Even without obvious sweating, the fluid loss with a fever is substantial. This is particularly true if you have any diarrhea. Every effort should be made to consume a generous amount of replacement fluids. Almost anything will do. However, if nothing else is taken except water you will not be replacing the salt lost in sweat or diarrhea. Alcoholic beverages have some psychological advantages but they will ultimately increase the water loss and this is not the time to impair your judgment by alcoholic excess. In addition, alcohol will make it difficult for your family and friends to assess objectively your state of well being.

If the temperature gets too high, then it must be lowered. Children under three years should not be allowed to get hotter than 103° F. since the possibility of serious convulsions is significant at higher temperatures. Confusion or delirium in older children and adults, when it is associated with a high temperature, should be treated promptly. The treatment is the same as for children, only the aspirin dosage varies: aspirin orally or by rectal suppository; and sponging with cool water or rubbing alcohol in a tub or in bed. The best places for sponging are the armpits and between the legs, but it is important to sponge the entire body.

Breathing Irregularities and Coughing

Unless breathing stops or requires a conscious effort, we don't normally pay it much attention. But there are other things that can go wrong in the respiratory mechanism between your nose and your lungs.

The subjects discussed below are concerned in some way with the respiratory process. Either normal or abnormal, trivial or life threatening, their discussion provides some perspective and orientation to the physiology of breathing.

COUGH

Most people cough frequently and many produce sputum (phlegm). This is part of the normal process of cleaning the lungs: 70 per cent of one-pack-a-day smokers have a persistent cough; 90 per cent of these cough up sputum (not saliva, but sputum, from the lungs). Almost one-quarter of the non-smokers cough on arising with the production of sputum.

Generally, coughing is a useful process. It cleans the tubes of the accumulated debris that gets down there during the night, clogging the system. The cough needs further attention when:

> it gets worse, suddenly or insidiously; or
> the non-productive cough becomes productive; or
> there is blood in the sputum.

Obviously, if it is part of another process, along with a fever or broken ribs, or a stab wound in the chest, then its perspective may be modified and your judgment should prevail. Like a fever, the presence of a cough requires an explanation. Unlike a fever, it may be normal and its cause trivial.

The explanation for a cough is almost a catalogue of the ills of mankind. Aside from the more serious problems (pneumonia, cancer, etc.) and the simple ones (cigarettes, cold air, etc.), the following are worthy of particular attention:

> The "nervous" cough is usually more severe when the anxiety increases. If the intensity or frequency of the cough varies with the tenseness of the situation, it is likely to have an anxious component to it. The simple association of an anxious component, however, does not establish that there is not any other cause.
>
> Any irritant will elicit a cough. Obviously, cigarette smoke will. Marijuana is not selected for its qualities of mildness and may often be more irritating than tobacco, but most people don't smoke twenty joints a day. Tear gas can certainly produce enough irritation to yield several days of post-exposure coughing.

The treatment of a cough is only rarely based on rational considerations. First, consider if you really want to suppress the process. Coughing is basically a protective reflex. You cough to eliminate something in your respiratory passages. If there are copious secretions or your cough produces some kind of sputum, it should probably not be suppressed unless the coughing is extremely painful or uncomfortable.

If you are going to treat a cough, there is certain information about medicines you should have.

Cough drops: The garden-variety cough, the nervous type, or a cough associated with a mild upper respiratory infection can often do well with the candy-type cough drop. These accomplish nothing more than soothing the irritated parts of your mouth and the accessible parts of your "throat." They get swallowed rather than inhaled. They have no effect whatever on the cough-producing mechanisms. Effective cough medications get transported either to your lungs to suppress the cough or to your brain to suppress the cough reflex. Cough drops do neither. This is not to say that they do not make your throat feel better, which they do, but only to note that they will accomplish nothing to resolve the cough process itself. They are simple, inexpensive (the expensive, medicinally flavored ones are not any better than the inexpensive candy-flavored kinds) and very convenient. They can be effective in reducing the tickling irritation present in the back of your throat.

The *cough medicines* have four basic constituents:

> Some *flavoring agent*. These agents taste good or medicinal, whichever you prefer. Many, particularly those called "elixirs," contain significant, or even substantial, amounts of alcohol. The alcohol has no therapeutic effectiveness in treating a cough but is thought by some to improve the flavor.
>
> An *expectorant*. This serves to liquify the sputum and make it easier to cough it up. Its value is based on the assumption that one is more likely to be comfortable if he can cough up the sputum, and that this medication will assist in that process. The former assumption seems reasonable; the latter is open to serious question. If it is useful to encourage expectoration, the simplest and most useful way to accomplish this is to increase fluid intake.
>
> An *antihistamine*. There is no logical reason for cough medicines to contain an antihistamine. They serve no useful purpose.
>
> A *cough suppressant*. Most cough suppressants are narcotics (though mild ones) and we are reasonably convinced that any dose large enough to significantly suppress a cough is probably large enough to produce some significant side effects, mostly drug dependence or sedation. If a cough needs suppression, these narcotics without the other constituents should do it, but the doses needed will require a prescription.

DIFFICULT BREATHING (Dyspnea)

Here we make the distinction between fast, hard breathing (the kind that follows a run up a flight of stairs) and dyspnea, the sensation of distress or suffocation which comes from the extremely unpleasant feeling of not getting enough air. The deep, rapid breathing which comes from exercises and is associated with conditioning, age, sex, etc., may be difficult but it is brief, resolves with rest and does not produce the agony of not getting enough air or of not being able to breathe.

The distinction is important because only the latter type is potentially serious.

The need for air is controlled by such things as your activity, your state of health (you need slightly more if you have a fever, for example), and how much oxygen is in the air you are breathing. When you exceed a certain level of activity or altitude, for example, no amount of increased breathing will enable you to get enough air quickly enough to overcome the sensation of not having enough. The treatment in these cases is decreased activity or lower altitude. The capacity of your lungs is more likely to be related to a chronic disease, but problems may emerge in a relatively acute or sudden way. Even in those with long-standing lung disease, some conditions can precipitate an episode of extreme discomfort in an otherwise stable situation. For example, the asthmatic exposed to tear gas is in serious trouble; for the patient with emphysema, a cold may have life-threatening implications.

COUGHING UP BLOOD (Hemoptysis)

It is important to make the distinction between coughing up blood, vomiting up blood, and spitting up blood. Not that one is any better or worse, but they are all different and mean different things. Most people don't differentiate them but it shouldn't be difficult if you pay attention to what you are doing when you are doing it—are you coughing, vomiting, or spitting?

If you still can't tell, you will have to take a look at the product of your efforts. Blood that comes from the lungs is usually mixed with sputum (thick and viscous) and tends to be frothy and bubbly, since it is also mixed with air. If it comes from the stomach, it may or may not have some food particles in it, and depending on how long it has been in your stomach, it will be dark red or brown in color. Blood in the stomach gets digested and is acted upon by stomach acids, so that, classically, it has the appearance of coffee grounds.

The source of the hemoptysis may be nothing more severe than a violent cough or it may be a manifestation of serious intrinsic disease of the lungs. It should not be neglected if it occurs more than once, particularly if it occurs in the presence of other symptoms such as fever, dyspnea, weight loss, chest pain, etc.

One exception is in the case of tear gas. Irritants can cause hemoptysis, particularly if they are associated with violent coughing. Normally, the treatment for tear gas (see Chapter 6) is better air, and the hemoptysis resolves with a bit of patience.

CYANOSIS (Bluish Color of the Skin)

The explanation for the blue lips, fingernails, ears, etc. is simple but requires some familiarity with physiology. The hemoglobin in the blood carries the oxygen. There are basically two kinds of hemoglobin; that with oxygen (oxygenated hemoglobin) and that without oxygen (unoxygenated hemoglobin). The oxygenated hemoglobin is red, the unoxygenated hemoglobin is much darker, almost blue. Blue color of the skin is entirely a function of the amount of unoxygenated hemoglobin in the small blood vessels of the skin.

Aside from all of the complex heart and lung diseases which cause cyanosis are these which warrant special consideration here.

Extreme cold will cause a constriction of the blood vessels in the skin and extremities and a relative stagnation of the blood supply. In a very short time the oxygen present is utilized, leaving unoxygenated hemoglobin and a blue color.

An unconscious patient may have enough brain damage to impair the normal respiratory mechanisms. The appearance of cyanosis in an unconscious patient is an emergency and requires immediate, definitive care.

SNEEZING

The primary purpose of sneezing appears to be as a cue to one's mother (or her equivalent) to say, "You are catching a cold . . . therefore you shouldn't do . . ." (fill in this space with whatever is appropriate at that time). This is an erroneous interpretation of a sneeze and should be wholly dismissed and disregarded.

At risk, however, of presenting a probably equally simplistic explanation, one should view sneezing as a normal mechanism for cleaning the nose. Since the nose gets stuffed more readily when you have a cold, you sneeze more often at that time. Sneezing is also occasionally a manifestation of an allergy.

BREATHING AT HIGH ALTITUDE

The major problem with high altitudes is that the air has less total oxygen than at sea level. Depending on the individual, and his conditioning and abruptness of exposure, the symptoms of the oxygen shortage vary. These symptoms may include headaches, nausea, dizziness, loss of appetite, fatigue and impaired judgment. These are all related to a shortage of the brain's oxygen supply.

HICCUPS

This may be a troublesome problem but is rarely serious. We cannot see the logic of any particular therapeutic effort with any of the standard home remedies, but it is innocuous to hold your breath, breathe into a paper bag, drink some water or belch.

In the event of protracted or disabling hiccups, various more elaborate forms of therapy may be needed, but in these cases, so too will a physician be necessary.

ASTHMA

A long list of things—a cold, unusual activity, pollens and dusts, emotional stress, cigarette smoke, etc.—may cause an asthmatic attack in susceptible people. Whatever causes the attack does so by causing a spasm of the small air passages in the lungs.

Various drugs and therapeutic maneuvers are useful in preventing attacks and in treating them once they have started. The drugs are potent and usually require some adjustment of dosage depending on the individual and the frequency and severity of the attacks. A physician is almost always going to be needed to manipulate the drug treatment.

Drugs, however, should be used only as a last resort. If you can identify a cause it should be excluded as much as possible from your environment. Since emotions frequently play a major role in initiating or prolonging an attack, stressful situations should be avoided. At the earliest signs of an attack, rest and tranquillity may help to minimize its severity. A generous supply of fluids and the judicious use of one of the non-prescription inhalers may make it less severe.

Asthma tends to be a disease of children and its severity usually, but not always, decreases in adult life. Its reappearance in early adulthood is often related to cigarette smoking. Occasionally, it will occur spontaneously in an adult. Audible inspiratory or expiratory wheezing suggests that the problem is primarily asthmatic.

If you have asthma or a hereditary predisposition to it, you are likely to know it already and probably have some familiarity with the kinds of things that elicit an attack and what to do about it.

An increasingly common problem with asthmatics appears to be the serious attacks which follow exposure to the various toxic gases. Asthma and tear gas do not do well together. Tear gas is surely one of the most potent asthmatic stimuli of all. Regardless of whatever else precipitates your asthma attacks, it is very likely that tear gas will as well. It is for each individual to balance the severity of his asthma, and his response to what medications are available to him, against the importance of his participation in a particular event, the likelihood of the use of tear gas and the speed with which he can get out to good air or avoid getting trapped. If you have asthma it would be prudent during a demonstration to reevaluate continually your escape route possibilities as your location changes. The persistence of tear gas, which adheres to skin and clothing, will provide a continuing stimulus to prolongation of the asthmatic attack and tear gas asthma tends to be very severe.

HYPERVENTILATION

One of the simple problems of breathing which can appear to be dramatic and life threatening is the hyperventilation syndrome or overbreathing. Usually it is not a serious problem and its treatment is simple and uncomplicated.

In the extreme case, a young, tense and anxious person complains of sharp chest pain, thundering palpitations of the heart, numbness of the fingers and lips, and the inability to get enough air. He is frightened, sweating and breathing enormous quantities of air rapidly and deeply. This alone should suggest that you may be dealing with a hyperventilation syndrome, and simple home remedies which may produce a dramatic result should be tried.

The underlying cause is whatever elicits tension and anxiety, which results in overbreathing in a labile person. It may be difficult to convince your patient that the symptoms that follow are related to the overbreathing and *not* vice versa. If you breathe rapidly and deeply for about five minutes and then close your eyes and carefully stand up rapidly you will experience these symptoms. Overbreathing will not increase the oxygen in your blood (the blood is already saturated with oxygen) but the rapid and over-enthusiastic breathing of air will remove the small, but important amount of carbon dioxide in your blood and lungs. In the body carbon dioxide functions as an acid and is important in maintaining the delicate acid-alkali balance. Remove the carbon dioxide and you lose acid. Your fingers and lips may tingle or feel numb, your heart starts pounding, and your pulse increases. The symptoms produce increasing discomfort and you breathe even more as your anxiety increases.

The therapy is twofold. First is reassurance. The patient has to be talked down from an "air-trip." Second is a paper bag for rebreathing. Since the mechanism for the problem involves a loss of carbon dioxide, breathing into and from a paper bag will tend to increase the body's store of carbon dioxide and the symptoms, but not the cause, may be alleviated. At least the vicious cycle may be broken.

Sometimes the simple recognition of the nature of the problem will prevent its recurrence. More often, it tends to recur from time to time. As the individual develops various alternate mechanisms to deal with anxieties, these may replace the hyperventilation syndrome and not be as unpleasant and uncomfortable. In an occasional patient, sedation or tranquilizers are needed to break the episode.

Bleeding and Anemia

There are mystical associations with blood which elicit strange reactions to its sudden appearance and about which encyclopedias of old-wives' tales exist, commenting about its function, presence, absence, replacement, rejuvenation, restoration, or discussing aspects of the mystic properties which it is held to possess. A few words about the physiology of blood will not, we hope, dispel any of the romance but will possibly provide some perspective.

Blood is a suspension of a number of microscopic particles in a complex yellowish-colored solution called plasma. The red color of blood is created by hundreds of millions of red blood cells or red blood corpuscles. A much smaller number of other kinds of blood cells, the white blood cells (leucocytes) and platelets are also present in blood.

The plasma, in addition to providing the fluidity for the movement of the cells, contains a number of proteins with diverse functions. The two major functions are the transport of various substances from one place to another within the body and the initiation of a blood clot in the event that one of the arteries, capillaries, or veins is injured or broken. Serum is that part of plasma remaining after blood has clotted. The red cells are responsible for transport of oxygen to tissues and for the removal of carbon dioxide. The hemoglobin within the red cell actually carries the oxygen and carbon dioxide.

Hemoglobin is a pigment which gives the red blood cells their red color. When it is fully oxygenated, as in healthy arterial blood, it is a bright red; when it is carrying less oxygen as in venous blood, it is much darker, almost blue, in color. The white blood cells play a major role in the body's mechanisms to combat infection. The platelets participate with the plasma in the clotting of blood.

The life-threatening aspects of blood loss relate primarily to the failure of the oxygen transport mechanism when too little blood is present. Without oxygen, there is no survival.

BLEEDING

Except for menstrual periods, bleeding is always abnormal. It occurs as a result of either of two processes: an injury or some sort of damaged or diseased tissue; or an inability of the blood to clot following an insignificant or trivial injury to normal tissues.

The latter process is much less common. If it exists it is usually obvious in childhood and usually hereditary. Individuals so affected have enough experience to know to avoid potentially dangerous situations. On rare occasions an adult will spontaneously develop an inability to clot blood. The most suggestive clue is the appearance of bleeding in the skin or joints without any obvious injury.

The more common kind of bleeding, that from injured or damaged tissue, is not always visible. A bleeding ulcer, for example, can be just as troublesome as an open scalp wound. Usually the signs of obscure bleeding become apparent with the development of other symptoms (e.g., pain, diarrhea), but in any case, obscure or obvious, the symptoms of the loss of blood depend upon how much and how quickly blood is lost. A slowly leaking ulcer may halve your total hemoglobin concentration with the appearance of only minor symptoms of fatigue, but the equivalent loss of that much blood from a rapidly bleeding abdominal wound would be catastrophic. With slow blood loss the body has time to adjust to the bleeding wound and, even if the red cells and hemoglobin cannot be replaced quickly enough, at least the body can restore the volume of the blood by the slow synthesis of additional plasma, and a more dilute (anemic) blood at least prevents the onset of shock.

ANEMIA

Anemia is the consequence of an inadequate supply of hemoglobin in the red cells, or too few red cells each with a normal hemoglobin concentration. In the former there is an inability of the body to manufacture enough hemoglobin to keep up with normal destruction and loss. The latter is most likely due to loss of blood at a rate greater than the red blood cells can be replaced and fluids dilute the red cells in the blood.

Only a small fraction of the people who are chronically tired are anemic (despite the advertisements to the contrary), but most people who have significant anemia are chronically tired. The recognition of anemia is simple and fairly reliable. A pale or sallow complexion often won't help because many people have naturally light complexions and are not anemic. Judging complexion is obviously useless in dark-skinned people or whites with a sunburn. Better, look at the eyes or fingernails; check the color of the inside of the lower eyelid or press on a fingernail and note the return of color in the nail bed just beyond the moon shape at the base. A more useful measure of anemia can be obtained by comparing this color against that of a normal person.

Anemia will also be manifested by a number of other relatively non-specific but suggestive symptoms. Such things as an increased heart rate at rest, a decreased exercise tolerance, fatigue, shortness of breath, headaches, dizziness, loss of appetite, loss of libido and cessation of menses are all consistent with anemia. These symptoms are also consistent with any of a number of other things and are the ordinary warnings that something is wrong.

Be careful about oversimplifying anemia and its treatment. Usually, it is due to excessive blood loss (most commonly menstrual bleeding) and/or due to deficient dietary iron intake. Rarely, it is due to some other disease process. A reasonable diet with supplementary iron pills will usually resolve the problem, but other home remedies will be useless. If it isn't caused by blood loss or iron deficiency, then tampering with it will only delay the initiation of appropriate diagnosis and therapy for which you will need expert medical assistance.

Functions of the Brain

Loss of consciousness or a change in the level of consciousness is a dramatic, frightening, and potentially life-threatening event. Its cause may be obvious or obscure; its onset slow or abrupt; its outcome innocuous or fatal. In all cases it represents a major problem not only for a physician but even more so for a layman faced with an unconscious or confused person and with the responsibility of organizing some kind of assistance.

As with most other general areas discussed in this chapter, the scope of the subject is boundless. This is even more the case here, since we are brazen enough to deal with the subtleties of the human mind and ask that you do so also in evaluating the well-being of your friends and family. We will not be comprehensive and will not offer a course in neuroanatomy or behavioral psychology. We will be simplistic in our discussion of what you might encounter, and use common words to describe various kinds of activities of the brain. The list is more than a glossary but substantially less than an exhaustive discussion. The comments will be useful rather than scientific.

NERVOUSNESS

This term is used to describe anything from restlessness or anxiety to blatant psychosis. The manifestations can vary from the usual symptoms of anxiety, hyperactivity, tearfulness, changes in mood, depression, anger, or somatic symptoms such as an upset stomach, diarrhea, or headaches or even the change of sleep or behavior patterns. In severe forms it may cause more profound changes in habits and life style. Any of the characteristics can be mild or serious. In the extreme, a "nervous breakdown" can represent a totally disordered state of thinking with bizarre behavior or serious psychosis. Despite its vagueness we still think that the word "nervousness" is a useful term. Given some kind of context it always seems to transmit some information about what is troubling the patient.

ANXIETY

This is scientifically a more specific term, although it has several meanings and is frequently interchangeable with nervousness. Usually, but not always, one is anxious about something forthcoming: a specific event, an examination, an encounter. It is the very vague and uneasy feeling that you have when you are worried and insecure. It is what causes deep breathing, a choking sensation in the throat, butterflies in the stomach, sweaty palms, heart palpitations and the absolute conviction of immediate triumph or doom.

It is entirely normal. Everyone has anxious moments and it is a totally reasonable response to stress. It is only when anxiety becomes a way of life, a pattern, a preoccupation that it becomes so troublesome as to require some kind of assistance for its resolution.

DEPRESSION

A person who is depressed usually complains of the symptoms of his depression rather than of sadness. As with anxiety or nervousness, depression may be perfectly normal; in this case a response to a bad or unhappy situation. When it becomes excessive or when some of the associated symptoms become substantial or prolonged, it becomes more significant. What characterizes excessive depression depends on your own interpretation. Symptoms like change in sleep patterns or appetite, crying spells, persistent loss of energy or interest, a sensation of hopelessness, futility or despair, all suggest that a reasonable adjustment has not occurred. The development of symptoms establishes and reinforces a vicious cycle of symptoms, depression symptoms, etc. A bad sign is when a person seems depressed over an apparently trivial event with the reaction and duration all out of proportion to its importance or when there doesn't seem to be any precipitating event at all.

FAINTING

Fainting used to be a very fashionable thing to do in Victorian parlors. It is too bad that it has gone out of style because it certainly is a very elegant but harmless way to express intense emotion. The fact that it has gone out of style helps to establish its cause as emotional. This is not to say that it isn't real; an intense experience, anxiety, pain or the like easily causes rapid dilatation of the blood vessels in the periphery of the body (mostly the skin). The blood pools in these dilated vessels and there is just not enough to get up to the brain. The brain runs short of supplies very quickly and a faint ensues. That you fall down is fortunate, since the head is now at the same level as the rest of the body and the heart no longer has to pump the remaining blood up to the brain. After a few seconds or minutes of lying flat, the blood gets redistributed to where it belongs and the fainter awakens. With some skill it can all be a beautiful scene.

Not all fainting spells are emotional. Nowadays relatively few are. A faint has to be differentiated from scores of other things which can cause a sudden loss of consciousness. Usually, if its onset is abrupt, its duration is brief and the recovery is complete, you are dealing with a simple fainting spell.

A sudden prolonged irregularity in the heart rhythm may also produce a fainting spell. An epileptic fit may sometimes look like a faint.

In addition to the serious things which cause a sudden loss of consciousness, there are a handful of innocuous things, other than emotion, which can cause a simple faint. If you are lying down and suddenly stand up, your heart may not pump enough blood uphill to the brain fast enough and you may have a moment of dizziness or faint. This postural dizziness is more common in older people.

A number of other strange things can cause a fainting spell. One of the more unusual is micturition syncope—the fainting that occurs usually in young men while standing to urinate. The vulnerable men appear to have a particularly sensitive neural reflex between their bladder and their heart. Sometime between the initiation and termination of urination, they will have a slowing of their heart rate, an inadequate supply of blood to the brain, and they will collapse in a heap on the floor. It is, fortunately, rare.

Thus, any of a large number of things which cause a sudden loss of consciousness range from the benign to the fatal.

Usually, fainting is associated with an inadequate blood supply to the brain. If you are there when someone faints, let him lie there with his head down on the floor and his face turned to the side (so that he won't gag on anything if he vomits). Don't prop up his head, but it may help to prop up his legs. Check his pulse. If it is over 50 and he is breathing, loosen his collar, and adjust things to get him comfortable. If you're in a hurry, splash some cold water in his face or break a capsule of smelling salts in front of his nose. Don't give him anything to eat or drink until he is fully awake, and be reassured that if uncomplicated, the episode is brief. If the pulse is absent or very slow (less than 50) or if he is not breathing or if he is having a seizure, then you ought to treat as a cardiac or respiratory arrest (see Chapter 5) or as a seizure (see below).

HALLUCINATIONS, DELUSIONS, ILLUSIONS

For the sake of purity of thought hallucinations ought to be differentiated from delusions and illusions. If you see a leaf being blown by the wind and you think it is a mouse, this is an illusion. If there is no leaf or mouse, this is a hallucination. When you continue to think that there is a mouse despite the presentation of normally convincing evidence to the contrary, then you are having a delusion. Illusions are not usually a problem. Hallucinations and delusions are. Hallucinations, by the way, are usually auditory, not visual. You hear little men rather than see little bugs. The voices are usually threatening or accusatory and focus around feelings of inadequacy or guilt on the part of the victim.

DIZZINESS

The medical word is "vertigo" but, technically, vertigo means a sensation of movement, either the feeling of your moving in your surroundings or of things moving around you. Dizziness is the sensation of lightheadedness or giddiness. If you have persistent true vertigo (movement), there is likely to be something wrong with the equilibrium apparatus in the inner part of your ear. That assumes that you don't have an ear infection, a cold, or some other reason for being dizzy such as an overindulgence in alcohol or sea sickness. If dizziness persists and there is no obvious explanation for it, you ought to have it checked by a competent physician.

CONCUSSION

This term has no precise medical or scientific meaning and so means different things to different people. A general description of a head injury may be useful. When you have had a head injury of any sort, and there has been any loss of consciousness or any kind of neurological disability (e.g., headache, dizziness, confusion), we can say for our purpose here that there has been a concussion and not quibble about the details. The brain is an elaborate and delicate organ, and when it bounces around inside the relatively rigid skull, almost anything can happen. A concussion may follow something as serious as running your head through an automobile windshield or something as seemingly innocuous as banging your head on a low doorway. Wide variations in brain damage may occur depending on the circumstances of the injury. The head may be movable or relatively firmly fixed when it is hit. The injury may be in a relatively sensitive or innocuous location. There may be a fracture. There may be internal bleeding, bruising, a laceration, swelling, shifting of the contents of the brain, or an injury to that part of the brain opposite to where the trauma occurred as the brain smashes against the inside of the skull on the opposite side of the head.

The seriousness of the concussion is roughly proportional to the magnitude of the symptoms with which it is associated. But no head injury should be treated lightly, for some injuries with even minor symptoms can become serious. Anyone with a concussion should be observed carefully for at least a few days.

MIGRAINE

This is a specific kind of headache, different from the ordinary tension headache and usually easily identifiable. It is important to make the differentiation because the treatment is different. Migraine headaches recur with a variable frequency and tend to decrease with aging. Women have them more often than men, and usually start having them by the time they are in their twenties. There is a good chance that it runs in their family. It has a characteristic pattern for each person, is often associated with nausea, sensitivity to light, and is usually very severe and disabling. Some people have premonitory symptoms. The association with other neurological symptoms is not uncommon. In its classic form the migraine is relieved by the use of an ergot-like drug in the early stages of the headache. The mechanism of action of the ergot is unknown, but it is interesting to note that LSD is an ergot derivative.

PARANOIA

Simply having the feeling of being persecuted is not enough. The persistent feelings ought to be delusional to qualify as paranoid. That is, the feelings of persecution exist despite the fact that normally convincing evidence establishes that it just isn't so.

DELIRIUM

When a person is very sick, usually with some kind of infection and usually with a high fever, he may become delirious. His thinking is not right, his level of consciousness is depressed, he is restless, agitated, and disoriented. He may have illusions or hallucinations. The treatment is usually the treatment of the underlying disease.

EPILEPSY

There is a very wide spectrum of things called epilepsy and a varying amount of disability associated with it. In epilepsy there is some kind of episodic, transient dysfunction of the brain. It is often associated with a convulsion (also called a fit or a seizure) which is a spasmodic twitching of all or some parts of the body, and usually a loss of consciousness. Between seizure episodes patients are usually quite normal, unless they have suffered some kind of brain damage from the seizures, or the brain damage from some other source is causing the seizures, or they have injured themselves during one of their seizures. Good medications are available which are effective in controlling the frequency and/or the severity of the attacks.

Seizures tend to be dramatic but aren't always as serious as they appear. Some patients can sense an impending seizure and can take precautions to prevent any injury. Unfortunately, this is not usually the case. If you happen to be with a person when he has an epileptic seizure, there is quite a bit you can do to help, but not much you can do to terminate the seizure itself. First, make every effort to see that the patient does not injure himself. Don't attempt to restrain him or to stop the muscle twitching. Pad or protect his head or any part of his body that might get injured. Loosen any tight clothing. If you can, turn his head to one side so that if he vomits the vomitus will flow out of his mouth rather than back down into his lungs. If his jaw is rigid or if he is biting his tongue, it is useful to put a firm object like a rolled-up handkerchief between his teeth to prevent him from injuring his tongue or cheeks. Epileptics occasionally urinate or defecate during a seizure.

Most seizures are over within a few minutes. If they persist or get more severe, the patient should be transported to a hospital where drugs to terminate the episode can be administered. Usually, when the spasms subside the patient remains drowsy, weak, or unconscious for a period of time. He should be kept comfortable and allowed to rest until he is fully conscious and alert, since premature activity may provoke another attack.

Once the individual has recovered, it is important to determine if he has had seizures before or if this has been the first attack. If it is the first seizure, he should have a complete medical evaluation. The list of possibilities which produce seizures is a very long one and ranges from simple drug withdrawal to a complicated brain tumor. If the seizure is one of many, probably no medical assistance is necessary unless he has sustained an injury during the seizure or some other problem has arisen.

The most frequent causes of seizures in epileptic patients are:

> Failure to take prescribed anti-seizure drugs. Check to make sure he has his medications and has been taking them.
>
> Alcohol in excess. As a general rule, alcohol and epilepsy don't mix too well.
>
> Chaotic use of any of a number of drugs. Some patients will have a seizure when they discontinue a drug which they have been taking regularly over a prolonged period of time, a withdrawal phenomenon. A rum fit following the discontinuation of alcohol in a chronic alcoholic is a classic example. Sometimes excessive use of some drugs will cause a seizure.

SLEEP AND INSOMNIA

Sleep is much less a problem than insomnia. Although an occasional person may complain of inability to stay awake, far more have persistent difficulty with going to sleep. The problem of not being able to stay awake relates either to too little sleep or it relates to the specifics of what is happening, a dull book, a boring lecture, or uninspiring company.

Normal people have wide variations in the amount of sleep they need to comfortably sustain themselves and their activities. There is nothing sacred about eight hours a night, and many people do well on five hours while some need nine.

Older people usually need less than younger people. Everyone's inner clock is set a bit different. If you are short of sleep one night you can make part of that deficit up the next night but you will not catch up on it all, nor need you. Similarly, you cannot store up sleep in anticipation of an expected sleepless night.

Dreaming is an important part of sleeping. Everyone dreams when he is asleep, although the ability to recall dreams differs. Dream sleep apparently contributes more to your state of well being than just refreshing your subconscious mechanisms. People who have been deprived of their dream time in laboratory studies soon become anxious and uncomfortable, although they are permitted to sleep their normal number of total hours.

Insomnia can be a very unpleasant problem but a number of things which are thought of as insomnia are not that at all. Many people who complain of insomnia are getting an adequate amount of sleep but have multiple episodes of wakefulness during the night. The episodes are brief but, in total, they can be quite uncomfortable and can create the sensation of being awake all night. Other people who don't sleep comfortably at night take a number of cat-naps during the day. These naps, which can be quite restful, can cut into the need for the eight hours which is sought every night. Finally, some people who try to get eight hours of sleep may not need that much. They may awaken early or have trouble getting to sleep and are rightfully unhappy about the few hours they spend in bed without sleeping.

Real insomnia is usually caused by the tensions and anxieties of the insomniac's world. Early awakening is often suggestive of depression rather than anxiety. Occasionally, insomnia is caused by the injudicious use of stimulants such as coffee, tea, or various soft drinks (which all contain caffeine) or drugs such as the appetite suppressants (amphetamines). Occasionally, insomnia is caused by a real physical problem like pain or the need to awaken frequently to urinate. Rarely is it based on some organic problem that upsets the sleep-regulating center in the brain, but it would be extremely unlikely for this rare phenomenon to occur without some other evidence of brain damage or injury.

An occasional sleepless night will have no long-term consequences, either mental or physical. Although it may cause some transient discomfort and disruption of your life, it should not be a cause for concern. People who have chronic problems with sleeplessness should first consider the possibilities outlined above and then the possibilities of modifying the sources of the tensions and anxieties which create the insomnia. Recognizing the difficulties of accomplishing the latter, we realistically suggest some of the ways you might want to approach the insomnia.

> There are dozens of home remedies which have an occasional place in solving the problem for some people, some of the time. Hot milk, a bad book, soft music, ear plugs, warm baths, counting sheep, television movies, aspirin and sexual relations all have their place in inducing sleep and most are worth a try.

> A number of drugs are available without a prescription which are advertised as having sleep-inducing effects. Most contain scopolamine in small doses or are antihistamines and are based on one of the common side effects of antihistamines, sedation. They are mild and occasionally effective, though it is doubtful that they would solve the problems of most people with chronic insomnia.

> A number of specific drugs are excellent sedatives. These will induce comfortable and sound sleep in all but the most resistant people. The barbiturates and other drugs like chloral hydrate are safe and will not develop addiction in any, save the most neurotic personality. These drugs will require a prescription.

ALTERATIONS IN CONSCIOUSNESS

A fully conscious person is awake, aware of his surroundings, and able to respond to various stimuli. There is, of course, some variation; you may have your attention so narrowly focused on a single particular object that you are unaware of the surroundings, but you are probably no less conscious. Consciousness can lapse into inattentiveness. Daydreaming is a good example. When you are asleep you are, in a sense, unconscious. The state of sleep is characterized, however, by the fact that you can be aroused easily and that you respond to stimuli.

There is a big overlap in the various mildly altered states of consciousness: somnolence, confusion, delirium and the like. They are not separable, they don't move from one to another in an orderly sequence. They often overlap. A delirious patient is usually variably somnolent and hyperactive and always confused.

Beyond this is the stuporous patient. He has minimal mental and physical activity. He responds slowly, usually in a primitive way to various stimuli. He will withdraw from pain and may moan. He cannot be awakened. When there is no sensation and no response to any stimuli, then there is coma.

When the coma is profound, the normal reflexes may disappear and abnormal ones may be found. Sometimes a comatose patient can respond to a very painful stimulus. It may seem cruel but it is worth checking to see if he responds to something like your knuckle pressing firmly against his sternum (the breastbone) or your fingernail pressing against the root of his fingernail. Try these and see how painful either of them can be with relatively little pressure. Take a look at his eyes. If the pupils (the black spot in the center of the eye) are roughly equal in size, get a flashlight and check to see if the pupils constrict with light. They will in all but the most severe coma. While you are up around the eye, gently (please, gently) touch the cornea with the end of a clean tissue or handkerchief. The cornea is that transparent part of the eye which covers the colored part in the center. In all but the most deeply comatose patient, touching the cornea will elicit a vigorous blink. If there is no blink, close both of the patient's eyes and keep them closed (with tape if necessary so that they don't dry out) and hurry. This is another sign of deep and serious coma.

Functions of the Heart

The major purpose of the heart is to pump blood around the body, and since the time of William Harvey in 1628, there has been little dispute about this. Hearts may have difficulty with the soul, but these problems are rarely fatal. No one has died of a "broken heart" probably since the early part of the nineteenth century. The problems with the heart are usually related to its difficulties as a pump; it is either pumping too much, too little, too rapidly, too slowly, at too great or too little pressure, or it fails to sustain its activities continually. When it fails as a pump it cannot get blood to the tissues where it is needed and the various organs in the body will fail to survive without an adequate blood supply.

The heart is a muscle which is just a little different from the ordinary muscles all over the rest of the body. By contracting and relaxing and utilizing a series of valves which cause the blood to move in one direction only, it pumps the blood first to the lungs where the blood disposes of waste carbon dioxide and picks up a fresh supply of oxygen. From the lungs, the blood flows back to the heart where it gets pumped into the arteries and out into the general circulation. Some of the blood is diverted into the coronary arteries, those vessels which nourish the heart muscle itself. When one of these coronary arteries is occluded or obstructed, a portion of the heart muscle dies and you have a heart attack (see below).

The contraction of the heart muscle is not a voluntary activity. The heart muscle continues to operate spontaneously almost totally beyond your control and it is governed by a complex set of feedback mechanisms involving nerves, hormones, and receptors for blood pressure, oxygen content of the blood, blood concentration, and a number of other factors.

ARTERIES, CAPILLARIES, AND VEINS

Blood pumped from the heart flows into the arteries under a substantial head of pressure which is generated by the pumping of the heart. Since arterial blood is laden with oxygen, it is bright red in color, and since it is under high pressure, an artery, when cut, will spurt out blood. When you feel the pulse (the best place to feel it is on the inside of the wrist on the side toward the thumb), you are feeling the pressure of the heart pumping blood into one of the major arteries of the arm. Arterial injuries are potentially more serious than injuries to other blood vessels partly because the high pressure causes the loss of a large amount of blood quickly, partly because the arteries are few in number and large in caliber and carry a relatively large volume of blood, and partly because the interference with the flow of blood may result in a lack of oxygen to vital organs downstream. The major arteries branch out into smaller arteries and eventually into finer and more dispersed vessels to become capillaries. The capillaries are microscopically small blood vessels which actually come into direct contact with virtually every cell in the body. The exchange of oxygen, carbon dioxide, nutrients, and waste products between the cell and the blood occurs when the blood in the capillary comes into immediate contact with the cell. The capillary network is so interconnected and adaptable that damage to a single capillary does not cause serious problems. As the injured area heals, so does the capillary network.

The capillaries eventually merge with one another to become larger and larger channels called veins which carry the blood back to the heart. The blood in these vessels is higher in carbon dioxide content but lower in oxygen and appears much darker, almost blue. Since the pressure that forced the blood from the arteries through the small capillaries is by now almost entirely dissipated, the pressure in the veins is quite low and an injury to a vein is not as dramatic, nor as serious, as an injury to an artery. Veins are more plentiful than arteries, many are more superficially located just beneath the skin and, because of this, are more commonly injured. Unlike an artery, the function of an injured or occluded vein can usually be accommodated by the collateral circulation, that is, its function can be assumed by another vein which is nearby. Arteries, on the other hand, usually have a unique function and serve a particular area. It is unlikely that an alternate artery can rapidly take over the function of a major artery if it is obstructed or injured.

RATE AND RHYTHM: PALPITATIONS

The heart normally beats between about 50 and 110 times per minute. The rate varies with physical condition, activity, emotions, body temperature, and a number of other similar factors. Athletes in top physical condition usually have a slower rate, about 50–60 per minute. Some excitable and anxious people run around 100 most of the time, but even in these people with a rapid pulse, the rate will drop when they are asleep. A sleeping pulse over 100 suggests that something is wrong; sometimes the thyroid gland, which is partly responsible for metabolic activity, may be overactive. If someone checks your pulse when you are asleep and it is more than 100, the problem should be evaluated by a doctor.

The rhythm of the heart is usually quite regular. In some people there may be a slight, barely discernible variation in rhythm during the phases of respiration. This is of no consequence and is more commonly found in the very young and the very old. A pulse which is distinctly irregular is usually abnormal. Sometimes it represents a type of heart disease but it is occasionally due to overwork, insufficient rest, too much coffee, cigarettes, or stimulants. An irregular rhythm is less efficient than a normal one. If it persists, it should be treated, simply to increase the efficiency and decrease the work of the heart.

You will not usually be able to feel your normal heart beating. Some people like the reassurance that they get from knowing that their heart is beating, but they can be reassured simply by the observation that they are alive and, presumably, conscious. The heart will tend to its affairs without your conscious intervention, and your worrying or wondering about it will not improve its functions one whit. There are four conditions wherein you might be aware of the sensation of the pounding of your heart in your chest, or what is frequently called palpitations.

1. When you are lying in bed and your hand is under the pillow and your world is quiet, you may hear your own pulse, either from the pulse in your wrist or from the pulsation of the blood in the arteries around your ear or in your head. If you listen intently and really concentrate and worry about it, the pounding may increase and sound like a beating drum. This is perfectly normal and is of no consequence. If you need reassurance, you need only lift your head from the pillow and the sound will disappear. This does not mean that your heart has stopped beating; only that the resonating sounds can no longer be heard. Turn over and go back to sleep.

2. Anxious, tense, and emotional people may sometimes have the feeling of their heart pounding in their chest. This may be a manifestation of the hyperventilation syndrome (see Chapter 4) or it may be a vague kind of symptom associated with various other problems such as chest pain, or difficulty in breathing. If you concentrate on the rate and, more importantly, the rhythm of the beat and find them both to be normal, you can be reassured. A few minutes of quiet rest sitting down or, better, lying down, with the dissipation of the emotional tension or anxiety will often suffice.

3. Sometimes people can be aware of their heart pounding after vigorous exercise or after the excessive use of various

kinds of stimulants such as coffee (caffeine), tea (caffeine), various cola drinks (caffeine), too many cigarettes (nicotine), or one of the amphetamine drugs. The heart is actually responding normally in these cases to unusual stimulation.

4. Finally, an abnormally rapid or irregular heartbeat can sometimes be sensed by some people. If it is associated with shortness of breath, a sense of suffocation, dizziness, chest pain or chest pressure, or a sense of impending doom, the palpitations and the associated heart problem may be serious and you should have it checked promptly.

One type of abnormal heartbeat which is seen occasionally in people in their teens and twenties is a rhythm called paroxysmal atrial tachycardia (P.A.T.). In an episode of P.A.T. there is an abrupt onset of a very rapid heart rate for no apparent reason. The rate may be as slow as 140 per minute or as high as 250 beats per minute. This rapid rate may last for a few minutes or even for a few days or longer. It may be associated with no symptoms at all or very uncomfortable symptoms of weakness, dizziness, fainting, chest pain, or the development of the symptoms of heart failure (see below). It usually stops as suddenly as it starts but, when it persists, may require medications or other techniques for its termination. People who have these episodes often learn how to treat the abnormal rhythm themselves with such maneuvers as pressing on their eyeballs (carefully and gently), massaging the carotid artery in the neck (better check with a doctor first), inducing vomiting, or assuming various positions such as bending, squatting, or turning upside down. A particularly effective technique is breathing out forcefully with the windpipe closed, a process which can best be simulated by recalling the process in which you bear down when you defecate or have a baby. In general, P.A.T. is not serious. It rarely represents more than an uncomfortable nuisance.

BLOOD PRESSURE AND HIGH BLOOD PRESSURE (Hypertension)

The pressure of the blood in your arteries is not steady; it increases with the heartbeat and decreases when the heart rests. The familiar recording of the blood pressure is represented as one number over another. This notation indicates the systolic pressure (the upper number) during contraction of the heart, over the diastolic pressure (the lower number) during the relaxation phase.

Normal blood pressure varies with age, but this may be nothing more than an observation of the aging process itself. In general, a blood pressure greater than 140/90 is considered abnormal and, in general, the denominator, the diastolic pressure, is a more precise measure of the magnitude of the high blood pressure. If the blood pressure is high when the heart is relaxed, this can be thought of as a more ominous sign.

A single random measure of blood pressure is only useful if it is normal. If it is high, the measurement should be repeated after the patient has had a few minutes (at least fifteen) of quiet rest and a chance to catch his breath and calm himself. There is nothing quite like seeing a cute nurse, or hurrying to get to a late appointment, or a quick run up a flight of stairs or an anxious medical examination to raise the blood pressure. Chances are that the pressure will be much lower, or even normal, the second or third time it is measured.

High blood pressure may be totally asymptomatic or may be associated with any of a number of signs and symptoms questionably related to the blood pressure elevation. Occasionally persistent or frequent nosebleeds or recurrent headaches, particularly those present on awakening in the morning, may indicate high blood pressure. Sometimes the hypertension will be manifested by a vague sense of fatigue, dizziness, or nervousness, but most people who are tired, dizzy, or nervous don't have hypertension. Most often high blood pressure is found on a routine physical examination.

If the pressure is high, it should be treated. In about 5 per cent of people with hypertension, its cause can be identified and treatment usually results in a cure. Usually, the treatment to lower the high blood pressure in the remaining 95 per cent will have to continue indefinitely. Untreated, severe hypertension will eventually create major problems in the blood vessels and may cause serious kidney, eye, heart, and brain damage.

CHEST PAIN

Most episodes of chest pain are not heart attacks, but even a little chest pain can be a frightening event, since almost everyone knows and worries about a heart attack. Heart attacks are particularly uncommon in young people. A number of other things can cause chest pain. Most commonly there is no specific or identifiable cause for the pain. The episode of chest pain simply doesn't have any good physical reason or explanation. Sometimes there are muscle aches and pains, the kinds you may see spontaneously or associated with the flu or a viral upper respiratory infection. Occasionally, a specific infection in the lungs (pneumonia) or lung coverings (pleurisy) will cause chest pain. A broken or bruised rib (Chapter 5), hyperventilation (Chapter 4), anxiety (Chapter 4), heartburn (Chapter 4), a hiatus hernia (Chapter 4), and dozens of other things can do it.

Identifying the cause can be very difficult and may require laboratory studies, x-rays, electrocardiograms, and, occasionally, hospitalization. Certain kinds of clues, however, may provide some distinguishing features and help you to determine if the pain is serious. As with most other symptoms, the best clues are provided by a detailed evaluation of the pain itself and the characteristics of the pain or by noting the presence of any associated symptoms.

The pain which is associated with heart problems or a heart attack is called angina pectoris, or simply angina. Angina means pain, and angina pectoris is Latin for chest pain. When the heart is under stress, for whatever reason, one manifestation of the stress is pain. The stress can be caused by excessive demands on the heart relative to its capabilities, and its capabilities may be limited by factors like age, its own blood supply or its atherosclerosis, i.e., the accumulation of fatty material in the arteries. Classical angina is quite characteristic; a rather severe, sharp and crushing sensation in the left side of the chest or beneath the sternum which radiates up to the left shoulder down the left arm (sometimes the right shoulder or arm as well) or sometimes up into the neck or jaw. It is often accompanied by shortness of breath, a sense of suffocation, dizziness, nausea, or vomiting. It usually starts abruptly when you are putting the heart under the stress which elicits the symptoms; hard work, vigorous physical activity, or after a heavy meal. It tends to subside with rest.

As with all classical forms of disease, the classical pattern may not fit your atypical or unique heart, and the pattern of your angina pectoris may vary greatly from the textbook description. Not all chest pain is angina pectoris and not all angina pectoris is a heart attack. Although angina pectoris means the heart is under stress, not all stress leads to a heart attack wherein there is damage and death of part of the heart muscle. Distinguishing between angina with or without a heart attack usually requires the skill of experienced doctors and the evaluation of changes in an electrocardiogram. It is occasionally diagnosed by an astute patient who identifies a change in the usual pattern of his angina.

Other kinds of chest pain can also be significant. If the pain is associated with a fever, a severe cough (particularly if there is some blood in the sputum), or difficulty breathing, there is a good chance that you are dealing with something that needs medical evaluation. If any of the signs of shock (see Chapter 5) are present (e.g., profuse sweating, a cold, clammy feeling, loss of consciousness), or if the chest pains are associated with an irregular rhythm, immediate and emergency medical attention is necessary.

HEART ATTACKS (Coronary, Myocardial Infarction)

The muscle of the heart is provided with its blood supply, not from within the chambers of the heart itself, but through a group of small arteries in the wall of the heart, just as any organ needs to be provided with arterial blood. When one of these arteries, called a coronary artery, is occluded, or narrowed, or in a spasm, the blood supply to that portion of the heart is compromised. If the blood supply is inadequate for a long enough period of time, that segment of heart muscle will stop functioning and eventually die. This is a heart attack. It is also called a "coronary," implying an occlusion or disease of one of the coronary arteries. Technically, it is called a "myocardial infarction"; myocardium is the medical word for heart muscle and infarction describes the process of tissue death because of failure of blood supply.

Not all heart attacks are fatal. The outcome depends partly on the extent and location of the affected area. Some parts of the heart are more important and vulnerable than others. Sometimes a heart attack will produce an arrhythmia because the damaged tissue within the heart is that part which controls or transmits the internal electrical impulses which produce the rhythmic contraction of the heart. If the arrhythmia is severe enough, the heart will beat randomly (and ineffectively) or stop beating entirely and death rapidly ensues. Sometimes a critical section of muscle is damaged and the function of the heart as a pump is so severely compromised that it either pumps not at all (fatal) or so poorly that the remaining tissues of the body cannot be properly perfused (usually ultimately fatal).

Many heart attacks are compatible with reasonably normal activities and normal life expectancy. A heart attack is always serious and always requires treatment. The treatment will not cure the process but may have some effect on preventing complications and/or its recurrence.

ARTERIOSCLEROSIS AND ATHEROSCLEROSIS

These two terms are often thought of as synonymous; they are not. Arteriosclerosis is a more general word. It means hardening of the arteries but does not specify what it is that is producing the process. The most common form of hardening of the arteries is caused by atherosclerosis. In this disease, fatty material (atheroma) accumulates in the arteries, causing thickening of the walls of the vessel, loss of elasticity and, ultimately, a narrowing or occlusion of the blood vessel.

Atherosclerosis is by far the most common cause of heart attacks. The disease starts early in life but usually does not become a problem until the progression of years has enabled the process to deposit enough fat in the blood vessels to be significant. Autopsies performed on soldiers killed in combat show that at least three-quarters of them have significant atherosclerosis by the time they are of military age. The sum total of our biological and medical knowledge does not provide us with anything that can be done to prevent this.

Atherosclerosis and the associated heart attack are probably the result of the combined effect of a number of factors. Rarely, some single factor can be found which is responsible for the problem. Almost always, it is a combination of many processes occurring simultaneously, each contributing to a variable degree to the atherosclerotic process. Some predisposing factors are more important than others. A bad family history is important. If your ancestors die in auto accidents in their eighties, this is good. If they die of heart attacks in their forties, this is bad, and you are very vulnerable in your forties, although not invariably so. Your dietary habits influence the rapidity of the atherosclerotic process and may predispose you to early heart attacks. Obesity, high blood pressure, diabetes, and cigarette smoking are strong predisposing influences on the likelihood of an early and usually a severe heart attack. Less easily documented and probably only slightly less important are the roles of stress and activity.

It is probable that the tense, anxious, uptight individual is more coronary-prone, and it is also probable that the sedentary, slothful way of life is not too good for you. The relaxed athlete is probably better off.

None of these factors is absolute because heart attacks occur in young, lean, muscular, non-smoking, non-diabetic, calm, tranquil athletes with no family history of heart problems. The statistics are on your side if you meet these advantageous criteria, but statistics deal with large groups of people, not with individuals.

One thing is worth noting. Whatever prevention or treatment is undertaken, it is much more effective if it is started in younger, rather than older people. Preventive measures, particularly those outlined in the comments on diet below, are a lot of work and unproven or, at best, only marginally effective.

DIET AND HEART DISEASE

Chapter 7 discusses food and eating in some detail. Our discussion here deals specifically with that part of diet and nutrition related to heart disease.

Fat, in particular two forms of fat, cholesterol and triglycerides, is what is deposited in the arteries in heart disease. Both cholesterol and triglycerides are synthesized in your liver, but the total amount that you have within you depends, in part, on how much you eat. It is a great over-simplification to suggest that you merely decrease your intake of cholesterol and triglycerides. For one thing, you need some fat in your diet. Some types of fat are essential and cannot be synthesized by the body. These essential forms cannot be separated in your diet from the non-essential forms; you can't have one without the other. Furthermore, aside from some kind of laboratory prepared diet or a faddist diet, neither of which is usually very palatable, it is almost impossible to avoid some fat because significant amounts are present in many ordinary foods. Lest we condemn fat as the source of all evil, we should note that it is an exceptionally efficient source of energy (this is how humans store energy, depositing it as fat to be called forth at some later time when needed) and fat is an important factor in the taste of many foods.

When your fat consumption is decreased you can usually assume that the total amount of fat in your body is decreased. The details of what happens when you modify your diet, however, are complicated by factors such as the possible increase in synthesis of fat (the body makes its own from carbohydrates) when dietary fat intake is reduced; hereditary factors which control fat levels; confusion about the relationship of what we can measure in the blood and the meaning it has to heart disease; and the possible existence of various types of atherosclerosis, some of which may be more sensitive to dietary control than others.

It usually is difficult to change lifelong dietary patterns and it appears that efforts to make major changes in diet are only marginally justified by the remote likelihood of any rewards. The exceptions to this exist only when there is a terrible history of early death from heart disease in your family; if you have had a heart attack (or angina) and you are under fifty; or if you have one of the types of blood fat abnormalities which are particularly amenable to control by dietary manipulation.

Unquestionably, the single most important dietary factor in controlling heart disease is weight reduction. You have to get down to your good lean weight. Without weight reduction, any other dietary manipulations are probably a total waste of time.

For most people, two good rules of eating are to avoid excessive dietary extremes, and to cut down on the obviously bad foods which are either laden with animal fat or with table sugar. Five simple changes to make in your diet which require little effort and with which you can probably spare your heart and arteries much grief and stress are: 1) The yolks of eggs are very high in cholesterol. Eggs should be limited to no more than two or three a week. 2) Cut away the visible fat on all meat and, if possible, switch to the white or lean meat rather than the red or fatty meat or switch from meat to chicken and fish. 3) Develop a taste for skim milk rather than whole milk. It is a different taste but once you get used to it, you will probably find that it is quite acceptable. 4) Eliminate or decrease the intake of cheese and cheese products. 5) Decrease or eliminate the use of table sugar and those products which have a high content of sugar.

If you are determined and very highly motivated, there are a number of specialized restricted diets that are available from organizations like the American Heart Association. We remind you again, however, of the apparent importance of obesity, smoking, exercise, genetics, and emotional turmoil.

HEART FAILURE

Heart failure does not mean the stoppage of the heart but, rather, its inability to successfully accomplish its task. The symptoms are related to insufficient blood supply in some organs and to the accumulation of pools of blood in other organs. Swelling of the legs or edema is due to this pooling of blood (it requires a lot of heart work to pump the blood back uphill all the way from the feet). Edema used to be called "dropsy," a less scientific but much more descriptive term. Difficulty in breathing is due to accumulation of fluid in the lungs in heart failure. A general decrease in exercise tolerance and fatigue is due to the poor reserve of the heart and its inability to respond to extra demands.

Heart failure can be treated but cannot be cured except in most unusual circumstances. Most commonly the problem is atherosclerosis.

HEART MURMURS

A heart murmur is not a disease but a noise, which may mean that something is wrong with your heart. It is one of the things that a doctor listens for with his stethoscope. Normally, as the heart pumps blood, the valves in the heart control the direction of flow and close with a simple lub-dub sound. There are no murmurs or extraneous noises. If one of the valves is abnormal or diseased or if the heart has a congenital defect or a hole between two of the chambers, there is a good likelihood that extra sounds will appear. The extra sounds or noises have characteristic qualities in terms of where they can be heard, when in the cardiac cycle, and what they sound like. These characteristics may make it possible to identify the abnormality simply from the sound of the murmur which is associated with it.

Innocent murmurs, those not associated with any significant disease or abnormality, are not uncommon in young people. They represent a vigorous flow of blood through a normal heart. All murmurs should be carefully evaluated, for they may represent a congenital abnormality, damage to a valve caused by rheumatic fever or, in older people, damage caused by arteriosclerosis. The newer surgical techniques can often completely relieve the problems caused by a faulty valve or congenital abnormality.

Intestinal Functions

The entire function of the intestinal tract is based on a long, thin, sophisticated tube. What goes in at one end (the mouth) gets processed, digested, and absorbed. A few things get added to the contents of the tube on the way. In general, what is not needed, not wanted, or not absorbable, along with a few things that the wisdom of the body decides to get rid of, are discarded at the other end of the tube (the anus).

When food is eaten, chewed, and swallowed it goes into the esophagus, which is nothing more than a passage through the chest. Its only significant function is to get the food from the mouth to the stomach. The stomach is a widened section of the intestinal tract located below the ribs in the upper left side of the abdomen. It processes the food briefly and passes it on to the small intestine, where the absorption of the various nutrients starts to take place. Different kinds of foods are efficiently absorbed at various places along the small intestine. More than 99 per cent of the carbohydrate and fat, and more than 97 per cent of the protein that you eat is absorbed in the intestinal system. Ultimately, what is left unabsorbed or non-absorbable is finally passed on to the large intestine, or colon, to be processed for excretion. The residue is gathered in the rectum until enough is present to create the sensation of fullness which is recognized by the brain (which tells you to empty your rectum). The fecal contents pass through the anus, the final part of the intestinal tract, and through the anal sphincter, a mechanism which holds things in place until you are ready to relax it and divest yourself of the contents of the rectum.

Three major organs contribute their efforts to the function of the system of the intestinal tract: the liver, the gall bladder, and the pancreas. The gall bladder and the pancreas secrete various substances into the small intestine. These substances have a number of functions, some of which act to assist in the breakdown of the food to its constituent particles or to assist in the absorption of the food constituents. Once absorbed, most of the nutrients are carried by the blood to the liver, which then processes them further in preparation for use by the other organs of the body.

Almost everything can go wrong in a system as sophisticated and complex as the gastrointestinal tract, and it is a wonder that it functions as well as it does. Fortunately, when something goes wrong in the intestinal tract, it usually is not serious.

Recognition should be made of the fact that the gastrointestinal tract is a very accessible organ and is subject to the influence of many and varied stimuli which can affect it profoundly. The gastrointestinal tract has to contend with wide variations of quality, quantity, and cleanliness of food and the variations in frequency and regularity with which you eat, in addition to other distractions which occur while you eat. The accessibility of the intestinal tract and the frequency with which we deal with the conscious intake and output from it make it an obvious target for all the emotional ills of mankind. It is a remarkably adaptable but an ultimately fragile system. You needn't be too careful with it, but if you abuse it, it may break down.

DYSPHAGIA

Dysphagia is difficulty in swallowing. It doesn't happen very often, but if you have difficulty getting your food down once you swallow, there is usually a good reason for it and it should be checked out. Dysphagia has to be differentiated from globus hystericus. Globus, the sensation of tightness or a lump in the throat, is quite independent of swallowing, and when it exists is present all the time. It is frequently associated with the sensation of difficulty in breathing and it almost invariably occurs in an emotional, anxious, or hysterical patient. It is not associated with any physical abnormality. Although it can be very disabling, its treatment is the treatment of the underlying emotional problem.

HEARTBURN

Heartburn is the strange feeling of a burning sensation underneath the sternum (breastbone) which is described endlessly on TV commercials. Its cause is often obscure, its treatment sometimes difficult and its presence the butt of many predictable jokes. The burning sensation is really in the esophagus and is sometimes related to distention of the esophagus or reflux of some of the acidic contents of the stomach back and up into the esophagus, or bulging of a portion of the stomach into the esophagus (hiatus hernia). There is no question of its relationship to certain types of food in some individuals, but that is unfortunately not the only explanation. If it persists and doesn't seem related to a particular food or type of food, it warrants a careful investigation.

ANOREXIA

This is the medical word for loss of appetite. Usually, when you lose your appetite, there is a good reason for it. You have a cold or a headache or an examination or a fight with your wife, or something like it. For brief periods it poses no problem. Even prolonged anorexia or fasting need not be a problem if people who have no appetite would continue to consume fluids, and after a while, a bit of salt. You would be in serious trouble within a few days without fluid intake but, depending on your weight and how much fat you have on you, you can go for weeks or even months without any significant food intake. The problem, then, is rarely the consequences of anorexia, but the cause. If the cause is obvious then your attention should be directed to that. If the cause is not apparent, then you may be dealing with a significant physical or emotional disease which probably deserves further evaluation if it persists. How long you want to wait to see if it goes away depends on your individual reaction to it, how intense it is, and your own threshold for the discomfort that it causes. It is rare indeed for the physical form of anorexia to persist for a very long time without the underlying disease showing itself in one way or another. It doesn't usually take a great deal of insight to appreciate or recognize that often your loss of appetite may be due to an emotional cause and it is not always that obscure. You don't always need a psychiatrist to recognize common mild anxiety or depression or some kind of situation which is creating an emotional stress in your life. The anorexia in these cases is secondary. In its most severe emotional form, an unusual syndrome called anorexia nervosa, which occurs almost exclusively in young women, the voluntary avoidance of food eventually leads to malnutrition, starvation, and ultimately, death.

INDIGESTION

This is another one of those words that mean almost anything you or the television commercials want it to mean, all of them unpleasant. It may be the kind of upset stomach that some people have after eating or drinking too much or the "wrong things," it may be a bloated sensation with gas and belching, it may be heartburn or a sense of abdominal pressure, or it may be flatulence. Its causes are equally varied. Some of the almost predictable causes vindicate your mother's warnings about eating; your intemperate eating habits, too much, too quickly, excess fatty foods, or coffee, or spicy foods or alcoholic beverages. It can be associated with certain kinds of foods that just don't get on well with certain individuals. It is possible, of course, to have significant symptoms of a serious disease and to pass it off as a little bit of indigestion. In this case again you have to rely on the persistence and intensity and pattern of the symptoms to alert you that something may be wrong. It is impossible to generalize, but perhaps the various problems described in this section and in Chapter 5 (abdominal injuries and abdominal pain) will help establish some perspective for you.

PTOMAINE POISONING

Ptomaine, technically, is a group of chemicals that get formed in decaying meat. This is rarely the cause of food poisoning and most people with "ptomaine poisoning" don't really have food poisoning at all. They usually have one or more of the kinds of things lumped under and discussed as indigestion.

This is not to say that food poisoning doesn't exist. Most often it is caused by some kind of bacteria in food. The bacteria can produce a poisonous substance or toxin like botulinum or ptomaine or any of a large number of other variably toxic substances. If you ingest the food with the toxin already in it, you are likely to develop symptoms within the first twenty-four hours. If you ingest the food with the organism, and the toxin is produced in your intestinal tract, then you probably won't develop symptoms for two or three days while the toxin is being manufactured. This is a little academic because in both cases you are probably getting a little bit of both the organism and the toxin in varying proportions. What you do about your case of food poisoning depends on how sick you are and the likely cause. For mild or short-term symptoms, you can get by with gentle self-indulgence and generous fluid replacement. More severe or protracted symptoms are going to require some kind of analysis of the probable cause, which means some kind of medical intervention and, possibly, hospitalization.

Not all kinds of food poisoning are caused by toxins produced by bacteria. Some foods are poisonous all by themselves. People still kill themselves in significant numbers (more than 100 per year) in this country by eating poisonous, wild mushrooms. A great many more get very sick but recover. The experts tell us that there is no good way of telling which of the mushroom varieties is poisonous and which is safe. Short of trying it out on the neighbor's cat (which seems cruel), we would suggest that you confine your edible mushrooms to those purchased at the nearby grocery store.

NAUSEA AND VOMITING

Nausea is what you feel like just before you vomit, although it does not always result in vomiting. (Some people get nauseated even when the subject is discussed.) There are some interesting things about vomiting which you probably didn't notice the last time you vomited. Surprisingly, it seems that your stomach plays a very passive role in the whole process. Most of the force comes from a violent contraction of the muscles in your abdominal wall; feel it next time. You probably also didn't notice that vomiting is accompanied by profuse sweating and the copious production of saliva and nasal mucus. This all is consistent with the view that vomiting is a systemic reaction not confined to your stomach. It involves all of you. (Simple regurgitation of food, like what babies do, doesn't count.) Furthermore, vomiting doesn't always come from an upset stomach, nor does it always mean that something is wrong with your intestinal system. Many other processes will produce nausea and vomiting in a perfectly well-ordered stomach. The nausea of pregnancy is a good example.

Persistent vomiting can be more than simply unpleasant. You should be aware of three possible consequences. (1) You can lose a lot of fluid very quickly and become seriously dehydrated in almost no time at all. It may seem foolish to suggest that you consume fluids if you are going to vomit them right back up, but it is worth a try. Drink what you enjoy drinking (non-alcoholic, please) and try taking it slowly in very small sips, like a teaspoon every five minutes if you want to watch the clock. For reasons unknown, cold carbonated or uncarbonated cola drinks have a particularly soothing effect and are probably worth a try. Sucking ice chips is also effective. (2) Aspiration, getting some of the vomited material back down the wrong tube and breathed into your lungs, is a serious problem. This occurs most commonly in people who are not fully conscious while they are vomiting. For this reason it is always suggested that you keep an unconscious person with his head turned toward one side, so that if he does vomit it will drain out rather than collect in the back of his mouth ready to flow back down to his lungs when he takes his next deep breath. If the vomitus gets into your lungs it will surely establish a chemical pneumonia which is difficult to treat, and it will tear up the insides of your lungs because the stomach contents are very acid and the lungs are very fragile. (3) If you vomit hard enough and with enough violence, you can literally break something. You can burst a blood vessel or perforate your stomach or esophagus. This kind of thing happens mostly in alcoholics who vomit a lot, but can conceivably happen to anyone. The sudden appearance of bright red blood in the vomitus or the sudden onset of severe chest or abdominal pain should justify a rapid trip to the hospital.

If you can manage it, take a look at what you have just vomited. Usually it is what you just ate. Notice the peas. If it has been more than a few hours since your last meal, there probably won't be much food there unless your entire gastrointestinal system has slowed down and some of the food is in your stomach for an excessively long time. The presence of blood should be a source of concern. Blood will appear anywhere from bright red if it is fresh, to the appearance and consistency of coffee grounds if it has been in your stomach for any length of time and the stomach acid has had a chance to act on it. The appearance of blood can mean a lot of different things; the two most common are gastritis (an inflammation of the stomach, which is probably why you are vomiting anyway) and ulcers. In either case, it isn't a good thing and you ought to check with a doctor. Finally, if you start vomiting some greenish material you are vomiting bile (the material secreted through your gall bladder into the small intestine). Its appearance is not serious in itself but only suggests that you have been vomiting a lot for a long time.

ULCERS

Here ulcers refer to those in the stomach or small intestine, although technically an ulcer is an erosion of any surface. The intestinal system has two very closely related types of ulcers; those in the stomach (gastric ulcers) and those in the first part of the small intestine (duodenal ulcers). Differentiation is not always easy or even possible, and both types can be called peptic ulcers.

It makes sense that ulcers should occur in this area. The stomach produces a very strong acid and other potent gastric juices which are necessary for the normal processes of digestion. It is not unreasonable for the stomach to start to digest itself as effectively as it does a small chunk of beef steak. Meat is meat and the gastric juices aren't very discriminatory. We don't all have ulcers though, and we don't all have our stomachs digested away. This is probably due to a mucus covering over the inside lining of the stomach. If the lining is not intact or properly distributed, or if it is otherwise abnormal, part of the surface of the wall gets exposed to the acid and gastric juices and gets eroded. That is an oversimplification of an unusually complicated process. It doesn't explain a number of things but it is useful in thinking about ulcers and the paradox of why we still have any stomachs at all.

The symptoms of an ulcer may be indistinguishable from those of indigestion (burning, gas, vomiting, belching, etc.). Ulcers are usually, but not always, painful, and there is a predictable quality to the pain, its location, and its time of occurrence. It most frequently occurs when the stomach is empty. Food, almost any kind, buffers the acid in the stomach and neutralizes it. Thus, ulcer patients are frequently awakened by pain in the middle of the night. A glass of milk, a piece of bread or a few crackers, or a dose of an antacid promptly relieves the pain.

The frightening thing about an ulcer is the bleeding. Bleeding is not always obvious, nor dangerous, but it can be both. Vomiting bright red blood or partly digested blood is not uncommon in a briskly bleeding ulcer. The generous bleeding is usually due to erosion of the ulcer into a large blood vessel. If the blood doesn't get vomited it continues its way down the intestinal tract and finally gets mixed with the feces. The digestive process turns it tar black in color. The blood is an intestinal irritant and there might be some diarrhea. Loose, tarry black stools should be assumed to be due to bleeding somewhere in the intestinal system, and they signal the need for prompt and definitive medical attention.

One other characteristic of ulcers is their variable activity over a period of weeks or months. They get better or worse. Antacids do more than just relieve the pain. By neutralizing the acid they permit the normal healing process to patch things up. Along with a bland diet and rest (emotional stress increases stomach acid production) the regular dosing of your stomach with antacids will be effective in resolving the problem. Most people don't take their antacids frequently enough. The stomach can produce an enormous amount of acid and the antacid effectiveness is probably very brief. One or two tablespoons every hour around the clock should be satisfactory; this is obviously impossible for reasons of time, taste, and side effects. It is a worthy goal, however.

ABDOMINAL PAIN

When you consider what is located in the abdomen (the stomach, intestines, liver, pancreas, gall bladder, appendix, kidneys, ovaries, uterus, bladder, a lot of miscellaneous connective tissue and the major blood vessels going to and from the heart and the lower half of the body), it is not surprising that identification of the source of pain that appears somewhere in the abdomen can be a difficult diagnostic challenge. Add to this the fact that usually the pain does not occur directly over the organ which is producing the pain, that most problems within the abdomen do not produce symptoms which are unique or characteristic of any particular organ, that what looks like a characteristic pattern may always be something else after all, that there is an enormously wide variability in the reaction to pain from one individual to another, that occasional problems with organs outside the abdomen (e.g., the heart) may produce symptoms in the abdomen, and that overriding it all is the striking emotional content wrapped up inside everyone's belly, and it is not surprising that sometimes it is difficult to tell what is going on and when something is serious. The presence of a few clues, however, will tip you off that the problem is severe enough to have a physician take a look at it. If there is a fever (more than 100°); persistence of the symptoms for more than twenty-four hours; unusually severe pain (you will have to define that yourself); other symptoms such as vomiting, bleeding, or painful urination; or if there is a good cause (like an automobile accident); or if the abdominal wall is very tender to touch or board-like rigid, you may possibly have more than a trivial problem.

APPENDICITIS

The appendix is a small sac which sticks out from the last part of the small intestine. It is a dead-end and serves no function at all. It can only cause trouble if it gets inflamed or infected. Sometimes a bit of partially digested food gets caught in the opening, or the appendix twists on itself and kinks, or it gets infected or something else goes wrong and you have a case of appendicitis. What usually starts as a little inflammation causes some swelling which interferes with the blood supply to the appendix. This causes gangrene and death of the local tissue. Untended, an inflamed appendix has a good chance of bursting with leakage of all its infected contents into the abdomen. A little localized infection becomes a lot of diffuse infection. The symptoms of appendicitis can be typical but aren't always so. It should start first as pain, either in the middle of the upper part of the abdomen or around the navel. With time, the pain starts to migrate down toward the right lower corner of your abdomen, you lose your appetite, may start to vomit and develop a fever. (The pain almost always comes before the other symptoms.) The abdominal wall becomes rigid and tender. If all these are present you probably have appendicitis. Other things can cause the same pattern, however, and appendicitis can appear with other patterns of symptoms.

There are some interesting sidelights about appendicitis. This is one of those diseases which tends to be more common in people of upper socio-economic levels. As food consumption goes down, its frequency decreases. It is rare with famine or prolonged malnutrition. It seems also to be a disappearing disease. For reasons unknown, it is not as common today, food or income aside, as it was a generation ago.

It usually takes surgery to cure it, but it is a simple and safe surgical procedure.

MILK ALLERGY

The kind of milk allergy described here is not really an allergy such as is seen in infants, it is a sensitivity. Discussion is warranted because it appears to be quite a bit more common than anyone had previously thought and its mechanism is now starting to be understood.

In many parts of the world milk is only used for the very youngest children or not at all. A lot of very well-intentioned charitable agencies abroad get very upset when the milk they are distributing gets used to whitewash the house or gets fed to the pigs. The reason becomes clear when we realize that as many as 60 to 90 per cent of adult Asians and black Africans (and many older children) have no mechanism for absorbing the specific sugar which is present in milk. Infants usually cope, but the defect becomes more significant with aging. Adults and sensitive children develop stomach cramps and diarrhea when they consume milk and usually quickly learn to avoid it. About 5 per cent of white Americans have the same defective mechanism. Small amounts of milk such as are present in bread, or coffee, are not troublesome, but most older children and adults in the world get sick when they consume milk directly.

The sugar in milk, lactose, is broken down to its constituent parts in the intestinal tract prior to absorption. If the enzyme (called lactase) which is responsible for the breakdown is not present in the intestinal wall, the lactose does not get absorbed and its presence causes diarrhea. It is hard to specify that the absence of lactase is a defect, since most people don't have it. Lactase enzyme is absent for a good reason but we simply have not yet determined what the reason is. If you are one of those 5 per cent of white Americans or are of Asian or African descent, this may explain why you don't like milk or why you like it but occasionally get cramps and diarrhea.

GAS, BELCHING, AND FLATULENCE

Most of the gas in your intestinal tract is swallowed. Swallowing air is perfectly normal, particularly when you eat certain kinds of food or you eat in a particular way. Some people swallow more than others. They tend to be anxious people and swallow air along with their saliva or just unconsciously. Some of the gas in your intestinal tract is produced by the normal chemical processes of digestion or absorption of the food you eat. Some foods cause a lot more gas than others. Beans really do cause more gas. (This is one of those myths that have been substantiated by good research. The good research seems to have been a by-product of the space age. The problem of the control of the gases in a space capsule has suddenly made it very important to find out what is in normal flatus—intestinal gas—and what increases it and what makes it more or less unpleasant.)

When gas is in your intestinal tract there are only two places for it to go, up or down. Most of it goes down and certainly that part of it which gets beyond your stomach almost surely goes down. Belched gas is always swallowed air or that which is consumed in carbonated beverages and the like. Some people are very discomforted by belching. There is no easy way to break the habit of air swallowing, but in extreme cases you can try keeping your teeth separated by a pencil or some other object. It is extremely difficult to swallow anything unless your teeth are together. This usually is not worth the trouble and it is better to practice at belching quietly and take some solace in understanding the mechanism that provides you with this problem.

Swallowed air that moves downward, along with the small amount of gas that gets formed in the intestinal tract, gets passed as flatus. Sometimes the process of moving it downward and the presence of a bloated feeling of intestinal gas is very uncomfortable. A fantastic array of remedies have been created to deal with the problem, none of which is notably successful, and relatively little, save calm reassurance, can be offered the unhappy patient who suffers from "gas."

So delicate is the sensory mechanism of the rectum and anus that it can differentiate whether the contents of the rectum are gas, liquid, or solid. The passage of gas is a very important physiologic mechanism and the rare individual who cannot make this differentiation is a very uncomfortable person.

BORBORYGMI

This is a magnificent word which is what doctors use to describe the gurgling, bubbling abdominal sounds that are always present and are sometimes disconcertingly loud. It is simply the sounds made by air and fluid moving along the ever-churning intestinal tract; gas bubbling through the fluid. It is not necessarily a sign of hunger.

CONSTIPATION

Constipation is rarely life-threatening. There is so much variation in the bowel habits of individuals that what constitutes constipation has to be defined in terms of the habits of the individual. There is nothing sacred or healthy or necessary or desirable or important about a daily bowel movement. The preoccupation that people have with the successful achievement of this momentous ritual is probably the major cause of constipation. Our toilet-trained society with a heritage of the medicinal value of purgatives is so preoccupied with this almost religious symbol that it overuses laxatives with consummate devotion. The regular use of laxatives decreases the tone and sensation of the large intestine and the intestine soon becomes dependent on laxatives to initiate defecation. The failure to achieve a comfortable bowel movement today should be viewed as an unusual opportunity for tomorrow.

Constipation is a significant problem and should be treated in people who are bedridden, debilitated, or dehydrated. Prolonged bed rest or lack of activity slows down the normal movement of the intestinal tract and dehydration can prevent the formation of normal stools.

Occasionally, the appearance of constipation in an individual who is otherwise untroubled with his bowels may represent a significant or serious disease of the bowel and, in this case, should be investigated. Constipation commonly occurs in people who are traveling. Studies of this phenomenon are consistent with the view that emotional intensity frequently is manifested as disturbances of gastrointestinal function.

DIARRHEA

Diarrhea is the passage of excessively frequent or excessively liquid stools or a combination thereof. Unlike constipation, diarrhea is usually a sign of significant disease of intestinal function. Usually the sudden appearance of diarrhea suggests a viral infection or the consumption of bad food (see ptomaine poisoning). If the diarrhea persists or recurs frequently, it should be evaluated. Unless very severe or prolonged, it does not require any particular therapy other than fluid replacement. Unfortunately, the best therapy involves the use of opium derivatives and requires a prescription. (Heroin users, and even those using methadone, have a serious problem with constipation because the opiates are so effective at slowing down the activity of the bowel.)

Dysentery is a word which is frequently used synonymously with severe diarrhea. Technically, the word is used in association with a particular kind of bacterial disease (bacillary dysentery) or a particular kind of parasitic infestation (amebic dysentery). This technicality should not prevent you from using the word any way you like.

As we have noted, bloody diarrhea requires prompt medical evaluation.

Skin and Hair

We ought to treat our skin with more respect, but we take it for granted and it gets abused and neglected until it catches something which is painful, ugly, or itching. One of its remarkable features is that it tolerates this abuse so well. It is also waterproof, impermeable to foreign bodies, bacteria, viruses and other objectionable things; able to excrete things like sweat and to grow hair; it is flexible and soft; comfortable;

able to hold things in place; heals very rapidly; is able to regenerate itself; and it fits rather well, regardless of your size or shape or how fast you are growing.

It is made up of two parts, the relatively thin epidermis on the surface, and a much thicker layer called the dermis underneath. The epidermis, or the surface skin, is the part which is involved in a first-degree burn. Both the epidermis and dermis underneath are involved in a second-degree burn. The sweat glands and hair follicles originate in the dermis. Beneath these two layers of skin usually is a layer of fat, the thickness of which depends on your sex, the part of the body, and how heavy you are. This fat layer covers the underlying muscles. When both the layers of skin and the underlying tissues are involved in a burn, it is called a third-degree burn.

SWEATING

Everybody sweats to regulate his body temperature. As the sweat evaporates from your skin, it creates a small cooling effect. Without sweating, your body temperature would continually rise as a result of the body metabolism and you would rapidly die of heat prostration unless some other mechanism could be developed to cool your body.

An apparently second major but unfortunate function of sweating is to make you uncomfortable on hot, humid days when you sweat more and the sweat doesn't evaporate as fast as you'd like it to. It accumulates in puddles under your arms and in other places and after a while starts to smell.

There are two kinds of sweat. One is a watery kind which is mostly a salt-water solution. The other is a thicker more viscous secretion. The former is more widely distributed over the skin and is more common; the thicker viscous sweat is more specialized. The highest density of the watery sweat glands is on the palms of the hands, the soles of the feet and, less so, in the armpits. The watery sweat is the type that gets produced by heat, fever, exercise, and emotional excitement. This is the sweat which cools as it evaporates. The nature of the thick viscous type of sweat varies from one part of the body to another, since it usually has a particular kind of local function. It is what provides the distinctive odors that characterize the armpits, the genitalia and the breasts, and there are even special kinds of sweat for the nose and the eyelids. Even the wax in your ear is a concentrated sweat solution. Both the watery and the viscous sweat glands are present in varying proportions all over your body. The watery sweat glands account for the volume and the viscous sweat glands account for the local and unique characteristics of the sweat.

Some people simply sweat more than others. This is another of those characteristics that you are born with, and the sooner you adapt to it the more fortunate you are. There is relatively little that will change it but a few things will make it more tolerable. Some specific medications can decrease the amount of sweat produced, but the side effects of these drugs, a dry mouth, blurred vision, palpitations and hot skin, are uncomfortable enough to assure that most people would rather sweat than take these drugs.

The simplest, and by far the most effective way to deal with sweat is to wash it off with any kind of ordinary soap and water. This removes the odoriferous secretions and prevents their accumulation. Ordinary skin bacteria will then have less opportunity to utilize the sweat as a substrate for the production of still more unpleasant odors. Some kinds of antibacterial soap will tend to decrease the skin's bacteria slightly and retard the production of the odors but recent reports suggest that the antibacterial constituents may be harmful when used excessively. Deodorants may have some similar antibacterial activity but for the most part do nothing more than cover the odor with a more acceptable one. They function primarily as a perfume. (Deodorants should be distinguished from antiperspirants.) Talc or other drying powders will absorb the moisture and thereby decrease the activity of the bacteria. Locally applied antibiotics may temporarily decrease the skin's bacteria but they have a way of causing skin irritation and, if they are used for a prolonged period, may be more trouble than they are worth.

Antiperspirants are technically different from deodorants. An antiperspirant will be labeled as such. These products appear to actually decrease the production of sweat, although exactly how they do this is not really known. Most, but not all, of the antiperspirants contain some kind of aluminum salt. They can be reasonably effective in small areas of high sweat discomfort, like the armpits.

ITCHING

Itching has to be defined operationally in terms of scratching. It is the sensation which produces the desire to scratch and the sensation on the skin which is relieved by scratching. Pain occurs all over; itching is a unique phenomenon and occurs only on the skin.

The proper treatment for an itch, however, may not necessarily be to scratch. What to do about an itch depends on its cause. The cause may be a skin problem or a complication of any of a number of minor or serious diseases which are unrelated to the skin. A good firm scratch with sharp fingernails will solve many of your problems, but not all, and may make the itching worse. Continuous scratching of a continuous itch will sometimes establish a vicious cycle. As you scratch you get further irritation of the skin and dilatation of the local blood vessels. As the vessels dilate, the itch sensation invariably gets worse. This dilatation of the blood vessels may well be the reason for increased itching in some people at night when they are in bed. Aside from giving them more time to think about their problem, rest allows the skin vessels to dilate and the itching sensation becomes more severe.

The treatment of an itch has tried the best of men's minds and a severe continuous itch can defy the most elaborate therapeutic efforts known to medicine. Common sense says to find the cause of the itch and remove it. Sometimes, as in poison ivy, the cause is obvious, but too late; the poison is on the skin, the damage has been done, and you have to try something more elaborate. A simple and effective remedy is to establish a counterirritant which simply "fools the brain." The brain tends to concentrate on only one kind of unpleasant sensation at a time. Ordinary pain can often be relieved by applying a mild irritant to the skin such as liniment or a mustard plaster. Similarly, gentle pinching of the skin in an area adjacent to the itch will frequently provide some transient relief. Cold baths or compresses or towels will accomplish the same thing and will also constrict the local blood vessels. The effect of a cooling medication such as calamine lotion is based on the same process. Some medications, such as the antihistamine drugs, will relieve itching of an uncommon allergic reaction (like hives) and various other kinds of lotions and salves will often be helpful. In general, these medications will need a prescription, and if the itch is that bad, or that uncomfortable or that disabling, it probably is a good idea to get some medical advice on the subject anyway.

RASHES

Rashes are not so simple. They belong to the science and art of dermatology and it isn't easy to make useful generalizations. Consider the color, shape, size, and distribution of a rash; whether it appears flat or raised as bumps, pimples, nodules, wheals, vesicles, or pustules; if it itches or not, has crusts, or scales, is growing smaller or getting bigger, getting deeper or higher; if it contains fluid or blood and what is your best guess about its cause. Any combination will do. Your problem is to decide whether to ignore it, treat it yourself, or get to a physician for more elaborate therapy.

If the rash is associated with a fever or some other signs of systemic illness (e.g., headache, vomiting, diarrhea), then it obviously involves more than just the skin and it would be wise to get a doctor to tell you what it is. If it persists and you don't know what caused it (you might know, for example, that you've been digging up your patch of poison ivy or that you are allergic to the enzymes in the laundry soap you've been using), and particularly if it seems to be getting worse, you would also be wise to have a doctor see it. Finally, if it is very uncomfortable and your home remedies don't relieve it, a doctor may be able to pull something off his shelf and give you at least some relief.

There's a fair chance, though, that the average or even well-trained and competent physician will not be able to identify the rash specifically, and treatment may be nothing more than trial and error with previously proven medication. That's fair as long as he's honest about it. You may need a skin specialist but usually the rash is gone by the time you get to see him. You can help the evaluation by doing some of your own careful observation and by not putting anything on the rash before you go to see a doctor. The subtleties of shade and delicacy of its appearance may be lost through a layer of skin cream.

HAIR

As far as one can tell, the only function of hair is cosmetic. It had a more useful function for our primeval ancestors but nowadays its problems can be grouped into these categories:

> too little,
> too much,
> too curly,
> too straight,
> the wrong color,
> or its distribution in the wrong places.

Since all of these factors are primarily determined by your genetic characteristics (i.e., your parents), there is very little that anyone can do about most hair problems. Hair can be shaved, dyed, straightened, or curled but the new hair that grows in, inexorably, will be exactly like the old hair. Nothing you do on the surface of the skin affects its growth or its characteristics. Like fingernails, hair is dead tissue, and any manipulation of the end of the hair (or at the end of the fingernail, for that matter) has no effect on what happens down at the base of the hair follicle where it is being formed.

Too much hair is sometimes a very distressing cosmetic problem, particularly facial hair in women. This is a problem that runs in families; if your mother was a bit hairy, you will probably tend in that direction yourself. We can recommend only three ways of getting rid of unwanted hair.

> *Shaving.* Assuming the source of concern is facial hair, shaving can create more emotional discomfort than it solves. Although most American women shave their armpits and legs, many are reluctant to shave their faces because of the fear that the new hair will grow in bristly and stiff. This is simply not true. Shaving will not change the basic characteristics of the hair. The new growth will have the sensation of being bristly, but only because it is short. As it gets longer, it will get soft again. Shaving is fine but you have to be willing to keep ahead of it.
>
> *Depilatories.* These will dissolve the hair on the skin surface. Some of the depilatory preparations can be moderately irritating to the skin, particularly on sensitive areas like the face. You will have to experiment a little to see what your skin can tolerate. The new growth of hair after using a depilatory will feel just as bristly as if you shaved it off, but it too gets softer as it gets longer.
>
> *Electrolysis.* This is the only certain solution. A tiny electrode which is placed into the skin burns out and destroys the hair root. However, electrolysis is usually uncomfortable, expensive, time-consuming and, unfortunately, there are some practitioners of this delicate art who are poorly trained, unskilled operators and a few who are outright frauds.

At the other end of the hair spectrum is baldness. There is nothing that can be done to get hair to grow where there is none growing. Some success in regrowing hair has been achieved with hair transplants, a very costly, time-consuming, and uncomfortable procedure. This process assumes that you have some scalp hair on the sides or on the back of your head which can be transplanted to the top of your head. Hair growing elsewhere on the body has neither the density nor characteristics of scalp hair and its transplantation to your head would be a cosmetic disaster. Many people have gotten very rich deceiving bald people into thinking that their potions, treatments, massages, vitamin pills, and hormones will get hair to grow when there isn't any. You could spend the family fortune on these worthless cures, but you will not grow any hair.

It may be of some interest to know that hair grows faster in warm weather and that it appears to grow faster with increased sexual desires. The latter observation was made by a meticulous island lighthouse keeper who shaved daily with an electric razor and weighed the shavings collected. There was a reproducible and unambiguous increase in the weight of the shaved hair before and during the few days of his intermittent visits to his friends on the mainland.

Dandruff probably rates as the winner of the hair preparation advertising derby. Everyone has some continuous scaling and flaking of the superficial layers of skin all over the body, and the scalp is no different. The normal small flakes of skin, the normal oily secretions of the scalp, and the normal amount of dust and debris which collect in anyone's hair combine and cause dandruff. There is no cure for dandruff, but sometimes, when the rate of production of the flaky material seems to be getting excessive, it needs some kind of control.

The best control is with the regular use of any shampoo. None is better than any other. If you live in an area with soft water, any ordinary soap will do as well and will be a lot less expensive. There is no reason why hair cannot be shampooed every day if necessary; this process has no deleterious effect on the hair, scalp, skull, or the brain underneath it. As with acne treatment (see the section on acne in Chapter 5), washing will remove the oils and secretions on the scalp but that is exactly what you are trying to do. The severity of dandruff ranges widely and people who swear by some magic potion or another are usually applying an ordinary shampoo about the same time that their dandruff is getting better by itself.

If the dandruff is really excessive and itchy, the various kinds of medications, basically similar to those used to treat acne, can be used. Something containing drying agents like sulfur and/or salicylic acid may be tried. If a daily shampoo won't control the dandruff, these medications might be worth a try.

4 Medical Emergencies

Shock

There are some significant differences between the medical or technical use of the word "shock" and the general impression of what shock is. The ambiguity adds something to the mysticism of medicine, particularly since shock is one of those words that transmits a specific concept in a precise medical setting and yet is only vaguely defined itself. (Medicine is more art and less science than most physicians would like to admit.)

The best understanding of what happens when someone is in shock requires a little biology and physiology. The heart pumps the blood throughout the body. If, for whatever reason, the various tissues of the body are not being perfused with an adequate supply of blood, a state of shock may develop. There are multiple possible causes for this defective tissue perfusion, and the extent to which tissue perfusion must be diminished before the state of shock is present depends on a wide variety of circumstances.

What are some of the problems which might produce shock? Some of the potentially less serious causes include:

• Intense or prolonged emotional experiences can sometimes produce shock. Emotional stress can occasionally initiate a complex set of automatic reflexes involving the blood vessels and the heartbeat. These reflexes can modify the blood flow to the brain and the resultant inadequate oxygenation can cause a faint or transient period of shock.

• An ordinary fainting spell (technically called syncope) is the simplest form of shock.

• Not too dissimilar from the emotional reaction is the

surprise effect of an injury where the victim is "stunned." This can produce shock and may be the single most important immediate factor in shock following an injury. It is not directly related to the type of injury.

These forms of shock are usually not serious in themselves. They are brief and the collapse associated with them usually is sufficient to readjust the blood flow and initiate the spontaneous recovery process. The treatment is the same as that for a faint.

Shock can be extremely serious, or even fatal, when it occurs in certain circumstances.

- When someone has a heart attack, the heart does not pump adequately and shock sometimes is produced. The combination of a heart attack and the failing circulation resulting from the shock can be irreversible and fatal.
- Profuse and rapid blood loss produces shock because there simply isn't enough blood remaining in the body to pump to the vital organs like the brain and the heart. If there has been a substantial blood loss, for whatever reason, shock may persist even if the bleeding has stopped, unless the blood can be replaced or appropriate treatment can be started promptly.
- A severe burn is often associated with shock. Here a number of factors are contributory; the pain, the fright and emotional stress, and the rapid and profuse loss of fluid from the burned area are all responsible for the production and prolongation of the state of shock.
- Certain types of severe infections produce shock.
- Some head injuries or brain damage are characteristically associated with shock.

How do you know when you are dealing with shock? Simple unconsciousness is not a good sign. Not everyone who is unconscious is in shock and not everyone who is in shock is unconscious. Look at the patient and touch him. If he is in shock, he looks pale and uncomfortable. His skin feels cold and clammy. He is sweating. He may be restless or confused or unconscious. Take his pulse. Someone in shock has a pulse which feels "thready"; it feels weak, small, and rapid. The conscious patient in shock usually is nauseated and, whether he is conscious or not, he may be vomiting. He feels sick, he looks sick, and everything appears desperate. The situation is an emergency. Untreated, he is likely to die.

Ideally, it is good to know why he is in shock, for definitive therapy depends upon it. But chances are you won't be administering definitive therapy. There are a number of simple things that you can and should do while arrangements are being made for the patient's transportation to a hospital. First, make sure that the patient is lying flat on the ground. Don't prop his head up on a pillow. In fact, if it is convenient, and he is not bleeding from a head wound, prop up his feet and legs to keep his head below the rest of his body. He is likely to vomit anything he eats or drinks. Don't give him anything to drink even if he is thirsty. Any bleeding should be controlled. The persistent loss of blood will increase the severity of shock. Simple pressure with your finger, hand, or anything else will usually stop the bleeding. Keep the patient warm and comfortable, particularly if he has been exposed to cold water or weather. If there is an injured or burned arm or leg, local cooling, if possible, may decrease the loss of fluids from that area. If you have sophisticated equipment for intravenous infusions (see Chapter 8), start an infusion of saline. If oxygen is available, run about six liters a minute through a face mask.

Use your common sense, your good judgment, and enlist the aid of anyone available to arrange for the patient's prompt and proper transport to a hospital.

Head Injuries

The head is designed to protect the brain (which is enclosed within the skull), and to house the sensory organs; the eyes, the ears, and the nose (which transmit messages to the brain through carefully placed openings in the skull). Somewhere within the brain are the intellect, the memory, the personality, the imagination, possibly the soul, and a nervous system which is so incredibly sophisticated and complex that it defies our remotest dreams of understanding, controlling, or duplicating.

An injury to the head can damage the brain in basically the following ways:

- The force of the impact can damage the brain by producing swelling, brain tissue destruction, and microscopic bleeding within the brain itself.
- The skull may be fractured, and the broken fragments may be pushed down into the brain, damaging or destroying the underlying tissue.
- A forceful blow can damage a blood vessel in the brain, damaging or compromising the circulation to a specific part of the brain and injuring or irritating the region around the bleeding.
- A head injury can result in the formation of a blood clot under the skull which compresses the brain within the rigid skull itself.

The extent of the damage depends on the severity of the blow and the location of the injury. Fortunately, the most vital areas of the brain, the areas controlling breathing and the heartbeat, are located in a relatively protected region, but a well-placed and strategic blow to the head can damage them just as well as the more accessible, easily injured areas.

Don't ignore any injury to the head, no matter how trivial it may appear. Any blow can kill. It's hard to ignore a cracked skull produced by the full force of a club or by the toe of a military boot, but it is unfortunately human nature to ignore a skull injury when it is associated with other more obvious injuries. If you fall down a flight of stairs and break your arm, it is obvious and easily and adequately treated. But the fact that you struck your head on virtually every step, and that you are dazed and confused and have a brain concussion (see Chapter 4) is too often ignored. People tend naturally and reflexly to protect their heads when they sense impending injury, but frequently, the protection is incomplete, too late, or inadequate. Many automobile accidents are associated with unrecognized head injuries and the dazed, confused state of the victim is often mistakenly attributed to shock. Shock may be present as well, but don't let the more obvious injuries distract you from the subtle ones.

In the majority of head injuries, the skull itself absorbs most of the force of the blow and the brain is relatively spared. In an uncomplicated skull injury, with no bleeding, no fractured skull, and no other injury, warning signs that the brain may be injured are often obvious, but frequently very subtle or obscure. If the victim cannot clearly and accurately describe the events associated with his injury, he should be carefully and responsibly observed by someone with the primary responsibility for taking care of him. The victim's activity should be restricted for at least twenty-four hours, and he should not be left alone. Watch for the following warning signs:

Excessive sleepiness or difficulty awakening him: Don't confuse this with normal sleep. Anyone who receives a head injury should be awakened every one or two hours to determine his state of consciousness. If he is unusually lethargic, if his rate of speech is retarded, if he is not arousable, or if it is increasingly difficult to awaken him, get medical attention immediately.

Any variability in the state of consciousness suggests increasing pressure on the brain. Periods of drowsiness interrupted by alertness and lucidity and then drowsiness again is an ominous sign and should be watched with caution. Anyone who is unconscious for more than a few seconds after a head injury should probably get complete medical evaluation.

Unusual or irrational behavior may be a warning. Take into account the circumstances of the moment, and the frequently associated excitement and anxiety after a confrontation and an injury.

Vomiting in the absence of any obvious cause suggests

increased pressure on the brain. While pursuing more definite therapy, be certain that the victim is placed on his side so that he doesn't choke on his vomitus, particularly if he is drowsy or lethargic.

Persistent or severe headaches should alert you to trouble. This is difficult to evaluate because some headache is likely and expected after any head injury. But an ordinary headache tends to gradually decrease and not intensify with time, and the intensity of the headache should be roughly commensurate with the severity of the injury. Treat the headache with an ice pack, a cool wet towel, or aspirins if necessary, but nothing stronger than this. If these measures are ineffective in controlling the symptoms, medical attention is probably warranted.

Unusual and persistent restlessness is often associated with the irrational behavior and may be a sign of increased pressure on the brain.

Any change in vision, particularly double vision or blurred vision, is an important sign and medical attention should be sought if it persists.

Any muscle weakness in the arm or leg, or asymmetry of the face, a drooping eye or one side of the mouth, and any asymmetric tingling or numbness in the extremities suggests possible brain damage. Don't delay getting medical attention.

All of the above signs do not require any particular medical training to observe. What is needed is a patient and, if possible, a concerned friend who can make objective judgments about the victim's behavior and state of consciousness. There are other more objective criteria which should be evaluated regularly, particularly in doubtful situations. They require only a little more training and experience.

Check the pupils regularly. The pupil is the small black circle inside the colored ring in the center of the eye. The pupils should be the same size in both eyes and should shrink in size when you shine a light in them. If the pupils are of unequal size or don't react appropriately to light (by constricting rapidly), this may be a sign of increased brain pressure and medical attention is urgently needed.

The *pulse rate* is a good sign of increasing pressure on the brain. Check the pulse and if it falls below 60 per minute or increases to above 100 per minute when it had previously been normal and there is no obvious cause for the increased rate such as pain, anxiety, excitement, or activity, this could mean increasing pressure.

A watery or bloody discharge from the ears or from the nose may indicate leaking of spinal fluid and medical attention is necessary immediately.

Irregular, slow, and deep breathing often is an indication of increased pressure on the brain and an ominous sign of trouble.

Just as it is frequently possible to ignore head injuries in the presence of more obvious trauma such as a broken arm, it is often possible to ignore other more subtle injuries to the rest of the body when the victim has been kicked in the head. Don't forget to check for abdominal or chest trauma when someone has a head injury and treat these problems accordingly. Associated injuries may be very subtle and difficult to evaluate when the victim is drowsy and confused as a result of his head wound.

Neck and spine injuries can occur just as readily as a head injury in a fight or automobile accident. Be alert to a possible broken neck or spine if there is pain in this region or if the victim is conscious and is paralyzed, unable to move his arms or legs or both. If the victim is unconscious and even if a broken neck or spine is a remote possibility, you should make every effort to move the victim as little as possible and to immobilize the head and neck with pillows, clothing, stones or whatever is available. If the victim has to be moved, at least three people are necessary. All three should stand on the same side, place their hands under the victim and lift together.

Don't let the fear of a neck injury, and the required immobilization of the victim, immobilize you as well. Broken necks or spines are pretty rare, and if the victim can move his fingers or toes and has no back or neck pain, you don't have to leave him in a contorted position in the middle of the road, wondering if it's all right to move him.

There will usually be some painful and tender swelling at the site of a head injury. If there is bleeding, treat it as you would any laceration (see Chapter 5). Keep in mind that scalp lacerations bleed profusely; much more so than a similar cut on the arm or hand. Profuse bleeding is usually not as ominous as it looks initially. A man with clotted and dried blood streaming down his face from a small or trivial scalp laceration creates a frightening impression often far out of proportion to the severity of his wound. It can be evaluated much more objectively when the blood is washed from his face and hair.

A skull fracture can sometimes be very hard to detect. If you can feel crackling bones in the region of the injury it is reasonable to assume that the skull is fractured. But sometimes the skull can be fractured without the bone shattering or the fragments displaced or depressed, and in the presence of the swelling and bleeding, the only certain method to determine if the skull is fractured is to get x-rays. If no fracture is present and the laceration and bleeding are controlled, the head often feels better with an ice pack or a cold wet towel placed on it. Do not give any sedatives, analgesics, psychotropic drugs or alcohol to anyone with a head injury. Give no medications for pain, except perhaps aspirin, if the victim is lucid, alert, and has a headache. Food and fluids should not be forced and may be kept to a minimum for the first twenty-four hours or until his condition is stable and satisfactory.

There are some late and subtle sequels to head injuries which should be watched for. There can be a seemingly normal, uncomplicated recovery from even a slight or trivial head injury and some days or even weeks later changes begin to appear which should alert you to trouble. These can include slight but definite personality changes, confusion, and increasing somnolence. Further tests may be necessary to rule out a slowly expanding subdural hematoma. This is a blood clot within the skull which compresses the brain.

FRACTURED JAW

The jaw is like a door with the hinges located below and slightly in front of the ears. You can feel it move when you open your mouth. If you get in a fight and are hit in the face, a fractured or dislocated jaw is not unusual. If the bones are displaced, you may not be able to open or close your jaw and medical attention is needed promptly. If the bone is broken but the fragments are not displaced and the jaw is not dislocated, the situation is not quite as urgent and emergency care can probably be delayed until it is more convenient, but not for more than twenty-four hours.

The jaw should be supported closed with a temporary bandage. Pain can be a problem, since oral medication can't be taken because chewing is impossible and swallowing is difficult. The injury should be checked and treated as soon as is practical. Too much talking or other mouth activity will undoubtedly make matters worse.

FACIAL INJURIES

The face is particularly vulnerable to injury. It is the target of most direct blows from an angry assailant, and usually is the part of the body which goes through the front window of a car first when it stops suddenly.

Cuts and bruises of the face are like cuts and bruises everywhere else (see Chapter 5) except for a few major differences. The face is very vascular, it is well supplied with blood vessels and it bleeds profusely when it is cut, just like the scalp and the hands. A laceration on the face, even a small one, can be a major problem, and the repair must be done by competent hands with meticulous attention to details to avoid unsightly scars.

A forceful blow to the face can fracture some of the small

and fragile bones around and behind the eyes (see Chapter 5), the nose, or the cheeks. There is usually swelling, tenderness, and pain in the area of the fracture. A facial fracture has to be checked promptly by an experienced doctor to make sure there are no complications, but sometimes it may be necessary or desirable for him to delay definitive treatment until the swelling has subsided. There is no cast to put on, but the displaced fragments can do a lot of damage getting pushed into the eye, the sinuses, or even into the brain. An ice pack and aspirins will reduce the swelling and pain.

SEIZURES

See Chapter 4.

NOSEBLEEDS

See Chapter 6.

TOOTHACHES

See Chapter 6.

Eye Injuries

FOREIGN BODIES

Usually, the irritation of a foreign body in the eye provokes tearing and this protective mechanism washes out most particles very nicely. Therefore, the first thing to do when you feel something in your eye is to close your eye and let the natural protective fluids take their course. *Don't rub your eye.* Plain common sense should tell you that rubbing a small sliver of anything in that delicate area is almost certain to cause trouble. Resist the urge to rub, even if rubbing feels good, because it invariably promotes further irritation, often makes the foreign body less accessible, and rarely helps to get rid of the offending irritant.

If tears alone don't work, get a friend to do the following:

Have the patient look up and fix his sight on some specific object to keep the eye from wandering. Place your finger just beneath the eye and gently pull the lower lid down. If you see the foreign body on the inside of the lower lid, it can easily be removed by touching it with the tip of a clean handkerchief or a gauze pad.

If you haven't found the foreign body on the inside of the lower lid, while you have the lower lid pulled out and the inside exposed, look at the white part of the eye (the sclera). Have the patient look up to his right and up to his left. You can then release the lower lid. Gently hold the upper lid up as far as you can while he looks down and to the lower right and left. If you spot the particle on the sclera, you can get it off with a handkerchief or gauze pad but you will need to be more careful and use a delicate touch. Any frontal assault on the eye will elicit a blink and you will have to start all over again. Best to approach it from the side and sneak up on it, staying out of the line of sight of the pupil in the center. Don't scrape the particle off the sclera. If gentle brushing does not get it off, then there is a chance that the particle is imbedded in the sclera and expert attention may be needed to get it out. If this is the case, patch the eye (tape an eye patch, gauze pad, or clean handkerchief over the closed eye). This will cut down on the blinking and the irritation that may result.

If you still have not found the irritating particle, you will have to have a look under the upper lid. This requires a little more skill and patience but gets easier with practice. Gently grasp the upper lashes and pull the upper lid away from the eye. Do this three or four times, to stimulate the flow of tears. If you do not find the particle, have the patient look down, again focusing on something specific, like his knee (you have to keep the eye from wandering). To turn the upper lid over so you can have a look beneath you will need a small object such as a wooden match stick or even a hairpin. Have a gauze pad or a clean handkerchief ready. Place the match stick (or whatever) across the outside of the upper lid and with the other hand, gently pull the upper lashes and the eyelid away from the eye. Rotate the lid over the match stick. Once the lid has been turned inside out, gently remove the match stick by pulling it out sideways across the eye. Hold the lid open and everted by pressing the lashes gently against the upper eye or eyebrow. The patient must continue to look down, because if he looks up, the lid will flip back down again and you will have to start all over. A little practice will help you master this delicate but simple task. Now that the lid is up and over, most foreign bodies on the lid will be visible and can easily be removed by touching them with the clean handkerchief or gauze pad. If you don't see anything, it probably is worthwhile to gently rub a moist cotton applicator stick across the exposed lid in case the offending particle is a sliver of glass or a cigarette ash and not easily visible. The lid can easily be returned to normal by having the patient look upward.

If the foreign body is still not located, and the patient's eye is still irritated, the offending particle may be located on the cornea (the very delicate and transparent dark area in the center of the eye) and may not be visible. This could mean trouble. Sometimes it may be spotted by examining the cornea with a good strong flashlight illuminating the eye from the side. Generally speaking, it is not a good idea to fool with a corneal foreign body yourself. The risk of scratching the cornea and scarring it is already significant without adding your inexperienced touch to the problem. If you see something on the cornea, or if you don't find the offending particle and the eye is still irritated, or if you think you have removed the foreign body and the irritation persists, there may be another particle you missed. If you can you should:

> Place a drop of a local anesthetic (0.5% pontocaine) in the eye to relieve the pain.
>
> Place some antibiotic eye ointment into the eye. (Have the patient look up, pull the lower lid down, and squeeze the ointment into the pouch which is opened. Then close the eye.)
>
> Patch the eye closed. Never put an anesthetic in the eye unless you plan to patch it. The eye's major protective mechanism is its blink which sweeps away the vast majority of the particles that get into the eye. Anesthetize the eye and you lose the protection. If it is uncomfortable enough to anesthetize it, it needs an eye patch.
>
> Have the eye examined by a competent ophthalmologist (eye doctor) within twenty-four hours.

Looking for foreign bodies in eyes can still be a frustrating experience. The foreign body may have been washed or blinked away, but the irritation it has caused may persist and the pain may continue for hours. If the pain persists too long or gets worse, it is likely that something is still in the eye.

BLACK EYE (Periorbital Ecchymosis)

A black eye is very common, usually very embarrassing, but almost always of no consequence and generally nothing to worry about. Any blow to the side of the face, to the region around the eye, or to the nose (as with a fist or a doorknob) may cause some damage or break some of the small blood vessels in this area. The blood tends to collect in the loose skin surrounding the eye and unfortunately remains there for a long period of time. As the blood slowly gets reabsorbed into the system, the "black eye" gradually turns from purple to green to a yellow orange in a period of about two weeks.

In the first few hours, an ice pack will help to stop the bleeding and minimize the swelling. After twelve to twenty-four hours, warm heat applied in any reasonable fashion will hasten the reabsorption of the blood and decrease the swelling. Nothing much else need be done and anything else will probably do more harm than good.

BLUNT INJURY TO THE EYE (Contusions of the Globe)

A good sock in the eye may result in a black eye and nothing more than that, but you should remember that the eye is a highly complex and extremely delicate organ. While a black eye is the result of broken vessels under the skin around the eye, the small capillaries inside the eye and the bones of the skull around and behind the eye are sensitive also and may well be torn or injured when subjected to any strong force.

Three problems complicate and confuse the evaluation of the eye injuries resulting from a direct blow to this region. First, there may be no external manifestations of the injury and the patient may not notice anything wrong. Second, the injury or the bleeding may not appear for days or even weeks after the blow was received. Finally, it is important to remember that a very small injury in a crucial area can sometimes produce a devastating blindness.

Our intent is to alert you to the problems which sometimes occur when the eye is injured. If you are at all concerned about an eye injury, you should have it examined by a competent eye doctor as soon as practical.

LACERATION OF THE EYELIDS

If you get a cut on your eyelid, you can expect it to bleed profusely for a long time. It is hard to get it to stop bleeding since you cannot very well put a tourniquet on your eye, and all you can sensibly do is put some gentle pressure on the laceration and be very patient. The degree of bleeding is often so profuse as to provoke alarm, but the bleeding is generally no problem unless the blood is bright red and comes out in gentle spurts. The spurting means a cut artery. Arterial bleeding will need a stitch or two to get it under control. If a lacerated eyelid does not get sewn up with proper care and exquisite attention to detail, the cosmetic result may be regrettable.

A cut eyelid may be the external manifestation of more serious and less obvious injury to the delicate structures within the eyelid or to the eye itself. A complete careful eye examination is essential after the lacerated lid has been treated.

Chest Injuries

RIB AND STERNUM FRACTURES

A broken rib or sternum (the breastbone) has unusual significance not because of the broken bone itself, but because of the major organs which are adjacent to or just under the ribs. Serious complications can result from what may appear to be a relatively trivial injury. The ribs form a firm but relatively flexible cage which protect the heart and lungs from injury. They are attached in the front to the sternum and in the back to the spine. If you press, kick, or strike hard enough, or if you fall far enough, the ribs can easily be broken and the underlying heart and lungs may be damaged. It does not take too much to break a rib. A strong blow with a club will do it. Getting thrown against a steering wheel in a car accident can and often does break the sternum or a few ribs. A fit of coughing in unusual circumstances may break a rib.

The broken rib is usually nothing to get too worked up about, and often nothing has to be done except to limit activity and take something for the pain. If you have a broken rib, you will usually find that certain positions or activities will increase the pain and you will be more comfortable sitting quietly or in some particular position. The most comfortable position is probably best for you. One does not have to be totally immobilized unless the pain is very severe, but usually it is best to keep activity to a minimum initially. Aspirin may help relieve the pain but you will probably need something stronger like codeine. The pain is usually due to pressure of the broken rib fragments on a nerve which lies just adjacent to the broken rib, and if the pain cannot be relieved with codeine it may be necessary to inject a local anesthetic around the nerve to get relief. This injection can be a little tricky, because in the process of injecting an anesthetic around the nerve, it is very easy to puncture the lung with the needle and do much more harm than good. An ice pack may give some relief during the first twenty-four hours, or until the swelling is down. After that, heat is advised for some added comfort.

A common practice in the past was to strap the chest with tape or a tight cloth binder. This immobilized the broken rib margins, as one would immobilize a fractured leg or finger, and thus tended to decrease the pain. It also immobilized the lung, however, on the side of the fracture, and thus decreased the aeration of the lung and favored the development of pneumonia. Most experts no longer recommend binding or strapping broken ribs, except for brief periods when activity or position cannot be restricted.

Rib fractures are not to be taken lightly. In some instances, they can cause serious problems with major complications and you should be alert for any of the following problems:

Some pain on breathing is to be expected, since the fractured and painful rib moves with each breath and you cannot stop breathing for too long. However, if the chest pain is very severe, or it does not seem localized to the area of the broken rib, or if the pain radiates to the shoulder or is localized in the shoulder region, or if there is marked shortness of breath with a sensation of smothering and an inability to get a deep breath, then there is a possibility of a pneumothorax (see below). The broken edges of the rib may have punctured the lung and allowed the lung or part of it to collapse. The seriousness of this problem depends on how much of the lung has collapsed and how much is therefore non-functioning. In any case, an x-ray is necessary to evaluate the severity, and competent medical treatment is urgent if any of these problems is present.

Coughing up blood when you have a fractured rib indicates that the lung has probably been damaged by the fracture. Such coughing is usually transient, but it may indicate serious lung damage and should not be ignored. An x-ray and competent medical advice as soon as possible is recommended.

Multiple rib fractures are a lot more serious than just one or two broken ribs. If you somehow manage to break a set of ribs (as few as four, five, or six ribs), the whole side of the chest becomes essentially non-functioning, even if you haven't damaged the lung. You need the expansion of the ribs and the chest wall to pull air into the lungs when you take a breath in. With the ribs broken, the chest wall is likely to get sucked in rather than expand out when you breath in. This is a serious and potentially a fatal problem. If you see a man whose chest has been pushed in for whatever reason, and he has multiple broken ribs, he will probably be in shock (see Chapter 4) and he needs emergency medical attention. The side of the chest has to be immobilized to decrease the paradoxical and ineffective movement of the broken ribs. Press a towel tightly against the broken ribs and tape it firmly in place (or if you can pull the collapsed chest wall out and hold it in place) until the victim can be taken to a hospital.

Fractures of the sternum (breastbone) are similar to fractures of the ribs, but there are some important differences. This fracture can be suspected if the blow is directly to the front of the chest, as when a driver gets thrown against the steering wheel in an auto accident or if someone steps on your chest when you are flat on your back. If the blow or pressure is strong enough to break the sternum, it is likely to have caused some damage to the heart, which lies just beneath it. The heart injury can be anything from trivial to catastrophic, and complete evaluation of the heart with an electrocardiogram is necessary to determine the extent of the injury. If the bone is broken and displaced, the diagnosis is obvious. However, the sternum may be broken and the two fragments may be perfectly aligned. If there is pain, particularly if it is associated with tenderness on the sternum, a fracture is probable. Treatment is the same as for fractured ribs, with more attention paid to possible heart damage.

CHEST CONTUSION AND COMPRESSION

Serious damage can be done to the organs within the chest after rib cage compression even in the absence of any rib or sternum fracture. The ribs are flexible (less so in older people), and heavy blows to the chest can do a lot of internal damage without breaking any ribs. Sudden forced compression of the chest can produce a wave of destruction internally, breaking blood vessels, damaging the heart or the lungs as the ribs and the chest whip back to their normal position. If, after heavy or repeated blows to the chest (a) the victim appears restless, or (b) is having trouble breathing, or (c) has persistent chest pain, he should be treated as if he were in shock. A complete medical evaluation is necessary to determine the extent of damage to the heart and lungs.

PNEUMOTHORAX (Collapse of the Lung)

A pneumothorax literally means air in the chest. The significance of a pneumothorax and its potential danger lie in the fact that the air accumulates within the chest, but not inside the lungs. A pocket of air in the chest prevents the lungs from expanding fully.

A pneumothorax can occur spontaneously with no evident cause. It seems to be a problem more frequently seen in smokers and it does occur more often in people who have had a pneumothorax before. If you develop a sudden onset of persistent and sharp chest pain with shortness of breath and pain on breathing or moving, a spontaneous pneumothorax is a good possibility. A pneumothorax can occur after a heavy bout of coughing and can frequently be a problem associated with a fractured rib.

There usually is a moderate amount of pain when air leaks out of the lung into the chest to form a pneumothorax. It hurts so much to breathe that the patient almost holds his breath or breathes slowly and cautiously. This doesn't help because he is already short of breath from the collapsed lung and the shallow breathing makes this worse, making him anxious and restless with pain and producing a sense of suffocation. Best to relieve the pain as soon as possible; codeine, if you have it available, is probably a good drug to start with. It may not be strong enough, but codeine, as well as anything stronger, will need a prescription.

If you suspect a pneumothorax, an x-ray will almost certainly be necessary to determine the extent of the collapse and the need for further treatment. The administration of oxygen may help to relieve the restlessness and breathlessness. If the pneumothorax is extensive and the lung is seriously collapsed, it is sometimes necessary to withdraw the air pocket with a needle or syringe to allow the lung to re-expand.

A tension pneumothorax is even more serious and, untreated, is rapidly fatal. This can occur when air leaks out of the lung into the chest via a "check valve" injury of the lung. Air escapes from the lung into the chest with each breath in, and enlarges the pneumothorax, gradually increasing the pressure on the lung and further collapsing it. The patient is desperately uncomfortable, gasping for air but increasingly breathless with each breath. The best and sometimes life-saving procedure is to insert a large needle between the ribs into the chest, and allow the pocket of air which is under increasing pressure to escape. This permits the lung to re-expand. Sometimes you don't have time to get to a hospital or wait for an x-ray. The patient is gasping for air and may be dying. If you suspect a tension pneumothorax and the patient is getting worse, you may be able to save his life by putting a hypodermic needle into the side of the chest just above a rib about four inches down from the armpit on the side which is painful. Don't try it unless he is really in distress, clearly getting worse and you "know what you are doing." If you hear air hissing out, you have done the right thing. If you don't hear hissing and there is no improvement, remove the needle and get the patient to a hospital. Codeine for pain, and oxygen, if available, to relieve the shortness of breath will help.

STAB WOUNDS AND BULLET WOUNDS OF THE CHEST

Treatment for either a stab or a bullet wound of the chest is generally the same, except that a bullet frequently (but not always) remains in the chest and may have to be removed, and the weapon producing a stab wound usually (but not always) is removed.

A stab wound may take many unusual and unexpected forms. It is not always caused by a stiletto brandished by a "wild man with fire in his eyes," but may be anything from a hat pin or an ice pick to an icicle or an umbrella. It may be intentional or inadvertent, as when a man falls against a sharp picket fence or gets pushed through a glass window.

If the stab wound or the bullet manages to hit the heart or some important blood vessel, the wound is usually fatal. For a major wound, there is little that one can do in first-aid conditions. Often very little can be done, for that matter, in an operating room of a fully equipped hospital. Many, if not most stab wounds or bullets in the chest do not fatally injure the heart or major arteries, and although any chest wound is a potentially serious injury, it is not necessarily fatal.

It is a rare chest wound that does not require the facilities of a large hospital for treatment. The circumstances requiring anonymity, secrecy, or privacy would have to be overwhelming and extremely vital to keep a man with a chest wound away from the hospital. An extremely well equipped aid station with trained personnel might be a satisfactory alternative, but little else will do. Your decision to treat a man with a chest wound outside of a hospital may be a fatal decision, and there probably is no other type of injury in which there is so much a need for modern hospital facilities.

There are a number of things which can and must be done for the man with a penetrating wound of the chest. As always, there are also many well-intentioned things which are done to help but which inadvertently do more harm than good and are better left undone.

> For a bullet or stab wound in which the penetrating object has been removed, the wound site should be covered with a sterile bandage, a Telfa℞ dressing or petrolatum gauze if available, and a firm pressure dressing should be placed over the wound. You should try to seal off the hole to prevent air from leaking in or out. If you don't have anything fancy to seal the hole, some Scotch Tape may help temporarily.

> There is some controversy as to whether a knife or penetrating object should be removed immediately or if it is best left in place and removed at the hospital. So much depends on the nature of the wound, the type and size of the weapon, the location of the wound, and the condition of the victim that no generalization can be made with certainty. For example, if a small hat pin is stuck in the skin between the ribs, it probably should be removed before it gets pushed in deeper. If a sharp ice pick is pushed deep into the front of a man's chest and seems to pulsate with each heartbeat, it probably should not be removed since it often makes a puncture path into the heart or the muscle and seals the hole, preventing bleeding, much as you might see when you push a skewer into a piece of beef. If you remove the pick, you might provoke some bleeding, and it should not be removed except under very controlled conditions. Needless to say, you should go to particular efforts to make sure it is not pushed farther in or knocked around. If a man falls

against a sharp spike, you may find that you may not be able to remove the spike if it is wedged tightly in between two ribs. Probably best to leave it alone.

You have to use a lot of judgment, intuition, and knowledge of anatomy to make this decision. If you cannot decide, if the victim is relatively comfortable and cooperative, and if you can leave the knife undisturbed in its place, it is generally best to leave it where it is and let them remove it at the hospital, where there is access to blood transfusions, x-rays, operating rooms, and skilled personnel.

The victim will usually be in pain, will be anxious, and agitated, particularly if he is in shock (see Chapter 4). He should be kept at rest with minimal activity and disturbed as little as possible. The best treatment for the anxiety, fear, and agitation is gentle and persuasive reassurance. Don't panic, and if you are frightened or upset, don't let the victim know it. It might be hard and dishonest to deceive him but it is clearly to his advantage to rest quietly until he can be taken to a hospital. If the pain is severe, small doses of analgesics can be given, but remember that large doses depress breathing and this is very undesirable in the presence of a chest wound. If necessary, gentle manual restraints can be applied to prevent the victim from hurting himself, but unless applied carefully, they can serve to agitate him even more and frighten him into more thrashing and restlessness.

Nothing by mouth is a good rule of thumb for all severe injuries and chest wounds in particular. With the victim in shock, in pain, bleeding, etc., the stomach is poorly equipped to handle or digest anything it receives, and most food, fluid, or medicine taken by mouth will be vomited up. The disadvantages of vomiting or retching with a fresh chest wound, a bullet in the lung, or a hat pin in the heart are painfully clear. An empty stomach is a distinct advantage. If the victim starts vomiting, roll him gently on his side so he won't choke on the material vomited. No medications should be given by mouth. Pills are of no help sitting unabsorbed in the stomach or vomited up. No alcohol, no coffee, no stimulants are needed or justified.

Make sure the victim is able to breathe. The bullet or knife may have penetrated part of the lung and he may be choking on fluid or blood in his air passages. If you have access to oxygen, this will usually help relieve the sense of smothering which often makes the victim so restless and uncomfortable.

Treat for shock.

Do not try to remove any bullet or foreign body which is imbedded under the skin.

Get the victim to the hospital with as little extraneous movement as possible and as fast as possible.

Abdominal Injuries

When a man is having abdominal pain, the cause is sometimes obvious but the diagnosis may require the sophisticated facilities of a modern medical center. The treatment may also be simple: a laxative or antacid, but sometimes the problem persists despite the best that medicine has to offer.

This section is not a comprehensive treatise on pains in the abdomen, but offers rather some guidelines and advice for its management. Unfortunately, there is no substitute for experience. The advice of a competent doctor is usually necessary if things don't sort out promptly after simple measures are attempted.

We tried to draw up a list of all the things which could reasonably be the cause of abdominal pain, and we stopped after we had listed fifty-three. There are other causes, but this was enough to make the point. There is a vast catalogue of things which can go wrong inside the abdomen. What follows are some of the clues which should alert you to a significant or serious abnormality, suggestions for some things you might try and some things to avoid. These clues are intended as an aid to help you determine the source of your pain and whether further investigation is warranted.

- Abdominal pain seldom occurs alone. It is almost always present with varying degrees of nausea, loss of appetite, or vomiting and sometimes diarrhea. Constipation is usually more subtle and may go unnoticed for days.
- If the vomitus contains the remains of your last meal, this is usually no cause for alarm. Clear vomitus usually comes from the stomach. Green and bitter-tasting vomitus is usually bile from the gall bladder and indicates only that you have been vomiting for a long time. Yellow vomitus may be an indication of obstruction in the small intestine. If the vomitus has a fecal odor or appearance, it indicates an obstruction in the colon or an abnormal connection between the colon and the stomach—a distinctly abnormal condition.
- If the vomitus contains blood, either liquid or in the form of blood clots, it should not be ignored. When blood stays in the stomach for a while, the acid and gastric juices turn the blood black and the vomitus has the appearance of coffee grounds. It may mean an ulcer but it certainly indicates bleeding and must be checked.
- Bleeding anywhere in the intestinal tract will produce blood in the stools. Then stools may be red, indicating fresh bleeding from low down (usually from hemorrhoids, or a polyp), or the stools may contain blood clots or may be black, suggesting a bleeding point higher up. Blood in the intestinal tract usually produces diarrhea and the stools have a powerful odor. Curiously, bleeding is not always associated with abdominal pain.
- If the abdominal pain is on the right side, is associated

with loss of appetite, light-colored stools and dark urine, see the section on *hepatitis* (Chapter 5).

- An inflamed appendix usually starts off with pain in the midline just below the ribs and is usually associated with nausea and vomiting. Only later does it characteristically move to the right side lower down. But pain of appendicitis can present in any combination and location. The typical characteristic features seen in the textbook may not fit your atypical appendix, and the symptoms and pattern vary tremendously.

- If the pain is on your flank (on the side just below or under the ribs) or in your back and is associated with burning or discomfort on urinating, or frequent urination, this may be an indication of a kidney infection (see Chapter 5).

- It probably is not a good idea to take any medicine for the abdominal pain. If it is too severe for you to be comfortable and you feel too sick to be stoic, then you should have it checked. You should avoid medication, not to see how tough you are, but to prevent your distorting or changing or covering up the pattern of pain which may be important in determining what is wrong. Aspirin should be avoided since it frequently upsets the stomach, and you don't need that. Any strong pain medication may give you relief and allow you to get some rest, but the appendix is still inflamed or the ulcer is still irritated and both can perforate while you are resting in comfort.

- Don't take any laxatives or enemas. Constipation as the cause of abdominal pain is pretty unusual, particularly in young people. If you are having abdominal pain, a "good cleaning out" is not what you need. A laxative can do a great deal of harm if you have an intestinal obstruction. Don't feel there is anything wrong if you don't have a good bowel movement every day; every two or three days is quite normal for some people (see Chapter 4).

- It is probably not a good idea to take any antibiotics. They may combat an infection, but that's rarely the problem.

After you take an antibiotic, you make it very difficult to sort out exactly what the problem was. Antibiotics may be useful later when the diagnosis is more definitely established, but not initially.

- If the onset of the pain is sudden or rather abrupt and reaches its maximum intensity shortly after it starts, this would tend to indicate a more serious abnormality than a pain which gradually builds up to its maximum over the course of a few hours. However, the latter pattern, the gradually increasing pain, is not necessarily a trivial one to be ignored.
- It is unusual for significant abdominal pain to be the result of "something you ate." Spoiled or contaminated food usually produces nausea, vomiting, and diarrhea, and pain is not a major feature.
- If flank pain is extreme and severe and radiates down to the groin and occurs in waves, it may indicate a kidney stone. Burning on urination and blood in the urine are usually present.

NON-PENETRATING ABDOMINAL INJURIES

Abdominal injuries are usually a result of a fight, an auto accident, or some form of violence. The injury may be so severe that bleeding and damage to the internal organs may lead to shock and death before any treatment can be given. A lacerated liver or a ruptured spleen are not uncommon. The internal damage done by a club in the solar plexus, or the toe of a boot into a man's flank or groin depends on a number of factors:

> the severity of the blow;
>
> the size and shape of the striking object. A sharp or small object can produce severe but localized damage, whereas a flat or blunt object may produce more widespread but less severe injuries;
>
> the ability of the victim to respond to the blow, his state of preparedness, how much warning he has, his ability to

ward off or deflect the blow, and, most important, his ability to tighten his abdominal muscles to reflexly protect his internal organs;

the strength of the abdominal muscles;

the presence of serious injuries elsewhere in the body.

As noted, the description of the injury itself may not indicate its severity since so many other factors are involved. There are some clues which should alert you to a serious problem:

Persistent pain which lasts longer than you would expect from the physical blow itself;

Pain located in a different area than the region of the injury;

Pain in either shoulder may sometimes indicate irritation of or injury to the diaphragm. This could be from a multitude of causes, but almost always indicates a serious problem;

Nausea and/or vomiting may be a reflex reaction to severe pain, but may indicate damage to the intestinal tract;

Vomiting up blood is an ominous sign and suggests damage to the stomach or intestinal tract. It should not be ignored.

Diarrhea or blood in the stools suggests damage to the lower intestinal tract and also should not be ignored;

Blood in the urine indicates kidney or bladder damage.

Fractures, Strains, and Sprains

A first-aid manual of fractures is inevitably a catalogue of the numerous bones in the body, how and where they break, what complications to expect, and what kind of cast to put on for how long. Rather than provide this kind of information which cannot be too helpful, this section will discuss some general ideas about fractures, how to tell when a bone is broken, and what to do about it.

The amount of force needed to break a bone is tremendously variable. It depends, among other things, on the age, sex, and size of the patient, and location of the bone. The bones can withstand a surprising amount of pressure and tension if they are protected. If you are alert for the stress, you can tense your muscles to protect a bone early enough or relax a limb that's about to be jolted. It may be possible to protect the bone and avoid a fracture. On the other hand, minor trauma can break a large bone if you are caught by surprise or if the force is applied to a particularly vulnerable position or in the right direction, and if the leverage is just right.

Without being too technical, clarifying some of the confusion about definitions is worthwhile. A *fracture* is a broken bone and a *dislocation* is a separation or displacement of two bones at a joint. What was formerly called a compound fracture is now called an *open fracture* and refers to a fracture where the broken ends of a bone pierce through the skin. A *closed fracture* or a simple fracture is one where the bone fragments do not cut through the skin. You may hear the doctors talk about transverse, oblique, or comminuted fractures. *Tranverse fractures* are straight or nearly straight breaks across a bone and generally heal easier because the broken fragments rest flat against each other. An *oblique fracture* or a *spiral fracture* is a twisted break and is often a more serious problem because there is less stability and the bone fragments tend to slide off one another as the muscles which are attached to the bones pull them together or apart. A *comminuted fracture* is a shattered bone with multiple fragments, the kind you might see with a bullet wound. A *greenstick fracture* is usually seen in children with softer and less brittle bones. This kind of fracture is similar to what you would see if you bend a soft piece of wood; the outer part tends to splinter but the wood or soft bone does not break all the way through.

Fractures have to be differentiated from sprains and strains. An x-ray is usually necessary to be certain. A *sprain* is an injury to the muscle ligaments, tendons, and soft tissues in the region of a joint. Muscles, ligaments, and tendons are attached to the bones and are the mechanisms for moving them and holding them in place. Ligaments, tendons, and small blood vessels are stretched and sometimes torn when an ankle or wrist is sprained. Swelling, pain, and tenderness can imitate a fracture. A *strain* is merely a muscle injury from overexertion or stretching. The common back injury is usually a strain.

Fractures in children are usually less of a problem than fractures in adults. Young bones heal very rapidly and almost always normally. Adults don't heal quite as fast or as well as children. Older people have even more brittle bones which tend to break easily and which often don't heal properly, or at all. Sometimes a metal pin or nail has to be inserted to hold non-healing bones together.

Most people who break a bone know it immediately. You can often hear the alarming sound of the bone cracking, or the limb is bent in the wrong direction, or the broken fragments of bone are sticking out of the skin. But you can break a bone with no displacement of the two fragments, or you can chip a small piece of bone off without seeing any abnormality, except perhaps a little swelling. When the question of a fracture is raised, you are ultimately going to need an x-ray. No amount of clinical judgment can replace an actual view of the displaced broken fragments on an x-ray. Even when a fracture is certain, an x-ray is necessary to determine the type of fracture and the location and alignment of the fragments.

Getting fractured bones back together is usually very simple. The broken fragments are replaced in the proper alignment and kept there until a bony bridge can form between the fragments and until the fracture is healed. Keeping the fragments aligned requires a plaster cast or a metal pin which sometimes has to be inserted inside the bone to add stability. When the bony bridge is as stable and as strong as ordinary bone, the cast can be removed and you can go about your normal business. The realignment of the broken fragments is essential for good healing. The patient with the broken bone can expect that this will be done satisfactorily by a doctor in the vast majority of cases.

If, after the injury, the bones are still aligned, there is no need to manipulate them and a cast can be applied with minimum discomfort. If the fragments are displaced they will have to be pushed, prodded, or coaxed back into proper position. In simple cases this can be done in the doctor's office or in a hospital emergency room. It will be painful but the pain will be brief and the doctor can give you a good dose of a pain medication or even light anesthesia. In complicated fractures or in those involving certain bones, the realignment will have to be done under general or spinal anesthesia. This means that you will be admitted to the hospital and the procedure will be done in an operating room. In this case you will have an open or closed reduction of the fracture. If it is closed, the doctor will use the anesthesia to put you to sleep so that he can manipulate the fragments without the excruciating pain this process causes. If it is an open reduction, the doctor will make an incision to view the bony fragments before putting them together. This is done when it is necessary to pin, wire, or nail the pieces together. If the bone fragments are penetrating the skin (an open fracture), you will probably need hospitalization to treat what is an extremely likely problem of infection of the bones and adjacent soft tissues.

First aid for a fracture is remarkably simple. Remove rings, bracelets, or other jewelry as soon as possible, for removing them later when swelling occurs may be difficult. Put a splint on to immobilize the broken bone. The mystique of splints is overstated. There is nothing mysterious about it and almost anything will do for a splint. A rolled up newspaper held in place with a belt, an ice cream stick for a broken finger, a ski pole or even a pillow wrapped firmly around a broken leg will do. Use your ingenuity. When a bone is broken, the muscles attached to the bone often go into spasm and displace the fragments even further. Any unnecessary movement will increase the separation and as the sharp edges drift farther apart, more of the adjacent soft tissue and blood vessels can be damaged.

Don't check for a fracture by having the victim "test his leg" or walk on it. Generally it is best to assume it is broken until proven otherwise. If the limb is quiet and undisturbed, there is usually little pain except for a feeling of fullness and pressure in the area of the break and some tenderness if you press your finger over the fracture itself. Pain reappears when there is any movement and it can be quite severe. If the fracture is open and the bone edges are visible through the skin, don't try to push them back. You stand an excellent chance of making things worse. Just cover it, keep it as clean as possible, and try to stop any bleeding. You can usually control the bleeding with a tourniquet above the bleeding point, but if it can be done without causing too much pain, it is probably much better to apply pressure to the bleeding site with gauze, a clean handkerchief or towel until the bleeding stops. If you are going to use a tourniquet, it should be tightened just enough to stop the bleeding. It probably is wise to release the tourniquet periodically, but if you do loosen it you should not be surprised if bleeding starts again. Something clean should be placed over the wound. Sometimes a fracture produces so much distortion and displacement of the limb that one is tempted to straighten it out before putting a splint on. Do this with much care and compassion, since it will hurt. When you straighten a broken limb you should pull out the broken and distal portion with a strong steady pull and someone should support the limb at the site of the fracture. Remember, when the bone breaks the muscles go into spasm and tend to pull the broken fragments over each other. The purpose of the strong steady pull is to stretch those tightened muscles to allow the bones to get back into place. You can do a lot of harm moving around and stretching broken legs and arms, so if you don't have to, leave the break alone and splint it the way it is to prevent unnecessary further displacement. Fractures of the ribs, the skull, or face do not have to be immobilized with a splint since they will normally immobilize themselves. It would be a test of anyone's ingenuity to put a splint on a skull fracture or a broken jaw.

Pain medications are usually not necessary after a fracture if the broken bone can be kept at rest and immobilized. In fact, nothing, neither liquid nor solid, should be consumed after an injury. Some degree of shock is usually present with major fractures and, among other things, shock slows down the digestive process. The patient will probably vomit whatever is consumed after an injury. Furthermore, if some broken bones have to be realigned in an operating room under general anesthesia, it has to be done on an empty stomach (at least four hours after eating). Don't eat anything after a serious injury.

A minor controversy in medicine concerns the treatment of strains and sprains. One school advocates ice packs and the other favors heat, hot packs, and hot water bottles. An apparently rational approach to treatment takes the best from both schools. Ice packs (a few ice cubes in a towel or a wet towel stored in the refrigerator) initially will help decrease the swelling and decrease the pain. Heat, applied after the swelling has decreased, usually in about twenty-four to forty-eight hours, will probably increase the circulation, promote more rapid healing and, most important, relieve muscle spasm. Rest for a few days and a supporting elastic bandage are usually all that is necessary for a sprain. If the sprain has ruptured a tendon, pain may be quite severe and a cast may be necessary to permit healing. If the pain is very severe, you will need an x-ray to rule out a fracture. A ruptured tendon can sometimes be heard as a "pop."

There are a few relatively unusual fractures which need special attention because of the potential difficulty or problems that they create:

Occasionally, a bone fragment will cut into a major artery which is adjacent to the broken bone and which supplies the blood to the limb distal to the break. If it is a closed fracture, the blood will leak into the soft tissues and the skin will be swollen, tight, and very soon, blue. The bleeding will stop when the pressure gets high enough. A potentially dangerous amount of blood can leak into the soft tissues of a broken leg. This blood loss and the pain can easily produce shock.

Other vital organs could be injured by a broken bone as well. Fortunately, there are relatively few vital organs adjacent to bones, but some are worth mentioning. A broken skull can damage the underlying brain, particularly if the skull fragments are depressed into the brain. A broken neck or, rarely, a broken back can so distort the spinal cord as to cause irreversible paralysis or even death. Nothing is more important to immobilize than a broken neck. Use anything your ingenuity will permit to keep the neck from moving any more than necessary.

A fracture that involves a joint such as the knee or elbow is serious and requires immediate emergency attention. It frequently results in interference to the blood supply to the limb beyond the break, and unfortunately this sometimes requires amputation.

After the fracture is x-rayed, diagnosed, aligned, and stabilized, the patient is sent home. The doctor, having performed according to the best of medical tradition, washes the plaster off his hands and puts the x-rays away. You are left with the cast for anywhere from three weeks to six months to patiently wait for the bones to heal themselves. The problems for the doctor occur early, the problems for the patient usually start when the doctor is finished.

The care and feeding of a cast is a problem most of us are not prepared for. Of course, the doctor will give you some advice (if he isn't too rushed or too tired). Most people learn how to manage their cast by trial and error or from their previously fractured friends who have also learned by trial and error. Simple things like buttoning your shirt or cutting up your food are major crises if you have a cast on your arm or hand. With a cast on your leg you may find that driving a car or taking a shower is impossible, and arrangements often have to be made far in advance to get the simplest things done.

First thing you must adjust to is the presence of this new and usually heavy appendage to your body. It soon becomes a member of your family. Your family, your friends, your roommates will soon become intimately involved with it and you will find them inquiring daily into its status and welfare.

Don't pressure your doctor into removing, lightening, or changing your cast any earlier than he thinks wise, just because you are miserable.

You have to be alert in the first twenty-four to forty-eight hours to the possibility that the cast is too tight. If the part of your limb farther down from the cast (the fingers or toes with a cast on your arm or leg) starts to throb or become blue or painful, don't wait until morning to have it checked. It may be too tight and may have to be removed or loosened. If it is too tight, it can cut off the circulation or injure a nerve and cause far greater and sometimes permanent damage than you had from the broken bones alone.

You can expect to have a variable amount of itching under the cast. It depends on how long the cast has to stay on and how dry or oily your skin usually is. Normally, the outer layer of the skin sheds off continually as new skin appears underneath to replace the old skin. The outer layer is washed or rubbed off without your realizing it. The same process goes on under your cast, but the flaking skin does not get washed or rubbed off. It may start itching. You have to come to terms fairly early with your itching because there isn't too much you can do about it. Most people find that the amount of itching is related to how much they think about it and the itching is normally best and most easily controlled with some sort of diversion. Your mind can usually cope with only one thing at a time and if you keep busy or distracted, the itching goes away. But it is real and can be annoying. Some clever people have devised a variety of methods to scratch beneath the cast, including wire hangers or hair pins. If you can squeeze something like this up under your cast, it may well be too loose, and you may end up injuring the skin. Some talcum powder, if you can get it under the cast, may help.

The cast will be hot shortly after it is put on as the plaster dries. If you notice that your broken arm, leg, or whatever gets warm once the plaster is thoroughly dried, particularly if the fracture was an open fracture or if you had to have an operation to get the fracture repaired, there is a possibility of an infection under the cast. If pain occurs also, you should have it checked. The cast will probably have to be removed and the wound examined for an infection.

Don't get the cast wet. Water will soften the plaster and a mushy cast gives you less support. Once a cast gets soft, its further destruction is inevitable. You can take a bath hanging your cast out of the tub or take a shower with the cast on the other side of the shower curtain. You can wrap the cast in plastic wrap and seal the ends with rubber bands. All this is ridiculous. The cast invariably gets wet, the bath is far from satisfying or satisfactory, and the half in–half out shower makes a mess of the bathroom. Your best bet is probably an old-fashioned sponge bath, with a washcloth and soap.

Don't hammer or bang anything with your cast. It is not a weapon, and it is not indestructible. Continual slapping or knocking the cast may relieve the itching temporarily, but it softens the plaster and you get less support.

You may have to alter your eating habits if you have an arm or hand in a cast and can't cut your food, unless you enjoy having someone do it for you. If not, stick to hamburgers instead of steaks or apples instead of oranges.

You may have to change the type of clothes you wear.

Wear clothes that don't need buttoning if this is a problem. A hook made from a wire hanger may help to pull on pants or even socks if you cannot reach down. Some clothes won't fit over a cast and you may need to cut up the seam of your pants leg or wear a short-sleeved shirt.

Sleeping with a cast can be messy. It will rip up your sheets, and you might try wrapping it in an old towel to keep it from wearing a hole in the mattress. If you need to hold the towel in place, don't use a tight rubber band or string which may cut off the circulation during the night. Wearing a cast on a water bed is asking for trouble.

Your common sense will have to determine whether you can or want to drive. It depends on what kind of car you drive, what kind of shift it has, what kind of cast you have, and what kind of driver you are. If the cast gets down to your right ankle and interferes with the gas pedal, driving is probably insane. If you have a standard shift and the cast puts your right arm at a right angle, you might be able to shift with your left hand while steering with your fractured and casted right arm, but we don't advise it. Use your judgment and good sense. Remember, you won't be able to move too rapidly with a cast on in case of an emergency and you won't be able to swerve or step on the brake if your cast gets in the way.

Try to avoid situations or circumstances which will damage your cast or further injure the fracture, which just wants to be left alone to quietly heal itself. Theoretically, there is no reason why you can't play basketball or go bicycling with a cast on your arm or play ping pong or go rowing with a cast on your leg. It just doesn't seem like good sense and you would be better off giving the bones a chance to heal rather than trying to prove how tough you are.

Cuts and Bruises

Cuts and bruises are very simple to take care of but very easy to mess up, and poor management of a simple wound can result in ugly scars or loss of function. We will try to point out some of the problems you may encounter and some of the pitfalls you should be aware of.

It is important to distinguish among a contusion, an abrasion, a laceration, and a puncture.

A *contusion* is a bruise that is a result of a blunt injury to the skin and to the tissue beneath the skin. The damage is primarily to the underlying tissues and not to the skin itself.

An *abrasion* is a skin wound usually produced by rubbing or scraping the skin, but with no actual penetration through the skin.

A *laceration* is the medical term for what is called a cut. If an incision is made in the skin by anything, anywhere, you have been lacerated. It may or may not go all the way through the skin.

A *puncture* is actually a special form of laceration. A tack or a nail produces a puncture, and the major difference between this and a laceration is that the puncture opening gets closed off by the skin above it when the tack or nail is removed.

Everyone knows what a *scratch* is.

Contusions are uncomfortable, and nothing need be done except to relieve the pain. Most people voluntarily limit the activity of the bruised arm or leg or whatever, simply because it hurts to move it. Cold packs or ice in a towel should be placed on the bruise for the first twenty-four to forty-eight hours. This will tend to diminish the swelling which adds to the pain. A hot water bottle, heating pad, or towel soaked in hot water can be used thereafter if the pain persists for more than a day or two. A black eye is a special form of a contusion. A bruise turns the skin blue initially as the blood accumulates under the skin in the area of the injury. As the blood is reabsorbed, the colors change generally from blue to green to yellow in about two to three weeks.

Sometimes the blow may be severe enough to produce a fracture to an underlying bone. If the trauma is forceful, if the pain is severe, if the bruise is just over a bone and a fracture is suspected, it probably will be necessary to get an x-ray.

An *abrasion* if it is very extensive can result in serious problems. The main problem is to remove all the debris (rocks, glass, dirt, and stones) which are not only on the skin but, more important, which have become embedded in and under the skin from the force of the injury. This may take some determined and prolonged scrubbing and can be quite uncomfortable. If you don't get all the debris out from under the skin it may produce permanent discoloration and tattooing. If scrubbing is too painful, you may need a doctor to apply a local anesthetic and finish the job. If the abrasion is extensive you might want to apply a light non-adherent gauze (petrolatum gauze) and then a dry clean dressing, but this is not necessary and the abrasion can be left dry, open to the air if you prefer. No antibiotic ointments should be used unless there is an obvious infection. Extensive abrasions, particularly those with debris under the skin, require tetanus toxoid.

The management of a *laceration* depends on its location, what produced the injury and how deep it goes, the presence of residual foreign bodies in the laceration, the time delay before treatment, the presence of infection and sometimes, the presence of other associated injuries. Most of the time, all that is needed is a Band-Aid. The body heals itself very well if left alone. But an extensive wound in a vital location needs all the help it can get, and, more important, it does not need fumbling hands making mistakes and bad decisions.

Even a deep laceration can be left alone; if it is kept clean, it should not get infected. No stitches, no doctors, no hospitals need be involved. The purpose of repairing the laceration or bringing the two cut edges into contact with each other with stitches (or sutures, as doctors call them) is to prevent or minimize ugly scarring, to promote faster healing and prevent or minimize infection. If the laceration is not too deep, not infected, not too jagged (if the edges are sharp), if the edges are naturally placed close to one another, and if no tendons, nerves, or arteries are involved underneath the cut skin, the repair can often be accomplished by bringing the two cut edges into firm contact with adhesive tape, or a few Band-Aids placed across rather than lengthwise along the incision. However, it isn't this simple if the laceration is too long or too deep, if it involves an area where the skin does not stretch or pull easily (like the shin), if any vital organs or structures are involved, or if you are concerned about scars resulting. In any of these cases, repair by a competent physician is probably necessary.

A laceration on your shoulder, even if it is a deep wound, is usually of no great consequence. The shoulder is not a crucial site and there are few vital organs involved. But a deep laceration of your thumb or the palm of the hand may cut vital nerves affecting your sense of touch or may cut important tendons controlling the movement of your fingers. If these are not repaired with absolute precision, you can be left with a poorly functioning hand which may be a serious and permanent disability, even if you aren't a pianist. All deep lacerations of the hand should be checked by a doctor. If serious damage is done to the nerves, blood vessels, or tendons, it may require the services of a surgeon with special training in hand surgery to prevent permanent disability.

Another crucial and unfortunately frequent location for a laceration is the face. The same problems as we noted for lacerations of the hand, the damage to nerves and tendons, are present, but the problem is complicated by the need for a cosmetically acceptable repair of the skin. A scar on the shoulder should not trouble most people but a scar, even a small one, on the forehead or on the cheek, may be regrettable for years to come. All facial lacerations should be repaired by a competent surgeon.

Two particularly difficult areas are cuts on the lips or cuts on the eyelids. Both require a meticulous repair to produce an acceptable result. The pink borders of the lip must be aligned exactly or else the lip will heal with an unnatural irregular scar. If the laceration is on an eyelid, special techniques must be utilized to prevent a drooping or a contracted lid. If the eyebrow is lacerated, the hair should not be shaved to repair the laceration, since the hair of the eyebrow sometimes grows back irregularly or not at all, and it sometimes fails to match the shape of the other eyebrow. These are simple problems which can occur with small, unimportant lacerations just as well as with major and extensive injuries. We mention these simple problems among many others, not because you are going to sew up someone's eyelid, but to point out when professional help is likely to be needed and to emphasize the need for competent surgical repair if a satisfactory result is to be obtained.

There are a few other problems you should be alerted to. The skin of the face and scalp is very rich in blood vessels, and any laceration to the face, and particularly to the scalp, usually bleeds profusely, even if it is a relatively small and simple one. Notice how generous and prolonged the bleeding is with even a tiny razor nick inflicted while shaving. A scalp laceration can be rather alarming and makes a good photograph in the local paper with blood streaming down the victim's face from a trivial cut on his scalp. A small scratch looks like a major head wound.

The bleeding can usually be stopped by applying pressure to the wound with a clean dressing—a handkerchief will do. If the hair is matted with blood, you can't see the laceration until the blood is washed out, and sometimes the hair in the small area around the laceration has to be shaved off. This hair grows back eventually but the hair directly over the scar does not.

A sharp cut with a knife or razor blade goes in and comes out not doing too much other damage en route either way. The skin is neatly separated, and when the two edges are brought together, they are in reasonably good approximation.

Jagged cuts may result when you put your hand through a glass window or fall on a picket fence. Sometimes some of the skin scrapes off on the glass or on the fence, and the laceration is not necessarily straight or smooth, or a segment of skin is missing. When the two edges are brought together, they don't fit too smoothly and repair of this kind of laceration often takes a little bit of imagination and artistry.

A major consideration depends on the cleanliness of the cutting edge. "Dirt" doesn't always appear in the form of a handful of soil from the garden or the dust under the bed. If you carve the Thanksgiving turkey with a clean knife, but cut your finger before the first cut, it is probably relatively clean. Once the fat and fibers from the turkey get onto the knife and then you cut the finger, you probably have a dirty laceration. Dirt can be small flecks of paint or little slivers of glass or rust rubbed off an old spike, or fat from the turkey. The necessity for recognizing the presence of the dirt cannot be overemphasized, and you should make every reasonable effort to get all the foreign matter out of the wound before it is closed.

Just below the skin is a layer of fat and non-specific connective tissue which varies in thickness, depending on the location of the laceration. If you have cut down to the fat beneath the skin you have gone pretty deep. Actually, the fat and tissues beneath the skin cannot be recognized easily because of the blood in the wound, but you may have a chance to see how deep you have gone when you wash it out. Below the fat can be anything from muscle to bone, and if you are down this far, you had better have a doctor look at it to see what else you might have injured. You may have slashed a tendon or a nerve. If the wound is bleeding profusely, if the blood is bright red (rather than dark, almost blue red) and is pumping or pulsatile, you have probably cut an artery and the bleeding will stop only with firm, steady, and prolonged pressure.

If an artery is bleeding and you are putting pressure over it, don't peek every few minutes or remove the bandage to see if it is still bleeding. It generally is. The release of the pressure will start the bleeding again and the blood loss may be substantial. Although local pressure is preferable, a tourniquet may be necessary to stop the bleeding. You can use your ingenuity and your common sense as to how to style and devise it. There is nothing very obscure or subtle about a tourniquet. It should be positioned between the bleeding point and the heart or simply higher up on the leg or arm than the point of bleeding. The tourniquet should be tightened until the bleeding stops, and probably should be loosened carefully periodically. If the pain from the tourniquet gets too uncomfortable, it may be loosened temporarily while someone holds pressure over the wound to prevent excessive bleeding.

Use your common sense in evaluating the severity of a deep laceration. There are no firm rules to adhere to, but if you are concerned, if things don't look right, if you are very uncomfortable, you should probably have the wound evaluated by a doctor rather than take the chance of some of the later and devastating complications which may develop.

"Foreign bodies" is a medical term for any particles which may be left behind in the laceration. Particularly troublesome are small slivers of glass which cannot be seen but oddly enough can be heard if you gently stroke a sterile needle through the laceration. Most foreign particles can be removed by irrigating the wound with copious quantities of sterile or at least clean water. You can sterilize water by boiling it, but don't pour boiling or very hot water over anything; let it cool first. Simply holding a cut finger under running tap water with the edges of the laceration kept open, will flush most debris out of most wounds very easily. If this is not practical, you can clean the wound by pouring water over it (not too hot!) or splashing the wound around in a bucket of clean, soapy water (use liquid kitchen soap). The best method is to direct a small jet of clean water into the spread open wound: a clean syringe is ideal. You don't want a needle on the syringe. Some affluent homes have jet sprays for cleaning teeth, and these are excellent for flushing particles out of wounds.

Infections don't usually present a problem for the first twenty-four to forty-eight hours after the injury, but some of the precautions noted thus far, if taken in the first few minutes, will go a long way to preventing infection a few days later.

Some wounds are obviously grossly contaminated and no amount of flushing or cleaning will prevent infection. If you cut yourself with a pitchfork that you use to turn the compost heap, the possibility of infection is high; you had better get a tetanus shot as an additional precaution, and most doctors would recommend an antibiotic to help destroy the bacteria which have set up housekeeping under your skin.

Not all infections or potential infections need antibiotics, however. The normal healthy individual is quite capable of ridding himself of most trivial or minor infections through his own defense mechanisms, and antibiotics would only be necessary if the infection is extensive or severe or if the focus of infection is loculated in a pocket of pus, or if the victim is not a normal healthy individual. Diabetics, alcoholics, older people, or those who have maintained a chronically inadequate diet are likely to develop serious infections from relatively trivial causes.

You should be alert to the possibility of an infection developing in a wound if you note any of the following: 1) *Pain* which seems to be increasing rather than decreasing as it would with normal wound healing, particularly if the pain is associated with *tenderness* or *swelling;* 2) any *pus* or *discharge* from the wound; 3) *fever,* usually higher than 100° F. suggests an infection; 4) *red streaks* or tenderness in the arm or leg above the site of the wound suggests an infection.

If any of these develop, you should probably have the wound checked and may need an antibiotic or may need to have the infected area opened and drained. If you decide to sit it out, and don't believe in medicines, you may get better slowly as the normal body mechanisms win their battle with the evil germs. The wound will often heal but occasionally does not. If it does heal, the chances of a scar remaining are greater. If you lose the battle the infection will continue to spread. Some people die from an untreated infection, and in the days before penicillin, this was a frequent "mode of exitus."

Unless you have cut an artery or have hemophilia, bleeding should stop in less than ten minutes. Actually, some brisk bleeding may be good since it helps to flush out foreign particles, but blood is a lot more expensive than water and excessive bleeding should be stopped regardless of how much good it may be doing. If you can elevate the lacerated hand or arm it may also help by decreasing some of the pressure in the veins. Excessive bleeding may cause shock and this may be a medical emergency.

ASSOCIATED INJURIES

If you accidentally cut yourself with a carving knife, all you have to worry about is the laceration. But nature and human beings are usually not that simple, and lacerations are often associated with other significant injuries. Depending on the injury, the resources and people available, you will have to make some decision as to who to take care of first and what to do first. Here are a few suggestions:

> First thing to check is if the victim is breathing and if his heart is beating. Precedence is given to this (see the section on cardiac resuscitation on pp. 163–170 to deal with this). A quick glance will usually make your decision, but don't start treating a lacerated arm when the victim is not breathing.

> Arterial bleeding—pumping bright red blood—requires immediate care. Don't worry about the tiny little pumpers, worry about the big ones. The big artery will only bleed for a short while and then it will stop when

there is too little blood left. Putting on a tourniquet is fast, simple, and definitive. Use a belt or a tie and then go on to other things as necessary. Non-arterial bleeding or small-artery bleeding usually can be controlled with pressure. Have the victim hold his own tourniquet or pressure pad if he can and you can then go on to take care of other things.

TETANUS

Tetanus still does occur in the 1970's but it is avoidable. Any laceration and particularly a puncture wound is fertile ground for the tetanus bacteria. (See the section on tetanus, pp. 170–173, for treatment and advice.)

DEALING WITH THE AUTHORITIES

Not all lacerations are due to carving the turkey or stepping on some broken glass at the beach. Sometimes people get in fights and stab each other. Sometimes people cut themselves when they put their hands through other people's windows or eyeglasses. People who don't use seat belts frequently leave their car through their front window. You should not delay or deny yourself needed medical care because of a possible confrontation with the authorities at the hospital, clinic, emergency room, or whatever. In most states, doctors are required by law to report any injury, stabbing, etc., caused by violence. Some doctors do and some don't report these incidents. Some forget to and some don't want to.

If you are uncomfortable about the possibility of discussing the incident with the police, you must weigh this against the difficulties, complications, and discomfort caused by the avoidance of treatment. Remember that you can use your good judgment in describing the incident. It is not a good idea to distort the basic nature of the injury (it is important for the doctor to know the cause of the wound), but the doctor should have no reason to question or cross-examine your description of how the wound was inflicted. (See Chapter 2, Your Medical Rights and Privileges.)

Burns

A burn can be as trivial as a first-degree sunburn or a second-degree blister on your finger from touching a hot stove. It can also be a devastating third-degree burn with its associated shock, scars, prolonged hospitalization, and frequent fatalities. Severe burns almost always are a combination of all types. Regardless of how much burn or how deep, it is always associated with a disproportionate amount of pain and discomfort and, with serious burns, an extraordinary amount of anxiety. Assuming the patient survives, the problem of scars and mutilation often complicates the recovery.

There are three main factors to consider when evaluating a burn. You can't make any judgment regarding the type of treatment, the necessity for hospitalization or medical evaluation, or the prognosis without evaluating 1) the depth of the burn, 2) the extent of the burn (i.e., how much skin area is involved), and 3) the location of the burn. It is also necessary to consider other important factors such as the age of the patient (older people and infants have a much more difficult time with a burn), the health of the patient (chronic illness or associated injuries substantially complicate recovery), and the amount of time elapsed between the burn and the initiation of therapy.

The depth of the burn. A burn is classified as a first-, second- or third-degree burn depending on its depth and not on its extent or on the amount of pain involved.

A first-degree burn involves just the outer surface of the skin, a sunburn, for example. Such burns will also result if your skin is exposed to (but not in direct contact with) a sudden burst of heat such as from a small explosion in your stove or a hydrogen bomb explosion in a neighboring city. The skin is red, dry, painful, and sensitive to touch. There is a variable amount of tingling and if you are white-skinned it turns pale when you press on it.

If the skin is swollen, puffy, weepy, or blistered, you may be dealing with a *second-degree burn*. This involves the tissue beneath the skin as well as the outer skin itself. The burn characteristically occurs, for example, when you touch a hot stove or spill boiling water on your skin. A severe sunburn can occasionally blister, producing second-degree burns, and a blast of heat close up usually results in a second-degree burn on the exposed skin.

The *third-degree burn* involves the skin and penetrates deep down to involve the tissue below the skin. It can involve any underlying tissue or organs depending on how serious the burn is. It is frequently, but not always, a fire burn, in which the skin is on fire and is cremated. Curiously but gratefully, the victim is often spared any severe local pain, because the nerves which transmit the pain from the skin are usually damaged or destroyed along with the skin. The patient will not complain of pain in the area of the burn but the margin of the third-degree burn is often second-degree and painful. The skin is usually dry, pale white or charred black; it is swollen and frequently broken open exposing the underlying tissues. A flame thrower or napalm usually produces a third-degree burn. Anyone whose clothes catch on fire and who can't get them off fast enough usually sustains a third-degree burn.

The extent of the burn. The area of skin involved in a second- or third-degree burn has to be measured carefully. It cannot be evaluated unless the affected clothing is removed and generally the measurement of the extent of the burn is less important as a first-aid measure than it becomes later when replacement of lost fluids becomes a critical factor and when the delicate management of a burned patient has to be controlled. The surface area of the victim's hand is equal to about 1 per cent of the total skin area, and using your own hand (don't touch), you can roughly estimate the extent of the burn. You can also roughly calculate the amount of burned skin based on the approximate "9 per cent estimates" of skin surface in a standard-sized adult. The head contains 9 per cent of the total skin surface area, the arms 9 per cent each, the legs 18 per cent each, the front and the back of the trunk 18 per cent each and the neck 1 per cent. Any second-degree burn which involves more than 10 to 15 per cent of the body surface area and any third-degree burn will likely be associated with shock.

The location of the burn. This is a critical factor. Shock is often present when the burn involves the head, face, hands, feet, or genitalia, even if it is of relatively small extent. The hands and feet are quite sensitive and burns in these areas are unusually painful. When the burns involve these areas, nursing care outside a hospital is often difficult and hospitalization may be necessary for even a relatively small burn.

If the victim has been trapped in a closed room or burning house, or if he has inhaled flames, hot air, or fumes, he probably has sustained some burn of the mucous membranes of his nose, throat, and probably his lungs. Hospitalization is usually necessary in anyone who has trouble speaking, swallowing, or breathing after a burn, or if the victim is hoarse or is wheezing. Patients with involvement of these organs often have problems with tissue swelling and fluid accumulation in the lungs and with associated problems of swallowing and breathing.

THE TREATMENT OF BURNS

The characteristic first-degree burn is the sunburn. Here, more than in most places, the prevention is much simpler than the treatment. Suntan lotions and creams have only a limited protective value and, while they help, they won't protect you against excessively prolonged exposure or an excessively hot sun. Sunburns are uncomfortable but not dangerous unless they are very extensive, or if they are associated with second-degree blistering. Severe sunburns often produce a low-grade fever and some headache. Two aspirins every three to four hours with generous fluid intake should alleviate both the fever and the headache. Some people are nauseated and thirsty due to the dehydration which is frequently present. Small and frequent sips of a cool drink (preferably nonalcoholic) should remedy this. Some people find sucking on chips of ice the best treatment for nausea and dehydration. Infants and children are entirely different cases, and the sunburned baby may have to be hospitalized for treatment of dehydration. High fever and a dry diaper are warning signs, and it may be necessary to administer intravenous fluids.

Although it probably has no effect on the healing process, cooling adds immeasurably to the patient's comfort. Whatever method is used is not as important as getting the heat out of the skin. Putting your burned finger in a cup of cold water is good. A cool bath is very pleasant relief for a sunburn. A clean towel soaked in ice water and placed on your face or chest will give substantial relief of the discomfort of a first-degree burn.

If the first-degree burn is dirty or contaminated, the skin should be washed very gently with a soapy water solution (liquid kitchen soap is convenient for making a solution) and then flushed with copious amounts of water. Do not put any salves, oils, grease, butter, or lubricants on the skin for a first-degree burn. We do not recommend any of the pain medications which are sprayed or applied onto the skin. They are expensive, their effect is temporary and, most serious, a significant number of people will have a reaction to the drugs which are the active ingredients. They are no more effective than the measures outlined above. If no complications occur and if re-exposure can be avoided, a first-degree burn should be comfortable in twelve to twenty-four hours and should heal satisfactorily with itching and skin peeling in about a week. The new skin is tanned but ready to be burned again.

For second-degree burns, when blisters, skin swelling, and weeping are present, the clothing over the burned area should be gently and carefully removed. The skin should be thoroughly cleaned with a soap solution and copiously rinsed with water. The loose scaling skin can be removed but the blisters *should not be opened* or drained. If they are accidentally broken, the covering skin should be left in place as an effective dressing. A single layer of a nonadherent lightly impregnated gauze such as petrolatum gauze (which can be obtained in most pharmacies) should cover the burn area, and this can be held in place with dry sterile gauze and a loosely wrapped elastic bandage. The dressing should be changed the next day and every two days thereafter, but if pain or fever develop or the dressings become wet or dirty, the burn should be examined more often. If fever develops or if pain and swelling increase, an infection is probably present and treatment with antibiotics may be necessary. A doctor should be consulted since the infection may spread and delay may seriously impede recovery. During the healing period it is best to avoid using the burned part if possible, and it is good to keep the area elevated and at rest. Don't forget to get a tetanus toxoid booster if you have been previously immunized. If not, a tetanus series is needed and, if the burn is seriously contaminated, your doctor may want to give you tetanus immune globulin for rapid protection. If your uncomplicated second-degree burn involves more than about 10 to 15 per cent of your body or any critical area (face, hands, genitalia, etc.), you should get some medical supervision.

All third-degree burns should be evaluated by competent physicians. Even a small burn may get infected, healing is slow, scars occur frequently, and surgery may be necessary. Most third-degree burns require hospitalization and usually require intravenous fluids and treatment for shock. A person with any but the most trivial third-degree burn should not be given anything to drink, since the stomach and intestines do not function very well with a patient in shock and he is likely to vomit. If transportation to a hospital is available don't fuss too much with the burns except to make the patient comfortable. If a delay is anticipated, remove the clothing and wrap the burns in a cool damp and clean dressing to prevent further contamination. If you can find one, simply wrap the patient up in a clean sheet. Don't put any grease, ointment or antiseptic on the burn prior to transportation to the hospital. It will only have to be removed, it delays things, and causes the patient some discomfort.

The pain associated with third-degree burns is difficult to assess. Generally the burn is not as painful as it looks to an anxious and sympathetic friend. As mentioned, most severe or third-degree burns are not very painful initially, and generally, if the burn is left alone, the pain is no great problem. Pain may occur in adjacent areas with second-degree burns and it may be quite severe. Pain should be anticipated, however, when moving the patient or changing dressings and some pain medication should be given beforehand if possible. Burn victims are restless, anxious, sometimes confused and delirious. This should not necessarily be interpreted as an indication of pain, but frequently a manifestation of shock and often a decrease in oxygen in the brain due to smoke or carbon monoxide inhalation. A sedative, oxygen or fresh air, and treatment for shock are more important than pain medication in these cases.

If the burn is due to contact with strong acid or alkali, then you should wash off the irritant with large quantities of clean water.

Bullet and Stab Wounds

In the old-fashioned and barbaric art of physical confrontation, people versus people, the good and the bad, cowboys and Indians, police versus demonstrators, them against us, the gun and the knife were acceptable modes of offense and defense and wounds from the bullet and the blade were common medical problems. Today we have more genteel and sophisticated techniques for dealing with the bad guys: tear gas and mace, rubber bullets and tranquilizer darts. Occasionally, the primitive instincts within us rise up and escape and we resort to guns and knives to settle our differences.

It seems that everyone has a gun in the house, and it seems that it is always accidentally being discharged when it is getting cleaned or at every noise in the night, or during some innocent hunting accident. Perhaps this is a subtle and effective method for dealing with the excess population, and we are selecting for an early demise those careless enough to clean their loaded guns or fire a gun at their housemates or hunting companions.

There are some technical aspects of bullet wounds which may be helpful in evaluating the severity of the problem.

Military weapons are usually very powerful, and the bullet travels at about 2,700 feet per second. The resultant wound is generally devastating, deep, and penetrating. Civilian weapons, the 22- or 38-caliber pistols, for example, produce lower-velocity missiles at about 700 feet per second with comparatively less damage. Hunting rifles are high-velocity weapons. Buckshot is intermediate and the velocity of the exiting pellets is about 1,300 feet per second. At long range, buckshot may produce nothing more than a bad stinging sensation, but at close range up to about 20 feet, the pellets can produce devastating damage because of their high velocity.

Most gunshot wounds are not painful at all. The wounded person notes a thump or stinging sensation initially and then feels warm blood oozing from the wound. Only later does pain develop as a result of the damage the bullet has done to nerves, bones, or soft tissue.

Shotgun wounds, however, are very uncomfortable. The pellets strike or penetrate the skin and produce a painful burning sensation.

The heat of a bullet is not enough to produce a burn, or hot enough to sterilize the bullet. A bullet wound is assumed to be contaminated with bacteria both from the bullet and from the clothes and skin as the missile enters the victim.

The problems created by a bullet or a knife are largely

related to the location of the wound and only secondarily to the health of the victim and the resources available to take care of the injury.

A bullet or knife wound can be fatal 1) if it hits a vital organ, such as the heart or the brain, and if the organ can no longer function effectively; or 2) if it severs a major artery, resulting in the victim's bleeding to death either internally or externally; or 3) if the missile or knife punctures or collapses a lung, compromising the victim's breathing (see Chapter 4). Many other factors, for example, the size of the knife or the location of the artery influence the outcome. Death can occur almost instantaneously or can occur slowly in a matter of hours or days, depending on the availability of medical assistance.

If the inflicted wound is not immediately fatal, and the victim survives the initial injury, there are many additional problems to be considered.

- Any wound to the head, the face or neck, or the chest and abdomen is potentially more serious than a wound elsewhere on the body such as the arm or leg. A bullet wound in the thigh or in the armpit can also be extremely dangerous if one of the major arteries is involved and internal bleeding results.
- A bullet-created fracture is difficult to manage, and healing is often delayed by the infection the bullet produces and because of the shattering effect a high-velocity missile has on the bone.
- The bullet wound may bleed profusely or not at all. If it is bleeding, you should apply pressure to stop it, but you must realize that the bleeding may continue internally from the damage within; you are merely covering up the external manifestation of the bleeding with pressure on the bullet hole. If it is an arm or leg wound, a tourniquet would be much better in controlling both the internal and external hemorrhage, but the tourniquet will probably have to be loosened periodically to permit some circulation to the damaged arm or leg.

- The victim of a gunshot or stab wound is usually frightened and angry. He is frightened if he has been caught and angry if he is innocent. A bullet or a stab wound is a frightening, dangerous, and upsetting incident for anyone. The stress of the moment often produces belligerent, combative, and obstreperous behavior, even with friends who are trying to help. Some of this is attributable to stress, but some of the unusual and difficult behavior may be due to a lack of oxygen or poor circulation if the bullet or knife has damaged the lungs or heart or the patient is in shock. There isn't much you can do except to try to prevent the victim from further injuring himself. Firm and gentle restraints and calm persistent reassurance may be all you can offer. Try not to let the victim know how upset you are.

A tetanus shot will be necessary for all bullet or knife wounds. If the victim has a massive wound which is obviously dirty and infected, or if he hasn't had a tetanus booster shot in ten years, then immunization with tetanus immune globulin or antitoxin may be necessary.

Almost every state has a law which requires the doctor to report gunshot wounds and most require reporting stab wounds as well. However, the doctor is not required to report anything more than the wounding. Anything else which you tell the doctor may be protected by the rule of confidentiality, unless the doctor feels that you represent a possible danger to yourself or the community. If you tell him you'll get the guy who shot you, don't be surprised if he tells this to the police.

Cardiac Arrest and Cardiac Massage

What was called artificial respiration a decade ago has been reevaluated, revised, and updated, and is now referred to as *cardiac resuscitation*. There are two main differences. First, it was recognized that the old technique of pushing air in and out of a man's chest was useless when his heart had stopped beating; this is usually the case when breathing has stopped. A heart which has stopped beating (or is "arrested") can frequently be induced to start again. At the very least, the effect of the beating heart could be temporarily reproduced by applying intermittent pressure to the appropriate area on the chest. Secondly, it was recognized that it was far more effective to blow air into a man's lungs than to push on his chest and let the air move in and out passively, as the former method recommended. The technique of cardiac resuscitation is simple to learn, and amazingly effective if the circumstances are favorable. The circumstances are rarely favorable, but if you are ever lucky enough to get the method to work, you will be overwhelmed with the personal sense of having made the difference.

We urge that before you jump on anyone's chest or attempt cardiac resuscitation, you thoroughly familiarize yourself with when to do it and when not to, how to do it and when to stop. It helps if you know what causes or predisposes the heart to stop beating, how to recognize it, what specifically you must do, and, often the most difficult decision, when to stop trying, recognizing that your efforts have not succeeded.

What causes a heart to stop beating and when do you try to resuscitate an arrested heart?

Almost any significant disease, illness, or injury can cause a cardiac arrest. Everyone dies eventually when his heart stops beating. It is the terminal event in every terminal illness. Its significance is not in this observation, however, but in the recognition of those cases where the termination of the heartbeat is sudden, accidental, or inadvertent, unrelated (relatively so) to the inexorable progression of another serious or fatal disease.

Even here, a list of the kinds of things which cause a sudden cardiac arrest is a long one, and not all patients with sudden cardiac arrests are candidates for resuscitation attempts. It is not always easy to make these distinctions, particularly in a stranger. The problem soon becomes theological, less how to do it and more when to do it. Our guideline is to try cardiac resuscitation on any young person who "dies" suddenly regardless of his state of health and on any older person who has a sudden cardiac arrest in the absence of obvious significant other disease which would likely cause his death in any event.

This guideline, though, is not particularly useful. The question of why not try it on anyone—"What do you have to lose?"—is not an idle one. The response relates partly to the futility of resuscitating a heart whose time has come, partly to the risk you take in resuscitating a heart when there has been irreversible brain damage (wherein the resuscitated heart beats in a body with no effective brain), and finally, in a major way, to the position you undertake in relation to what little dignity there is left in the natural process of dying.

Some examples will provide perspective. This list is not complete but includes some of the kinds of things which you could come upon in the street, with a stranger, or at home with a member of your family.

A victim with any *stab wound* or *gunshot wound*, particularly if it is inflicted to the chest or if it is associated with heavy blood loss and shock (see Chapter 5), is a candidate for resuscitation. Your chances for a successful resuscitation are negligible if the wound has injured the heart itself or any of the major blood vessels or organs inside the chest. The arrest is potentially much more likely to respond to your efforts if it is due primarily to shock or blood loss.

Electrocution causes death characteristically by producing a cardiac arrest and is one of the most likely things to respond to a resuscitation attempt because the heart is basically healthy: it stops beating for electrical reasons and can be easily restarted. The breathing and the brain are normal and there is no blood loss or impairment of blood flow. Electrocution is seldom produced by intentional execution any more. It is far more commonly seen when someone gets struck by lightning or even more commonly when someone comes into contact with a high-voltage power line. Many cardiac arrests are the result of home accidents, when someone uses a faulty piece of electrical equipment or reaches to turn off the radio while standing in the shower. By the way, be warned against rushing in to save your friend who has just electrocuted himself without first separating him from the source of electricity, or you too will have to be resuscitated when you reach out to help. Turn the power off or unplug the toaster which just dropped into the sink.

A heart attack frequently results in a cardiac arrest. It occurs much more commonly in someone who has a bad heart or has had a previous heart attack, and this should alert you if you know the victim. If a man has a cardiac arrest for no apparent reason, it is usually because he has had a heart attack.

A drug reaction may cause a cardiac arrest. It may be caused by either an overdose of a drug or an idiosyncratic reaction to a standard dose of a standard medication or the result of an unfortunate combination of medicines which place too great a strain on the heart. Some drugs are worse offenders than others. Shooting speed is probably the most hazardous and produces enormous demands on the heart.

An overdose of tear gas or mace in a sensitive individual, particularly someone with asthma or someone taking asthma medications, could conceivably produce a cardiac arrest.

Any severe chest injury or strong blow to the chest with or without broken ribs may damage the heart enough to cause it to stop beating. But keep in mind that sometimes an arrested heart can be resuscitated with a good thump of your closed fist across the front of the chest (see later).

Drowning or *asphyxia.*

Almost anything else which produces a severe physical or, rarely, emotional strain on an individual can stop the heart. An automobile accident in which the driver gets thrown against the steering wheel will cause a cardiac arrest. A person trapped in a smoke-filled room in a house on fire with too much carbon monoxide and too little oxygen may be a victim as well.

HOW DO YOU RECOGNIZE A CARDIAC ARREST?

Certain clues are strongly suggestive of a cardiac arrest, and you should look for these before you start resuscitation efforts or you will do a lot of harm to someone who is sound asleep or drunk or unconscious for some reason other than a cardiac arrest.

A cardiac arrest is almost always associated with a respiratory arrest, simultaneously, before, or after. If you stop breathing, your heart will soon stop beating, mostly for lack of oxygen. If your heart stops, your breathing will stop fairly soon also. This is useful for making a diagnosis of cardiac arrest and it is a critical consideration in your treatment (see below).

Remember that you have to act very fast. You must establish good effective blood circulation and some kind of effective breathing within three to five minutes. If it takes you longer than that to establish return of blood circulation and successful oxygenation, little is to be gained by your efforts.

- If you cannot feel a pulse at the wrist or you cannot hear the heart beating when you put your ear against the left side of a man's chest, this is good evidence to support your impression that he has had a cardiac arrest. This is useful only if you have had experience in feeling the pulse or listening to the heart and are sure you are feeling or listening correctly.
- The patient will be unresponsive to painful stimuli. If you are not sure, try pinching his skin, pushing your knuckle firmly down against his sternum (the breastbone, the middle bone in the center of the front part of your chest), or squeeze your thumbnail firmly against the crescent moon part of his fingernails. If he moves or withdraws he is not likely to have had a cardiac arrest.
- A cardiac arrest usually produces cyanosis, or a distinct blueness of the skin, best seen in the lips, cheeks, or tip of the nose and fingers. It is due to poorly oxygenated blood accumulating in the tissues. Although cyanosis is hard to see in black

people, and although other things can produce the same effect, generally it is a good sign that a person's blood is poorly oxygenated.
- Look at the patient's pupils (these are the black circular spots in the center of the eye). Examination of the pupils is usually not particularly rewarding and not worth the time, but if you have someone else available and a good flashlight, it is worth having him check the size of the pupils and whether or not they constrict (get smaller) when a light is flashed into them. If they are very widely dilated and unresponsive to light, the situation is ominous and further resuscitation efforts are often unrewarding. If they are relatively small and if they react to light, you still have a chance.
- The best way to tell if a man has stopped breathing is to hold a mirror or your glasses or some similar object to his nose or mouth and look for water vapor condensation. If he is not breathing, it doesn't necessarily mean his heart has stopped, but it is usually a good clue.

WHAT TO DO BEFORE RESUSCITATION

Think first. Don't bull your way into an impossible or dangerous situation without a few seconds of careful evaluation. So many factors have to be evaluated rapidly that the fifteen to thirty seconds spent quickly sizing up the patient, the circumstances, your resources, and any other available resources may prevent many serious errors from being made.
- Remember, you have only three to five minutes to restore blood flow to the brain before it is irreversibly damaged. The chances of success decrease rapidly the longer the delay, and the likelihood of success is negligible if more than about four minutes have elapsed since the cardiac arrest. Worse yet is that permanent brain damage usually occurs after a certain amount of time and you may successfully revive the heart but not the brain.
- Your greatest chance of success is if you witness the accident or injury, since only then can you initiate therapy

with an absolute minimum of delay. In the confusion, excitement, and chaos, however, your estimation of the time elapsed may be very inaccurate. If you have the presence of mind to look at your watch and make a mental note of the time, it may help greatly later.

- If you are alone, then you have to do it all yourself and the decisions follow in a logical sequence. If you are with others, you should take advantage of the team approach. This demands a leader, and if you cannot or will not accept the responsibility, make sure someone else does. A man's life is at stake and there is no excuse for allowing personal ego trips, rivalries, or animosities to interfere.
- The leader must assign certain tasks depending on each person's experience, maturity, state of mind, and availability. Get someone to go for help, whether it means knocking on someone's door to use the telephone, flagging down a passing car, or running back on the trail to the last camp site. Our experience indicates that frequently it is difficult to get someone to do this. Some people don't want to get involved, many have a morbid curiosity and don't want to miss the action, and some people don't want to leave a seriously injured or dying friend or relative because they are sincerely and justifiably concerned. The necessity for getting help quickly cannot be overemphasized and the leader has to decide how best to get it.

All this sounds very structured and formal: it never is and never can be so. You have to contend with a variety of circumstances from distraught relatives, multiple injuries, dangerous traffic, and the pattern does not flow according to schedule. The success of the effort depends on your intelligence, adaptability, skill, and luck.

ONCE YOU DECIDE TO ACT, WHAT DO YOU DO?

The die is cast and the man's heart has stopped beating. Now you must act quickly and decisively. All decisions are arbitrary and final: you will make mistakes in judgment and performance, but these can hardly be avoided.

- Place the patient flat on his back on a flat hard surface. You must be careful if there is an obvious fracture, particularly if you suspect a back or neck injury, but all other injuries are of secondary importance if the heart has stopped beating.
- A good hard thump across the front of the chest with a closed fist will sometimes get the heart started. It is simple, quick, and definitely worth a try. Check for a heartbeat or pulse before you start the full procedure.
- Loosen the collar and belt.
- Turn the patient's head to the side if he has vomited and clear his mouth and throat. Remove any foreign material and any false teeth if they are getting in the way. If he vomits again, turn his head to the side to let the vomitus drain out; otherwise he will choke on the vomitus and obstruct his airway and your efforts will be useless.
- It is probably best to remove the shirt, blouse, or underwear if you can easily do it. Don't waste time unbuttoning or looking for hooks. If you need to or can, cut off what clothes are in the way (not all will be in your way) or rip them open and push them aside. It would be nice to protect the privacy of your patient from the stares of passers-by, but that is low down on your list of important things to do and it generally is not feasible. Don't let Victorian virtues interfere with what you must do.
- There are two aspects to resuscitation. First is getting oxygen into the blood by blowing air into the lungs, and second is chest pressure to massage the heart and squeeze blood out of it into the circulation. Both these can be done by one person, but it is much easier and far more effective if performed by a team of two.
- *The mouth-to-mouth breathing* is done this way:

Kneel beside the victim at the level of his head.

In an unconscious subject the tongue falls back and obstructs the airway. There are many ways to get the tongue out of the way. Probably the easiest and fastest method is to tilt the head back, place one hand under the neck and gently lift up, allowing the head to fall back so the chin is pointing almost straight upward. You can place something under the shoulders such as a rolled up coat or a block of wood to maintain this position. Sometimes, just opening the airway by getting the tongue out of the way will allow resumption of spontaneous breathing. If there are two of you doing the resuscitation and one of you can devote full time to the breathing process, it will help to have someone grasp the patient's jaw way back below the ear and pull it forward (upward when the patient is on his back). This accomplishes the same thing as putting something under the shoulders to overextend the neck. It prevents the tongue from flopping back to clog up the airway and keeps it open for your respiratory efforts.

Pinch his nostrils closed and open his mouth. Take a deep breath and by tightly covering his mouth with yours, blow your air in his lungs. You will feel his lungs expand, see his chest rise, and hear the air passively blow out of his lungs after each breath. Blow as much air in as you would for a normal deep breath.

Don't blow as deeply for a child. For a baby, all you need is a small puff from your cheeks.

Don't get squeamish about placing your mouth over the mouth of some stranger. It can be unpleasant, particularly if he has vomited, but remember, you are saving his life and all other considerations are irrelevant. If you must, you can place a clean handkerchief between the two of you.

Repeat the cycle about twelve to fifteen times a minute for an adult and about twenty times a minute for a child. If you are doing both the cardiac massage and the mouth-to-mouth breathing, you will have to alternate the two.

The three most common errors in mouth-to-mouth resuscitation are: 1) air leaking out between your lips and the patient's, 2) either you don't open your mouth widely enough or his mouth closes to a small opening, and 3) during the process, the extension of the patient's neck, which is so important in keeping his tongue out of the way, tends to flatten out, obstructing the airway again. You may note that deep and methodical breathing like this, particularly if you are bent over, makes you dizzy and gives you numbness and a tingling sensation or a ringing in your ears. It is classical hyperventilation (Chapter 4), and all you can do is to breathe less deeply and a little slower unless you can get someone else to take over.

- *The cardiac massage* is done this way:

> The victim must be on a hard surface. If he is in a bed, you will do nothing except massage the mattress and springs. It is not necessary that the patient be removed from his bed if you can get a firm flat object between his chest and the mattress. A serving tray is good. If nothing like this is easily available, he will need to be taken out of bed and placed on his back on the floor.
>
> Kneel beside the victim at the level of his chest.
>
> Place the heel of one hand on the lower half of the sternum (breastbone) and place the second hand on top of the first.
>
> With both hands together, keep the arms straight and rock forward putting 60 to 100 pounds of pressure on the victim's chest, depressing the sternum about one and a half to two inches.
>
> Don't just let go, but let the chest resume its normal position in a rhythmic fashion. The force should be quick and even, and you should allow an approximately equal amount of time for the compression and relaxation

phases. What you accomplish with this maneuver is to squeeze the heart which is just beneath the sternum and thereby force the blood out into the circulation. As you let go, more blood enters the heart and it gets pumped out on the next compression.

Do this about sixty times a minute, about once a second.

Use only one hand for a child. For a baby, press gently over the lower half of the sternum with just two fingers about one hundred times a minute.

Once you start, do not stop for more than a few beats. You may have to stop to change position or to let someone else take over (it is very tiring, even if you are doing it properly) or to move the patient to a stretcher for transportation, but you should plan to continue massage while he is being moved. If you are alone, then you must perform both the mouth-to-mouth breathing as well as the cardiac massage. You cannot do them simultaneously, so you alternate. The recommended pattern is to compress the chest fifteen times and then quickly extend the neck and inflate the lungs twice. It is not as efficient, rather exhausting after a while, and clearly not as satisfactory as when done by a team of two.

WHAT TO DO NOW AND HOW LONG TO CONTINUE

Once you have started and you are reasonably satisfied that you are doing it properly, and all is going well, you really are obliged to continue until 1) the patient can be taken to a hospital or to some other appropriate facility, 2) the patient is resuscitated, he wakes up, and his heartbeat and breathing are apparently normal, or 3) there is no apparent response after persistent satisfactory efforts for a reasonable period of time and no help is available.

What a reasonable period of time is depends on all of the factors which we mentioned thus far. A reasonable period of time may be two or three hours in a sixteen-year-old boy who gets hit by lightning or may be twenty minutes in a seventy-five-year-old man who has had a heart attack. If help is on the way, it is best to keep trying. If no help is reasonably available, your chances of success after fifteen or twenty minutes with no spontaneous respiration or cardiac action are effectively nil.

Fatigue is a very realistic and important factor. Without help an individual might be able to continue for twenty minutes. A team alternating can persist for at least an hour.

If you are successful, you may be put in the ironic situation of trying to explain and justify to the victim, who is often a total stranger, what you have done. He may be confused, angry, or belligerent. His clothes may be torn off and he may have involuntarily urinated. He probably will have a pain in the chest from your cardiac massage and you may have broken some ribs in the process. He will be amnesic for the whole event from the time of his initial injury and frequently for some time thereafter, even though he may be awake. Be firm and reassuring, keep him comfortable and at rest until he can be taken to a hospital for evaluation.

A summary may provide a simple and effective reminder of the steps of cardiac resuscitation:

A—(A)irway opened
B—(B)reathing restored
C—(C)ardiac massage
D—(D)efinitive measures—(diagnosis, drugs, and defibrillation, which need the facilities of a well-equipped ambulance or hospital)

Tetanus (Lockjaw)

Tetanus is frequently a lethal disease. Despite modern methods of treatment, it is fatal in about 50 per cent of those afflicted. Most people know that stepping on a nail, particularly a rusty nail, may give you lockjaw, and when a child cuts his foot on the beach, nothing could strike more terror into the heart of an anxious mother. Tetanus is rare, but very serious. It is totally preventable with proper immunization. The fact that it exists at all in the United States is quiet testimony to the failure of one aspect of our medical care system, since we have no mechanism for reaching the people who get lost to the "routine" immunization procedures and no means to provide for regular booster immunizations.

The disease is the result of an infection with a bacterium, *clostridium tetani*. These bacteria are able to persist for many years, perhaps indefinitely, in a latent or spore form in dry soil or dirt. The bacteria become active when they get into and under the skin and when they enter a warm and moist environment. Since they grow only in an oxygen-free environment, the tetanus bacteria are most dangerous when they enter a wound beneath the skin. This is most likely with a puncture wound (a nail at the beach or a dirty hypodermic syringe) where the skin closes off the injured area and seals out any air. Any injury that breaks the skin, though, can cause tetanus, particularly if the injury is contaminated with any kind of dirty material.

The germs alone are a relatively minor problem and they can easily be controlled by an antibiotic such as penicillin. Before the germs can be eliminated by the antibiotic, however, they can produce enough of a deadly toxin (or poison) to cause the characteristic symptoms of tetanus. The tetanus toxin is one of the most potent poisons known to man. It paralyzes the nerve fibers leading to the muscles and affects nerve fibers in the spinal cord and the brain. It causes spasm of the muscles, including those of the jaws (lockjaw), and ultimately causes spasm of the muscles of breathing, resulting in death by suffocation. Antibiotics are ineffective in neutralizing the toxin, and the toxin continues to have an effect long after the bacteria are gone and the wound is healed. The poisonous effects of the tetanus toxin are not reversible.

There are two simple ways to protect yourself against tetanus. The first method, completely reliable and most effective, is immunization with tetanus toxoid. The second, and far less reliable, is the use of a tetanus antitoxin after an injury occurs.

When tetanus toxoid is injected, it stimulates the production of tetanus antibodies. The antibodies completely and rapidly neutralize the poison as it gets produced by the tetanus bacteria. The tetanus toxoid must be administered prior to any injury in order for it to be effective. It is given in a series of three shots at four to six week intervals. It does not give reliable protection until about six months after the third shot, but the protection then probably lasts for about ten years. (It may even be effective for your lifetime, but no one as yet knows for sure and it seems unwise to take a chance.) A single booster shot is suggested about every six to ten years. Almost everyone in the United States has had the basic tetanus toxoid series, but most people don't get their ten-year boosters as regularly as they should.

If you have never been immunized or if your immunization booster has gone too long to be reliable any more, you might need some additional protection when you step on a nail or cut yourself while turning the compost heap. An injection of tetanus antitoxin (which is the actual antibody to the toxin) given at the time of the injury can neutralize the tetanus toxin. You will need the antitoxin if:

> You have never been previously immunized with a tetanus toxoid series. (Most people have been when they were children or in the Armed Forces.)
>
> Your tetanus toxoid series was completed less than six months before the injury occurred.
>
> More than ten years have passed since completion of the tetanus toxoid series or last toxoid booster shot.
>
> In addition, most physicians recommend that antitoxin be given regardless of previous immunization if a wound

is extensive; is grossly contaminated, particularly if contaminated with soil; if treatment is delayed more than twenty-four hours after injury; or if the wound is sealed off from the air.

The tetanus antitoxin will give only temporary protection.

Tetanus, although rare, is most commonly seen in the United States in heroin addicts who are careless with their needles. Since tetanus is completely preventable and since it is so devastating in its effect, we strongly recommend tetanus toxoid immunization routinely for everyone, regardless of one's personal feeling about medication or immunization or one's religious beliefs.

5 Common Ailments

The Common Cold

The common cold is common, transient, and never fatal, is not affected by penicillin shots or vitamins, should not be confused with a strep throat or the flu, generally lasts for five to seven days regardless of what you do, is not caused by standing in drafts, getting your feet wet, not wearing a hat or rubbers in the rain, and cannot be cured or prevented by any known medications as of the time of this writing.

All of these statements are established medical facts and are not consistent with the "known facts" elaborated by your mother and ours. The frequency of the common cold and the frustration in treating it has created a vast collection of old-wives' tales, and a variety of therapeutic maneuvers ranging from drinking concoctions of tea laced with honey and whiskey to massive doses of vitamin C. It is rivaled only by the hiccup and the nosebleed in its number of imaginative and ineffective home remedies.

We do know a great deal about colds and a great deal of work continues to be done. Take heart—the conquest of the cold may occur in our lifetime. The vast majority, more than 95 per cent of colds, are caused by a virus. Penicillin and all the antibiotics, which are effective only against bacteria, are utterly useless in treatment of a cold. Moreover, they may be harmful when one considers the frequent side reactions which result from these potent drugs. There are three general families of viruses which cause the common cold and there are perhaps fifty different viruses in the three families which have been demonstrated to produce identical symptoms. This explains why colds can occur so frequently, why you don't develop natural immunity to the cold, and why it continues to be so impractical to vaccinate or immunize against the cold. There are too many viruses to make shots useful, and you may build up protection against one type of virus only to be struck down by another.

It is worthwhile to distinguish among a cold, a strep throat, and the flu. Usually the distinction is clinically impossible, but it may be important because a strep throat can be cured (by penicillin or another antibiotic) and an occasional untreated strep throat can result in a serious heart or kidney disease many years later. It is important to avoid treating all colds and sore throats with penicillin (much too risky and of no value) in the hope of curing the occasional strep throat. A throat culture will give you an answer, but this takes twenty-four hours and requires at least rudimentary laboratory facilities. Nevertheless, there are some general clues which may help you decide what to call your miseries. There is enormous variation in the symptoms.

	Cold	Strep throat	Flu
Fever*	usually low-grade, seldom above 101°	variable	maybe up to 104°
Nasal stuffiness	usually	infrequent	usually
Muscle aches	infrequent	infrequent	usually
Headaches	usually	infrequent	usually
Cough	sometimes	infrequent	usually
Chest pain	infrequent	infrequent	sometimes
Sore throat	often	always	sometimes
Earache	sometimes	often	infrequent

* All bets are off in children.

Most sore throats are viral, just like colds, and antibiotics can do nothing but harm. People who have the flu generally feel worse than those with only a cold. Fever, muscle aches, headaches, gastrointestinal symptoms, and a dry non-productive cough suggest influenza, or the flu. Like colds and most sore throats, the flu is also caused by a virus, and antibiotics offer no benefit. Flu shots tend to decrease the frequency of illness and probably decrease the severity of symptoms if you should get the flu anyway. The shots are useful because epidemics of the flu are sometimes due to a single specific influenza virus each year and the vaccine can be prepared specifically for the anticipated virus.

All of these illnesses are caused by germs, either bacteria or viruses. You cannot get a cold without being exposed to the virus. To catch a cold you must have been exposed to someone with a cold when he breathes, sneezes, or coughs on you. Whether or not the virus takes hold and you subsequently develop a cold depends on your resistance and a number of other less well understood biological factors. Some people insist that they get colds after standing in a draft or getting their feet wet. It is hard to refute this firmly held conviction. What is likely, however, is that they harbor the virus as a harmless inhabitant in their respiratory tract, the lung, nose, or throat. The virus produces disease only when the resistance is lowered, or other biological factors are altered. Probably the only factors which lower one's resistance are extreme fatigue and a chill. Cold wet fet alone probably won't do it. And a chill with or without fatigue won't do it either in the absence of the virus in the right spot at the right time.

There is no way to cure a cold. There are a number of things you can do, however, to make it more tolerable and make yourself more comfortable. The basis of the treatment is threefold. First, don't make it worse by unnecessary treatment. Second, do what you can to relieve the symptoms. Third, rest patiently and wait until the body can normally and naturally get rid of the virus and correct the damage the virus has done.

First, do no harm. Penicillin and antibiotics do no good and can produce needless, serious, and severe side reactions. We don't recommend them for any purpose except for a *proven* strep throat. If so, penicillin tablets for a full ten days are far safer than a penicillin shot. Large doses of vitamins, particularly vitamin C, have never been shown to do anything useful for a cold. Massive doses of vitamin C probably can't hurt, so if you want to spend your money and must take something, vitamin C is as harmless as almost anything.

Second, we suggest you take appropriate medications to relieve the symptoms of a cold. The great variety of products on the market attests to their ineffectiveness, for if there were anything really useful, the other products would rapidly disappear. We recommend the following:

> Aspirins in any form (generally the cheaper the better) will help relieve the headache, muscle aches, and soreness, will lower the fever of a cold or the flu, and will make the symptoms more tolerable. Take two aspirins every four hours as long as you feel it necessary. If they upset your stomach, you can try buffered aspirin or take the pills with some food, water, or milk.

> If you have a sore throat, gargle with warm salt water about every three or four hours. Try one or two teaspoons of salt in a glass of warm water. This is the cheapest and safest treatment, and none of the other lozenges, gargles, rinses, pills, or syrups are really very much better. The lozenges do have the advantage of portability, however. None of these treatments will cure your sore throat; they should be selected for cost, convenience, and flavor.

> Inexpensive therapy for a stuffed or running nose or a generally congested upper respiratory tract is available. The long-acting "cold" pills are effective but the price is outrageous and the pills contain many constituents which have obscure and doubtful therapeutic value. For example, most contain some kind of antihistamine, useful only if the nose is running because of an allergy. A cold

and an allergy are not the same thing, but the pills contain a little of a lot of things in an effort to cover every possibility. In so doing, they tend to cut down on the dose of each of the constituents, raise the price, and add to the risk of exposing you to a variety of unnecessary constituents (the antihistamine, for example, will tend to make you a bit drowsy).

Maximum effectiveness in treating a stuffed nose can be obtained by using a simple, non-prescription nose spray (like Neo-Synephrine ⅛ to ¼ per cent). If this is just too inconvenient, almost any of the "cold" pills will work, but the effect will not be as dramatic. A note of caution, however: prolonged use of nose spray will be associated with a diminution of its effectiveness (the development of a tolerance to it) and a tendency to "rebound" with more severe symptoms when the diminished effectiveness wears off after each dose. If you get hooked on a nose spray, you'll need progressively larger doses and obtain progressively smaller effect.

Most non-prescription cough medications are fairly ineffective and we don't recommend them unless the cough is driving you, your family, and the neighbors up the wall. If so, anything with codeine or one of the other mild narcotics, like dextrohydromorphinone, in it should suppress the cough relatively safely, but this usually means getting a prescription. The non-prescription cough syrups have less potency, but you may try them anyway. The syrup used to make Coca-Cola, oddly enough, may be effective in relieving the discomfort from the cough, but so are warm salt-water gargles. Neither does anything to suppress the cough itself.

Cough drops also have no direct effect on the cough. If they contain any cough suppressant at all (and many of them don't), the dose is too small to be effective. Their value, as Coca-Cola syrup or salt water gargle, derives entirely from the local soothing action they have on the back of your mouth and on accessible parts of your throat, where the cough originates. The liquid gets swallowed and, hopefully, not inhaled.

For the macerated tender nose suffering from too much rubbing or blowing, try any simple ointment which contains petrolatum.

Finally, try patience, fortitude, and other virtues. The body will rid itself of the virus and repair the damage if left to its own devices and if you are basically in good health. Most people feel better in about a week, almost regardless of what they do.

A non-puritan virtue is inactivity. Rest is very desirable simply because you'll feel better if you avoid the burdens of excessive or even normal activity. There is enormous variation in the amount of activity individuals consider normal. In general, a reduction in your own level of activity and certainly the avoidance of any heroic effort is recommended. The risk is the boredom, frustration, and anxiety of too little activity, and we have to assume that people have enough good judgment to achieve a reasonable personal compromise.

In general, the flu, as opposed to a cold, tends to last a bit longer and the recovery may be slower. Following the flu, you may not be "sick" in the classic sense of the word, but you won't feel quite right and you may not be back to normal for two to three weeks.

Hepatitis and Jaundice

Hepatitis has become the disease everyone points to when he describes the dangers of shooting anything. It is thought to be at the far end of the heroin and speed trail. The notoriety of hepatitis is only partly deserved because the inflammation is caused by any of a number of things; dirty needles are responsible only occasionally.

Hepatitis, an inflammation of the liver (*hepar* is Greek for liver), is the result of an infection which is produced by a virus which infects the liver. The common form of hepatitis is caused by one of two closely related viruses. Any other kind of hepatitis has to be qualified with some kind of adjective or it will be misunderstood. For example, the virus that causes infectious mononucleosis can cause mononucleosis hepatitis, and an occasional patient will have a toxic hepatitis due to a chemical or medication or a hepatitis due to some other unusual cause.

The two common types of viral hepatitis are more precisely specified as serum hepatitis and infectious hepatitis, but this terminology is disappearing as medical science is starting to understand more about the diseases and how the viruses damage the liver. There is a very fuzzy clinical distinction between the two and it isn't very important to expend a lot of effort in order to determine which one you have. They are indistinguishable except for the means by which they are transmitted.

One type, infectious hepatitis, is transmitted by ingesting food contaminated with hepatitis virus, usually from sewage contamination or by close contact with someone who has hepatitis. The second type, serum hepatitis, is transmitted via the blood, by using a dirty needle for a blood test, by getting a blood transfusion from someone who has hepatitis, or by sharing a needle with someone who has or had hepatitis.

The incubation period, or the delay between the time of infection and the appearance of symptoms, may distinguish between the two types of hepatitis if it isn't clear how you got infected. If, for example, you are living with someone who has hepatitis and simultaneously sharing a needle with someone else, the incubation period may give you some indication where it came from, but it isn't often important to find out. Infectious hepatitis is usually obvious within two to six weeks; serum hepatitis appears two to six months after exposure, but the distinction is far from accurate and it is often impossible to date the time of exposure or infection very accurately.

The concept of contaminated food or needles needs some clarification. In infectious hepatitis, the virus gets excreted in human feces. Sewage, for example, which is untreated or inadequately treated in sewage treatment facilities can and does infect shellfish in certain fishing areas, since the shellfish ingest the sewage and then carry the virus without getting sick. The shellfish are then contaminated and infectious when they are eaten. Contaminated food is not the only problem. Even under the most meticulous, finicky conditions, a person with hepatitis who is excreting the virus in his stools will probably spread the virus to his surroundings and is likely to have it on his hands. It is virtually impossible to avoid. That is why all of the children in a home for the mentally retarded will soon develop hepatitis. It may seem unpleasant, but infectious hepatitis is a disease of fecal-oral transmission.

In serum hepatitis, the disease is almost always transmitted by infected blood, and the fecal-oral route, although it occurs, is much less common. It takes very little blood to transmit the infection—as little as 1/1000th of a drop can do it. One drop of blood can infect a thousand people. The likelihood of disease transmission is proportional to the amount of blood and the concentration of virus in the blood. This is why a transfusion of a pint of blood is much more of a problem than a poorly sterilized needle or a random scratch with a contaminated needle.

The severity of the disease is tremendously variable and can range from no symptoms whatsoever (the only way to detect its presence is with positive blood tests), to a severe and rapidly fatal illness. There is no way of predicting what the outcome will be in any specific instance. However, the particularly mild or virulent forms tend to run in epidemics, and if you know where you got your hepatitis, you may expect that your case will be of similar severity. Fortunately, the mild form is much more common.

Unfortunately, hepatitis is not always an innocuous disease.

An occasional severe infection can be fatal, and rapidly so. An occasional less severe infection may be serious enough to destroy enough of the liver to leave the patient with a case of persistent liver failure which may be slowly fatal.

The symptoms, when they are present, are the same for both forms of the disease. The initial symptoms are vague and nonspecific before the appearance of the characteristic yellow jaundice. The early symptoms are a loss of appetite, fatigue, and a sense of weariness. This is usually followed or accompanied by nausea, occasional vomiting, diarrhea, vague moderate abdominal pain, and occasional pain and stiffness in the joints. The loss of appetite is quite striking and it is often accompanied by a curious definite and consistent loss of taste for cigarettes in smokers. There may be a low-grade fever.

These symptoms are general and nonspecific and may suggest hepatitis, but they can also suggest almost any form of low-grade illness, such as the flu and many diverse gastrointestinal diseases. The appearance of jaundice is often the tip-off that the liver is involved. Confirmation of the diagnosis is made with a number of blood tests; these tests are used to measure objectively the severity and the progress and resolution of the disease.

Jaundice is the yellow color which may appear in the skin and in the whites of the eyes. The yellow color is produced by a substance called bilirubin which gets deposited in the skin. Normally, bilirubin is produced by the regular breakdown of red blood cells. A healthy liver processes this waste product and excretes it through the gall bladder into the intestinal tract. The intestines break it down a little further and eventually it becomes the material which produces the brown color of normal feces. If the liver is damaged and cannot function properly, the bilirubin accumulates in the liver, leaks out into the blood instead of into the gall bladder, and gets deposited in the skin and eyes as a yellow pigment. Some of it gets excreted in the urine but very little is excreted with the feces. This explains the dark-colored urine and light-colored stools of liver disease. Eventually, as the liver gets better, the jaundice fades from the skin.

There's not a great deal you can do about hepatitis when you do get it. There is no specific treatment; you can only let the disease pursue its natural course and not do anything to make matters worse.

The traditional approach to treating hepatitis is an old-fashioned one, suggesting that we really have nothing more to offer than was available generations ago; lots of rest and lots of good food. Both modes of treatment are superficially good, sound advice, but are in fact offered without any scientific basis. There is no evidence that patients who rest in bed get better any faster than those who are obliged to get up and exercise regularly. Just as bed rest probably has no beneficial effect, it has not been shown that exercise is harmful or dangerous. However, it has always been our impression that with a quiet, uneventful convalescence, hepatitis often suddenly gets worse after some indiscretion or "overdoing it." While we don't recommend absolute rest in bed, we suggest that you avoid extremes of exertion and try to avoid getting fatigued. Get plenty of rest. This is unnecessary advice for the first week or two of the illness, simply because most people who have a significant degree of hepatitis don't feel much like getting up and doing anything, and rest generally suits them very well.

Another curious aspect of this disease is that most patients start to feel better in a few weeks, often before the blood tests show that the liver is on the way toward convalescence. It is during this period, when the patient starts to feel better but the liver is still damaged, that restricted activity and rest should be encouraged. Most people feel fine with decreased activity and do not appreciate how easily they fatigue with more than slight effort.

The second part of the nontreatment for hepatitis is plenty of good food. A good nourishing diet, it is said, helps the liver get better faster. Unfortunately, among the most common and most devastating symptoms of hepatitis, particularly in the early phases, is nausea, vomiting, and loss of appetite. The thought of food is enough to produce waves of nausea, and if you insist that the patient eat the recommended high-calorie, high-protein, low-fat nourishing diet, you are likely to provoke vomiting. The hepatitis patient who can keep anything down is lucky. Those who can't take any nourishment should probably best be hospitalized and given intravenous fluids. The patient should try to maintain generous fluid intake, particularly if there is a fever. A high-protein, low-fat diet is recommended, but we generally allow patients to select foods they like rather than insist on what is good but unappetizing. You can get some calories from hard candy, carbonated drinks, fruit juices, and soups, all of which are relatively easy to get down and keep down in the most nauseated stomach. Frequent small portions are less demanding. Supplementary vitamins should be added if the loss of appetite persists for more than a few weeks, but in this case, you should be under the supervision of a doctor and follow his advice.

Do not include alcohol in any form. Although it is hard to prove that alcohol delays convalescence or promotes recurrences of hepatitis, it seems very likely that this is the case since alcohol, even in small amounts, has a profound toxic effect on the liver, and the ailing liver needs all the help it can get without alcohol, even wine or beer, to do more damage.

One of the subtle benefits of the fatigue and the self-inflicted rest associated with hepatitis is the concomitant decrease in exposure of the infected person, the transmitter of the disease, to his relatives and friends at work and at school. Ordinary person-to-person transmission of hepatitis is unusual, and although patients with hepatitis are contagious as long as they have jaundice (and probably before the jaundice appears as well), it almost always takes fairly close and prolonged contact (with a breakdown of good hygiene) to transmit the virus and cause hepatitis.

To isolate patients with hepatitis when they are jaundiced

and when the disease becomes obvious is like closing the barn door about halfway when most, but not all, of the horses are gone, since the patient has been unsuspectingly excreting the virus for some time. When it is convenient it probably is a good idea for an infected person at home to have his own set of dishes and silverware which can be washed carefully and kept separately and, if possible, to restrict him to a toilet that no one else is using. At the very least, all members of the household, whether they are members of the family, roommates, lovers, or boarders, should use common sense and be careful about toilet habits, hand washing, personal hygiene and needle disposal. The closer and more intimate and more prolonged the exposure, the more likely is the transmission of the disease. Hepatitis is not a venereal disease so you needn't restrict sexual activity, except that fatigue, nausea, and the symptoms of hepatitis would normally impair satisfactory sexual relations. Remember that the virus is found in the feces and blood but not in the saliva.

Of much more utility than quarantine is the use of gamma globulin by intimates of the patient. The gamma globulin probably does not prevent the disease but does appear to diminish its intensity. It should be given as soon as possible to exposed household contacts or to people who have prolonged and close contact with a person who has hepatitis, particularly to those who are pregnant or who have a serious disease of their own. The gamma globulin is not necessary and of no value in people who have had a brief or transient contact with a hepatitis patient. Schoolteachers don't need it if one of the students gets hepatitis. You don't have to go to the doctor if you meet someone at a party with yellow eyes who later turns out to have hepatitis, even if you've touched him. (Gamma globulin is also useful if given to people who are traveling to an area where hepatitis is widespread and the possibility of consuming contaminated food is high.) The injection of gamma globulin is uncomfortable but useful enough to justify the discomfort.

Infectious Mononucleosis

Infectious mononucleosis (mono) is often confused with hepatitis. The early general symptoms are vaguely similar. Both hepatitis and mononucleosis occur in approximately the same age group and they both require a prolonged convalescence. Both are the result of a virus infection. The two diseases are very different, however. They shouldn't be confused, and they mean very different things. Hepatitis affects the liver; mononucleosis involves the blood and the lymph nodes. Mononucleosis is probably an infectious disease and is probably transmitted by an as yet unidentified virus.

Mononucleosis is frequently found in young people and most frequently in college students and military personnel. It may occur just as often among other groups or individuals as well, but people in dormitories and barracks are gathered together and their state of health is monitored so that it is easy to identify an outbreak or epidemic among them and difficult to do so among random people scattered throughout the general population. Among the groups of people gathered together it may occur in an epidemic or in isolated, sporadic cases which appear and disappear without any pattern. When an isolated or sporadic case appears, it frequently is attributed to the flu or a virus.

Much of the vagueness of the disease relates to the non-specific symptoms. They are in no way characteristic or unique and are similar to many different kinds of colds, flus, or upset stomachs. In a classical case, a recognizable pattern may sometimes be apparent. During the first three to five days, or as much as a week, there are non-specific symptoms of headache, a low-grade fever, and fatigue. The headache is often localized behind the eyes. A typical triad of symptoms occasionally suggests mononucleosis; a fever, a severe sore throat, and enlargement of the lymph nodes (lymph glands) in the neck. About the time some of these symptoms develop some of the blood tests start to become characteristic of the disease and can confirm the diagnosis.

The symptoms can then persist for anywhere from a week to months. Some of the later and persistent symptoms are similar to hepatitis. You may have a headache way out of proportion to the severity of the illness or to the magnitude of the fever.

The recovery is often associated with marked fatigue and malaise and fluctuating periods of improvement and relapse. The disease is rarely serious but almost always very unpleasant.

Mononucleosis is not particularly contagious, although much college folklore has been created around its mode of transmission. There is not very much more than anecdotes to establish scientifically that it is transmitted by kissing.

The treatment is directed entirely toward alleviating the symptoms rather than toward curing the disease. Warm salt water gargles or various throat lozenges may help relieve the severe sore throat. Aspirin is useful for both the headache and for lowering the fever. Rest is gratefully appreciated and most people don't feel much like doing anything that will take them very far from their bed. Antibiotics will not be of any value for the sore throat unless the inflamed tissues get infected with a bacteria entirely unrelated to the mononucleosis. Sometimes the spleen gets enlarged. You can't feel it but a doctor might be able to and should check to determine if there is any swelling. Those who have significant enlargement of their spleen should not get involved in too vigorous activity, particularly contact sports, until the spleen has returned to normal size. The enlarged spleen is particularly fragile and could be injured relatively easily with even minor trauma.

Recovery is almost always complete, although it may sometimes be very delayed.

Urinary Tract Infections

The urinary tract is a sophisticated and complex system which can be understood and explained in simple terms. Urine is produced in the two kidneys, located in your flanks just beneath the lower ribs. Blood flows through them and is, in effect, filtered. The urine, which contains much of the body's waste products, flows down from the kidneys through two long, narrow tubes, called ureters, into the bladder. The bladder is an expandable bag located low down in your abdomen in the midline. The bladder stores the urine until it is full and the sensation of fullness is evident. Urination is simply the process of opening the valves and draining the bladder. The urine flows to the outside world through a single tube called the urethra.

Although the urinary system and reproductive system are anatomically located in close proximity to one another and share some organs which have a dual function (e.g., the penis), the two systems are actually quite unrelated, and an abnormality or infection in one system only occasionally has a significant effect upon the other.

Infections in the urinary tract are almost always in the bladder or the kidneys and occur much more frequently in women than in men. The urethra in women is short and straight and empties near the front part of the vagina. In men it is longer and curved, passing through the penis. This difference in anatomy is responsible for the frequent infections which occur in the bladders of women and the relative infrequency in men. The bacteria can easily ascend into the bladder through the urethra from the skin in the region of the vagina, since this area is not, and cannot be, kept clean and sterile.

The symptoms of a urinary infection are hard to ignore in either sex. Frequent and painful or burning urination are common. Occasionally there will be some blood in the urine.

If the infection is in the bladder, there may be some pain in the region over the bladder, low and midline in the abdomen. If the infection is high up in the kidneys as well, some flank pain on the side or in the back below the ribs may also be present. These distinctions are not too reliable in differentiating bladder from kidney infections. Usually, urinary infections do not produce a fever, or only a mild, low-grade temperature elevation when the infection is confined to the bladder. The presence of a high fever (103°–104°) suggests a kidney infection. These points can often be misleading in differentiating the two. Children often have a high fever, and sometimes a very brief episode of symptoms associated with an infection of their urinary tract.

A careful look at a specimen of your urine will often help in making a diagnosis. If a urinary infection is present, you may note that the urine is cloudy rather than clear and sometimes appears dark or bloody.

You will probably need to and want to see a doctor the first time you have a urinary infection, but since it is so common in young women, no special tests other than a urinalysis, and possibly a urine culture, are necessary. If infections are particularly severe or recurrent despite normal precautions, you should have the entire urinary system checked carefully. Recurrent infections can mean anything from a kidney stone or a bladder polyp to a wide variety of major or minor abnormalities anywhere in the urinary tract. A urinary infection does not necessarily mean that there is anatomically anything wrong with some part of the urinary system, and very often no underlying abnormality is present or can be found.

Infections occur frequently during pregnancy (see Chapter 6), probably because of the pressure of the pregnant uterus on the ureters and the interference that this may create with the normal flow of urine. A frequent problem, perhaps the most frequent cause of cystitis (bladder infection), is "honeymoon cystitis" or the infection which occurs in women after intercourse. The irritation and manipulation in the region of the vagina allows the bacteria to swim up the very short female urethra, about a billion abreast, into the bladder to set up house and multiply. Frequently recurring urinary tract infections may occur in diabetes, and if no other cause is found for your problem, you should have the possibility of diabetes evaluated.

Urinary tract infections occur in men, albeit less frequently. When they do occur they more often represent an abnormality of the urinary system rather than a random infection. The symptoms in men are similar to those seen in women: painful burning during urination, and the urge to urinate frequently.

The treatment for uncomplicated urinary infections is usually simple and extremely effective. In about twenty-four to forty-eight hours after you start taking an antibiotic like one of the sulfa drugs (best and least expensive is 4 to 8 grams of sulfasoxazole—Gantrisin—a day), the symptoms are virtually gone. You should continue the sulfa drug for seven to ten days even if you are free of symptoms so that an early recurrence from inadequate treatment does not occur. It is necessary to supplement your fluid intake to increase the urine flow and "flush out" the kidneys, and to prevent crystallization of the antibiotic in the urinary tract. Some people can't take sulfa drugs; they may be allergic to them or have a wide variety of unpleasant reactions to sulfa. Sometimes the infection is insensitive or resistant to simple sulfa drugs, particularly if you have recurrent infections, and stronger antibiotics are needed. If you don't get substantial relief of your symptoms in a day or two with the sulfa drugs, it is best to check back with your doctor to make sure you are getting enough of the right antibiotic. Frequent and recurrent infections should be treated aggressively and early, before they cause too much trouble and complications.

Some problems related to the male genitalia may appear with symptoms which could be mistaken for urinary infections. Some of these are the venereal diseases which are discussed in more detail in Chapter 6. A few other non-venereal diseases are discussed here.

Non-specific urethritis (NSU) causes symptoms very much like gonorrhea; burning and pain on urination and a persistent uncomfortable discharge from the penis. It may be caused by sexual contact but the exact infectious agent has not been clearly identified. It may be transmitted from someone with no symptoms and no venereal disease or evident infection but it is not caused by an infection with the gonorrheal bacteria. Gonorrhea and NSU can be differentiated by examination of the penile discharge under a microscope. If the gonorrhea bacteria cannot be identified, the infection is presumed to be NSU. The difference is important mostly because of the epidemicity of gonorrhea (i.e., who else has it?) and the necessity of treating all possible contacts. If there is any doubt about the diagnosis, it is probably best to assume that the discharge is caused by gonorrhea, since the bacteria which probably produce NSU should be susceptible to any treatment you could give for gonorrhea, but not vice versa.

The prostate is a gland in men only which is located near the bladder at the base of the urethra on its way through the penis. An inflammation of the prostate occasionally occurs with symptoms of urinary frequency, painful urination, possibly a fever and with pain in the scrotum, rectum, or the area between the two. It is sometimes the result of excess sexual stimulation without ejaculation. This prostatic inflammation, which is called prostatitis, normally needs antibiotic treatment and sometimes is relieved with prostatic massage. It can often be made more comfortable with hot baths twice a day. The prostate gland tends to enlarge with aging, and as it does, may obstruct the urethra and create problems with the flow of the urine. The enlargement may produce infections in the sluggishly flowing urine and may actually produce a complete urinary obstruction which will probably require surgical removal for its relief. This is rare in men below age sixty.

Hemorrhoids

As man evolved from a four-legged to a two-legged animal and into the upright position, he probably developed hemorrhoids. (These are also known as "piles," but since hemorrhoids is not too hard to say or spell, and since piles is such a painful word, we'll stick with hemorrhoids.) The dilated veins at the far end of the gastrointestinal tract just outside or just inside the anus are an "error of evolution." Nature in its infinite wisdom neglected to provide adequate support at the anus for the veins. The veins distend, often as a result of standing too much or sitting too long (a common problem in bus and truck drivers) and frequently appear in healthy young women during pregnancy. They are probably a small price to pay for the benefits of walking on two feet. The veins fill with blood and if the fight against gravity to get the blood up and back to the heart is too prolonged, the blood collects in the dilated veins and stays there.

Hemorrhoids are a problem in pregnancy because the enlarging uterus containing the growing fetus causes some obstruction to the normal flow of blood back to the heart and the veins in the rectal area can't drain out normally. People who are chronically constipated and are always "straining" tend to push out the hemorrhoids. The vast number of people who use bathrooms as a library ought to reflect for a moment what they are doing to their hemorrhoids: as they relax, so too do the muscles around the anus. With the muscular support gone, the veins tend to dilate with blood, ultimately resulting in hemorrhoids.

Any condition which irritates the anal area may cause hemorrhoids or may cause pre-existing and asymptomatic hemorrhoids to flare up. Poor hygiene probably is a predisposing factor. Rough and irritating toilet paper may make hemorrhoids worse. Some foods (see below) may irritate the sensitive area of the rectum and anus. Finally, hemorrhoids may be a major problem among homosexuals or among those who prefer anal intercourse. It isn't at all clear why this sexual practice should provoke hemorrhoids except for the probable mechanical irritation of the normally present small veins.

Most people don't know or don't care about their hemorrhoids. The hemorrhoids often don't produce any symptoms, but if they do, one can expect either itching, bleeding, or pain. When hemorrhoids itch, one can easily get into the neverending itch-scratch cycle. They itch, and you scratch, causing further irritation and itching and more scratching ad infinitum. Don't scratch itchy hemorrhoids. Bleeding usually occurs with bowel movements or when wiping afterward. Usually it stops easily, but sometimes it persists and recurs so often that it may produce a serious anemia from the blood loss if not corrected. Most hemorrhoids don't produce any pain, but if they protrude far enough and long enough, they may start to hurt. If the blood inside the veins clots, the resulting thrombosed hemorrhoid can be very painful.

Treating hemorrhoids involves justifiable self-indulgence which is frowned upon in our acquisitive society. A sitz bath, which is nothing more than sitting in a warm tub frequently and for a long time, is probably the best thing you can do for swollen hemorrhoids. If the hemorrhoids itch, you can add a cupful of cornstarch to a tub of water. Common sense suggests that since hemorrhoids are aggravated by standing too long or straining too much, rest is an ideal treatment. Actually, if they are really swollen and painful, lying on your belly or on your side with a pillow under your hips may help relieve the discomfort. Aspirin helps to relieve the pain and inflammation. You have to do what you can to avoid constipation, and any ordinary laxative will do (but see Chapter 3). The simplest thing to do to keep the stools soft and moist is to drink a lot of fluids. Toilet papers are a menace to delicate hemorrhoids. They are irritating and more so when they shred up. If you can manage, if it is convenient, use a damp, soft cloth and a little mineral oil. Don't rub or wipe. Gentle dabbing and patting is better. Some authorities contend that some foods are bad for hemorrhoids. Aside from avoiding foods that are likely to make you constipated, you should avoid foods which may irritate the delicate lining of the rectum. The usually implicated foods fall into five convenient categories: seeds, strings, skins, stimulants (coffee, tea, alcohol), and spices, but we can't be convinced that there is any utility in making an issue out of avoiding these foods. It is not necessary to get too carried away with this aspect unless something in particular makes you uncomfortable. It's unusual to have to resort to suppositories or ointments since most people will get adequate relief from the suggestions already outlined. If your way of life doesn't permit you to sit in a hot tub often enough or to rest long enough to treat your aching hemorrhoids, you might want to try any of the commercially available suppositories or ointments. There is no reason to believe that any of them is any better or worse than any other, since the active ingredients in most products are similar. The suppositories, which are placed in the rectum, have a dubious benefit, since the medications are released up and inside the rectum and that is not where the problem is. The ointments give slight and temporary relief of itching, pain, and the inflammation of irritated tissues. You don't need anything which contains an antibiotic since infection is not a part of the problem, and the very idea of sterilizing the anus is absurd.

As a last resort, and only when the hemorrhoids are driving you up the wall with itching or pain or if bleeding persists, you might want to see a doctor and consider getting them removed. It's a simple operation and is extremely effective but you will be out of action for a week or two and, as with all operations, there is a small but definite risk involved. Hemorrhoids sometimes recur after surgery and a few people are left with annoying scars or strictures.

As with most of the ailments of man, the best treatment is prevention. For those of you already suffering, take solace in the fact that sometimes hemorrhoids get better if you leave them alone.

Traveler's Diarrhea

Diarrhea is a frequent and, some think, an almost inevitable part of foreign travel. No statistics are available, but we don't know anyone who has traveled abroad for an extended length of time who didn't have some gastrointestinal distress sometime in his travels. Some people probably avoid it, but they probably have sterilized, sanitized, boiled, and purified experiences. If you spend your time trying to avoid traveler's diarrhea, you will probably do little else.

Don't confuse diarrhea with dysentery. Diarrhea refers to loose and/or frequent bowel movements, but does not identify the cause. Dysentery is one of the causes of the diarrhea and there are many different things which can produce dysentery. (Check in Chapter 3 for further comments.)

The diarrhea is probably only partially related to the standard of living or the state of civilization of the country in which you are traveling. You can get diarrhea traveling in most civilized cities in the U.S. as well as in countries where personal hygiene and sanitation are poor.

Diarrhea may be caused by drinking contaminated water. Sometimes the water is simply contaminated with raw sewage. Sometimes you are drinking water which is obtained from the stream which drains the field where a herd of cows or goats are feeding, and one of the goats is sick. But there are other causes for the diarrhea and you can't always attribute it to the water. You may eat some fruits or vegetables which have been grown in a garden where human feces were used as fertilizer. In many parts of the world it is the best and the only fertilizer available, and its cost is reasonable. If you eat in restaurants or in homes of local people you can expect that the cook and those involved in the preparation of the food are not quite as finicky as you would be back home. A common cause for the diarrhea is not contaminated food or water, but food which may be a little too exotic for your gentle stomach, eating irregularly while shifting your time zones, or drinking too much local wine or beer, or drinking perfectly clean water from a perfectly dirty cup or drinking water which contains an unusual or different amount of minerals or different acidity than your system is used to. You may assiduously avoid the water only to get struck down by the local wine or the homemade pastry at the village bazaar.

Why aren't the native people sick from drinking the same water or eating the same foods? For one thing, in some more unsophisticated cultures, they are sick and they have chronic diarrhea which is so much a part of their lives, they take it for granted. Secondly, they have built up a tolerance to the "exotic foods" or the alkaline water with high mineral content. They have a tolerance to water laden with coliform bacteria and their intestinal tracts have a satisfactory symbiotic relationship with these germs. They would probably get sick eating and drinking your food back home.

Not all diarrhea is the simple "Montezuma's Revenge," or "tourista," or whatever you or the natives call it. Sometimes people get something serious like cholera. Some people get amebiasis, and there are a variety of other significant microorganisms which may be responsible for diarrhea. There are textbooks on parasites and worms which can settle somewhere in your intestinal tract and can produce diarrhea. Parasitic infestation is common in many parts of the world. Schistosomiasis, a parasitic disease, is the second most common disease in the world. It is rarely seen back in the sterile U.S.A.

Most of the significant infections or infestations can be cured but need specific and careful medical care. You should be alerted to the possibility of one of these unusual but serious diseases if the illness has any of the following characteristics:

> Beware if the diarrhea is unusually prolonged. Most people have "tourista" for a few days. The first day is usually the worst and it gradually gets better during the second or third day. If it is not getting better on day two or three, it may not be just "tourista."
>
> Extremely large quantities of diarrhea with frequent and copious liquid stools suggest possible cholera. There has

recently been a pandemic of cholera and it is common on the Indian subcontinent. Cholera needs intensive and urgent treatment.

Severe abdominal cramps and fever greater than 101° F. are unusual with ordinary traveler's diarrhea.

If you see blood in the stools, you should be alert to a serious intestinal illness, and simple diarrhea would be unlikely.

You may have some nausea and vomiting with simple diarrhea, but these should not be the predominant features. If the nausea is profound or if the vomiting persists, you probably have something serious and should get it treated.

We have a few simple suggestions which may help you to avoid getting diarrhea and contribute to the sterilization and purification of your journey.
- Don't drink the water, particularly outside of major cities. Sometimes you have to drink something or you may want to drink some water. If so, we suggest you have a clean canteen and add a water purification tablet (either iodine or chlorine) according to the instructions that come with the tablets. We hate the idea of adding chemicals to what seems to be fresh, clean, or palatable water, and if you don't add the chemicals you may sometimes get away with it. It depends on what's more important to you, a fresh drink of clean stream water or three days of diarrhea.
- It is best to stick with drinks which come out of a closed bottle or can rather than from a tap or spigot.
- Try to avoid too many intermediate containers. There is no sense in pouring clean Coca-Cola into a dirty cup when you can drink it out of the bottle, but don't let this get to be an obsession or it can make you into an obnoxious American tourist.
- As a rule of thumb, there is no reason why you should drink milk anywhere while abroad, unless you are a baby or a

growing child. Even children can do without it for weeks or months if they take a vitamin and mineral supplement. Adults do not need milk (despite the Dairy Council's ads), and drinking milk is too risky.

- Don't put dirty ice cubes into clean drinks. The ice is made from the local water which you were trying to avoid. It rarely comes out of clean ice cube trays from sterile freezers.
- If the water is obviously contaminated, if it's cloudy or dirty, or smells bad, or if it comes out of a still pond, you have to be particularly careful. Don't brush your teeth with it. Don't boil your water for cooking and then wash your cup in non-boiled water. Use your judgment; you can be careful without becoming religious about it.

The treatment of traveler's diarrhea is relatively simple. A number of drugs will decrease the diarrhea. Despite the fact that it requires a doctor's prescription and is relatively expensive, we recommend a prescription drug which, in the U.S., is called Lomotil. The main advantage of Lomotil is that it is a small pill, relatively easy to take when you are nauseated, and it is not a liquid as most of the other medications are. Liquids often spill, and the bottle often breaks on a trip. We recommend one or two tablets of Lomotil each time you have diarrhea, but no more than eight tablets in any twenty-four-hour period. What may be better still is to take one or two tablets when you get that queasy gurgling feeling in your stomach which indicates that diarrhea is imminent. The Lomotil may settle things down enough to save the day. A second-choice medicine, if you don't have Lomotil available, is tincture of opium. Take ten or fifteen drops. It can be repeated in two or three hours if necessary.

If diarrhea is excessive, you have to replace the fluids which you lose as a result. If not, you will soon be dehydrated and thirsty and this adds to the misery. Drink whatever you like, but naturally avoid the water, any alcohol, or anything which may act as a subtle laxative (mint tea, for example).

The Lomotil and the opium are not antibiotics and will not

cure anything. They simply slow down the overactive bowel. Some people swear by a medication known as Entero-Vioform which contains an antibiotic. As best as we can determine, this medication has no effect on the vast majority of diarrheas. The diarrheas are not due to a specific infection with anything. Careful scientific studies indicate that antibiotics have no discernible effect on traveler's diarrhea and we do not recommend antibiotics for their routine treatment.

All this must sound pretty discouraging for the preparing traveler. You can worry about it, which won't change anything, or you can ignore it, accept it, and relax, or you can stay home. You can travel with a trunk full of canned American foods and bottled U.S. water and perhaps avoid the diarrhea, but you won't have much fun, and where will you brush your teeth?

Vaginitis

A small vaginal discharge or vaginitis is normally present in all menstruating women regardless of personal hygiene. The amount of discharge varies tremendously and what is normal for one woman may be offensive and abnormal for another. There generally is no cause for concern unless the pattern or nature of the discharge changes or if it is associated with other symptoms which we will discuss later.

There are five types of vaginal discharges which can be unintentionally self-inflicted.

• Some women maintain what is called, for want of a better euphemism, "poor personal hygiene." Either they don't care, or the economic situation or their life style prevents regular bathing. Vaginitis can sometimes be attributed to this and nothing more. The best treatment is simply more frequent bathing and laundering.

• It has been suggested that tight-fitting non-ventilating undergarments also predispose to vaginal infections. This may be related to the preference of certain kinds of organisms (yeast, for example) for a hot, moist climate. A good case can be made for cotton (which absorbs moisture) rather than nylon underwear, and it may be useful to loosen up a bit and wear a size or two larger for a while.

• On the other end of the spectrum are the cleanliness and hygiene faddists. The douche bag and all the assorted douching paraphernalia are perfectly all right occasionally, but regular and frequent douching, particularly with all the chemicals and compounds available on the druggists' shelves, upsets the normal bacteria which maintain the status quo and which probably belong in the vagina. Frequent and indiscriminate douching is unnecessary, unnatural, probably unesthetic, usually a waste of time, and if carried to an extreme, can be dangerous. It does, however, have the advantage of simulating masturbation. Douching is okay in some situations but, like almost everything else, if it is excessive, it can cause trouble.

Many women who finally consult a doctor for treatment of an unpleasant vaginal discharge feel embarrassed by the odor and douche before they see him. It's much better not to. If you douche first it will make it virtually impossible for him to tell what is wrong.

• Another culprit is a virtual drugstoreful of deodorants, sprays, creams, jellies, pads, and powders used to pretty things up for whatever reason. Excessive or indiscriminate use of these things may result in a form of chemical vaginitis. When the subsequent discharge gets unpleasant, the natural inclination is to use more of whatever you've used and a deteriorating cycle is established which can only be broken when you empty the medicine chest of all the junk and let Mother Nature take over.

• A curious and occasional cause of a vaginal discharge is the careless forgetting of any of a variety of foreign bodies which are inserted into the vagina. These range from a forgotten tampon or a diaphragm or pessary to a wide and amazing variety of objects used for sexual stimulation. Sand is a particularly irritating and difficult foreign body to deal with. The discharge resulting from a leftover foreign body is usually pretty foul and often tinged with blood. It may take some long and hard thinking to remember what may be responsible for the discharge and it sometimes requires a doctor and special equipment to fetch it out.

There are specific forms of vaginal infections which are totally unrelated to the "self-inflicted" phenomena we have described. Some tend to occur more frequently during pregnancy, some may be a side effect of a medication you are taking for another reason and sometimes a vaginal discharge can be attributed to birth control pills. Among the more common infections are the following:

Trichomonas is one of the most common infectious causes of a vaginal discharge. The discharge is frothy or foamy yellow-white or greenish. It is associated with severe itching, tenderness, a burning sensation on the outside of the vagina, and often painful intercourse. Fortunately, a simple, safe, and highly effective treatment is available. Flagyl taken three times a day for ten days should control the infection. Persistent or recurrent infections may also require the insertion of one or two Flagyl tablets high in the vagina over the same ten-day period. Trichomonas most commonly occurs or recurs after sexual contact with a male carrier who is totally free of symptoms, in whom the disease is of no consequence, and who is unaware of his infection. If repeat intercourse is anticipated, an infected male partner should take the Flagyl also; one pill three times a day for ten days. If not, the infection will just bounce back and forth indefinitely.

Monilia itches, as do all types of vaginal infections. The discharge is distinctively thick, white and creamy or curdlike. This is the type of vaginitis which occurs most commonly as a side effect in women who are taking antibiotics. It can also occur frequently in women taking birth control pills, during pregnancy, and frequently in women with diabetes.

There are two ways to treat monilia infections of the

vagina. The old way, which is still extremely effective, is to apply a 1 to 2 per cent solution of gentian violet to the vagina and the surrounding areas on the outside skin. This usually brings rapid relief of the itching, and the treatment should be repeated every two days for a total of four applications. Unfortunately, as effective as this treatment is, it is extremely messy, and the gentian violet stains everything in sight: underwear, clothing, hands, skin, sheets. A more "modern" although not any more effective treatment now is mycostatin vaginal suppositories inserted every morning and at night for two weeks. It is more esthetically acceptable than the gentian violet, but for almost immediate relief of the itching, the gentian violet can't be beaten.

If this type of vaginitis recurs and you are not taking birth control pills or antibiotics and you are not pregnant, you may have diabetes and it would probably be wise to have this checked. Antibiotic treatment or birth control pills should be discontinued if you get monilia unless it is very essential that they be continued uninterrupted. If the antibiotics are necessary, the mycostatin suppositories may have to be continued for ten to fourteen days after the treatment with antibiotics is completed.

Hemophilus vaginitis produces a thin watery or grayish odorous discharge and is best treated with a sulfa drug, either in the form of a pill or a vaginal suppository. This type of vaginitis, like the trichomonas, requires treatment of the sexual partner (with sulfa pills) to prevent recurrence of the infection.

Nonspecific vaginitis. There are vaginal infections which unfortunately do not clearly fit any of the patterns which we have already described. They are probably due to either a combination of these infections, perhaps a viral infection, or maybe an ordinary harmless bacteria resulting in an atypical infection in an unusual location. Most of these infections can be treated with applications of a vaginal cream containing a sulfa drug.

Menstrual Problems

Dysmenorrhea, or painful menstrual periods, tends to occur more commonly in women whose mothers have had painful menses. This could indicate that there is a familial tendency, but also suggests that attitudes toward menstrual discomfort picked up from Mom when the periods first start play some role in causing the discomfort in later life.

Women who have dysmenorrhea know what it is. There is almost always pelvic pain, sometimes nausea, occasionally vomiting and, in some women, a variable degree of tiredness, depression, or tension. The pains, or cramps, are usually sharp, intermittent, and low in the abdomen and pelvic region although they may sometimes radiate to the vagina, the thighs, or the lower back region. The symptoms usually appear on the first day of the period and decrease rapidly thereafter.

Some amount of menstrual discomfort is noted by about half of all women. One woman in five is so uncomfortable that something has to be done about it. Only a small number, perhaps 3 per cent, are so disabled that they have to stay home from school or work or substantially modify their normal activities.

If menstruation makes you very uncomfortable, it probably is a good idea to see a gynecologist to make sure a number of other problems may not be causing the discomfort. The great majority of women with dysmenorrhea have that and nothing more; simply discomfort from the menstrual period itself.

The treatment is simple and effective. Emotional factors occasionally contribute to the discomfort, particularly the fatigue, depression, and tension in a substantial number of women. These are best treated with such old-fashioned medicines as reassurance (a recognition that it isn't due to something more serious) and exercise. Rarely is a tranquilizer or sedative necessary. Patent medications prepared for menstrual pain usually contain aspirin and some caffeine to act as a mild stimulant. The caffeine is about as much as you would get in a cup or two of coffee, and you pay a lot more for this form of caffeine and aspirin than you would pay for coffee and aspirin alone.

Aspirin is probably the most effective and safest medication for painful menses. You can take two or three tablets every four hours if necessary. If this doesn't relieve the pain, you should have a pelvic examination before you start on other medications.

The best treatment for about 80 per cent of women with menstrual pain is birth control pills. If normal ovulation is suppressed, as is done with the pill, the menstrual period which follows is almost always pain-free. It's an added bonus of the pill and often reason enough to take it even if you are not concerned about pregnancy.

Another kind of menstrual problem is menopause. The menopause slowly creeps up on you somewhere between the ages of forty to fifty-five. One's lifetime of ovulation and menstruation is a familial characteristic; you will probably stop menstruating at about the same age that your mother did. The menopause is an indication of the end of a woman's capacity to ovulate, and therefore, it signals the end of her childbearing potential. It does not signify a decrease in sexual interest, nor does it indicate an end to a woman's ability to achieve an orgasm (unless the psychiatric aspects of the menopause distort either partner's approach to sex).

For most women, the menopause is associated with trivial symptoms or often none at all. There is an irregularity of the normally regular menstrual cycle, occasional missed menstrual periods, scant menstrual flow, increasingly infrequent menses, and then a total cessation of menstrual periods. Some women have hot flashes, which usually last only a few minutes, but can be severe and annoying. Some women have troublesome personality changes: a combination of nervousness and depression, sometimes insomnia and irritability. Other women have a profound depression associated with the menopause (see chapter on psychiatry). It is probably not due to the menopause itself, but a result of and associated with a change in pattern of living. The children are grown up and have left, the problems of family are settled. The middle years are now evident, old age is imminent, and the ambitions and goals of youth are no longer realistic or feasible. If an American woman has not fulfilled her creative potential whether it be on the labor force or in the home, she may be prey to depression, pessimism and emotionally based physical complaints during menopause.

Some women welcome the menopause. It heralds an end to problems of menstruation and frees women of the boredom of birth control.

The treatment of an unpleasant menopause depends on the severity of the symptoms. Usually nothing is required except a physician's reassurance that all is well after his careful examination. Occasionally some women take tranquilizers or antidepressants for the nervousness and irritability of menopause, but we don't recommend these unless the psychiatric symptoms are severe or persistent or disabling. The symptoms, particularly the hot flashes, can be successfully treated with female hormones, or estrogens. If you take these continually you will need a careful pelvic and breast examination at least yearly to prevent some of the long-term side effects of hormones.

Hiccups

Hiccups are different things for different people. They can be trivial, annoying, and embarrassing. They usually are of no significance but they may rarely be a clue to a serious underlying problem. If the hiccups persist for a while, they can interfere with sleeping and eating. Fortunately, they almost always are transient, usually a source of amusement, and generally disappear spontaneously.

There are vast numbers of home remedies for hiccups. They

vary according to the ethnic and sociological background of the hiccupper and his friends. The great number of remedies attest to how ineffective each method is, but since they are relatively harmless and simple, you can try them each in turn until one works.

Do nothing. Some people enjoy the periodic muscle twitching and are disappointed when it stops.

Carbon dioxide inhalation. There are the "paper bag freaks" and the "breath-holding faddists." Breathing in and out of a paper bag produces an elevation of the carbon dioxide in the body and supposedly turns off the hiccups. So does holding your breath; but stop the bag breathing or breath holding when and if you get dizzy.

Hyperventilation or rapid deep breathing, slowly in and out, lowers, not raises, the carbon dioxide. It's the opposite of the above suggestion, but many people swear by it. Stop when you get dizzy; you will if you continue long enough. (The hyperventilation problems are discussed in Chapter 3.)

Pressure on the eyeballs. Place a finger on each eye and gently massage—not too hard, or it may injure your eye or be uncomfortable.

Swallow something that irritates the back of your throat, a piece of hard bread, a piece of an ice cube, whatever you have handy that is harmless and tolerable.

Rapidly drink a glass or two of cold water, taking a gasp of breath between each gulp.

Try pulling on your tongue. It's hard to grasp your tongue with your bare fingers (it's too slippery), so use a clean handkerchief for traction. Gently pull for about twenty to thirty seconds. The only way to prevent someone from pulling too hard on your tongue is to do it yourself.

If you startle the hiccupper with a loud noise, it will usually distract him but it rarely stops the hiccups.

Try swallowing a tablespoon of dry sugar. It's a new and novel approach—maybe more effective than the others and easy enough to try.

It's rather unpleasant, but hiccups can occasionally be stopped by inducing vomiting. If you are at this stage, you must be getting desperate and the hiccups have to be annoying you. The best and easiest way to induce vomiting is to stick your finger into the back of your throat and make yourself gag.

If the hiccups persist through this self-inflicted torture, there are dozens of less standard, variably effective remedies from standing on your head to concentrating intently on your throat while slowly breathing in and out. Try anything you like or whatever pleases you. You can ignore the hiccups for a while. If the hiccups aren't bothering you too much, try a good shot of whiskey and go to sleep. If you can't sleep, can't rest, can't eat, then you must see a doctor. There are a variety of prescription medications which often work very well in relieving hiccups and a number of sophisticated surgical techniques which are almost always successful. These obviously require a desperate and deteriorating situation.

Nosebleed

A nosebleed is a very mundane and a very unromantic problem, but if a nosebleed persists it can be very serious and can easily put you out of effective action until the bleeding has stopped. A nosebleed may occur after someone punches you in the face, or sometimes can occur spontaneously for no apparent reason. It can occur on cold, dry days when the delicate tissue inside the nose dries out and bleeds easily, or if you pick your nose with too much enthusiasm, or if you get something stuck in your nose, as children often do. A nosebleed may indicate a significant problem in your nose, like a polyp, or a serious underlying disease such as high blood pressure or leukemia. The vast majority of nosebleeds are not significant or serious, however, and are nothing more than a nuisance. Medical attention is necessary only if the nose won't stop bleeding or if the bleeding recurs frequently.

The treatment for nosebleed is something like the treatment for hiccups; everyone has his own home remedy and none of the remedies has any consistent or reliable value. However, some simple measures are worth trying and will make you more comfortable. We suspect that these may not play a major role in getting the blood to stop flowing, but may help to prevent things from getting worse.

> Sit still, stay calm, and be quiet. Walking around and talking does not help.

> A sitting position with the head thrown back is probably best. Some people find it more comfortable to lie back, but remember to keep the head and shoulders slightly elevated.

> Simple pressure on the nostrils with your fingers pressing the outer part of the nose against the central septum may be all that is necessary. Breathe through your mouth and release the fingers after a few minutes. You may be pleased to find that the bleeding has stopped.

> If the bleeding can't be controlled by pressing your nose closed with your fingers, place a little gauze in the bleeding nostril and press again. If you have handy some epinephrine (Adrenalin) 1:1000 solution or Neo-Synephrine (as in most nose drops and nasal sprays), soak the gauze in this solution before you insert it into the nostril. Don't be impatient.

> Three or four drops of one of the nasal decongestants (like Neo-Synephrine nose drops, ⅛ to ¼ per cent)

might be useful. These solutions work by shrinking the mucous membranes in your nose, and this may be beneficial in slowing down the bleeding.

A cold pack on the bridge of your nose may be worth a try. Put some crushed ice in a plastic or rubber bag across your nose while your head is resting. The ice constricts some of the blood vessels in the skin over the nose and hopefully constricts some of the blood vessels in the nose itself.

You can try a variety of your own home remedies as well, if you want to or if you have no luck with the more standard procedures. Almost everything has been recommended. Sucking on ice chips; the placement of blotting paper or a paper towel on (or under) your tongue; and the wedging of a gauze pad in the space between your upper teeth and your upper lip, are commonplace techniques of no conceivable value.

In any event, if you can get the bleeding to stop, you must resist the urge to blow your nose. Your nose will be stuffed, clogged, and very uncomfortable, but if you blow it you will have blown out the clot that has controlled the bleeding and you probably will have to start all over again when the bleeding resumes. Give the stuffed nose and the blood clot a few hours at least to get organized.

If all fails and if bleeding persists despite sensible efforts and unreasonable amounts of patience, some medical intervention will be necessary. There is a good chance that the bleeding will stop on the way to the hospital emergency room, but if it doesn't, someone will have to either cauterize the bleeding point or pack the nose with gauze. Either of these is an unpleasant process and should be avoided where possible.

If the bleeding is due to trauma, you should be alerted to some other possible problems. If there has been a blow to the nose, then the treatment outlined above may be appropriate.

However, if there is any possibility that the blow may have also resulted in a skull fracture and the bleeding is mixed with leaking clear fluid, nothing should be inserted into the nose and medical attention is necessary. The clear fluid is spinal fluid coming from within the skull and this is a serious problem. If the blow to the nose has resulted in a fracture of the nasal bones or of the cartilage inside the nose, there is usually some swelling, displacement, or distortion of the nose. There is usually more pain in the area, and medical attention will probably be necessary to stop the bleeding and to straighten the nose. If the nose is broken and the bleeding has stopped and if there is no gross obstruction to breathing, the nose can be straightened and the fracture corrected later, at your convenience. Don't neglect other trauma to the face or head simply because you are distracted by the obvious flow of blood from the nose. (Chapter 4 discusses other considerations in head injuries.)

Earaches

For our purposes, the ear should be considered as having four parts. The part that you see on the side of your head, commonly called the ear, is only its external part. Most of the ear is inside your head. The outer part technically is called the pinna or the auricle. The canal which opens into the pinna is called the external canal. At the inside end of the external canal is a thin, delicate membrane, the tympanic membrane or eardrum, which separates the external canal from the middle ear. The middle ear contains the mechanisms which initiate the conversion of sounds into nerve impulses. The inner ear, even farther inside your head, contains the tiny balancing mechanisms, the semicircular canals, and the final mechanisms for converting the sound into the nerve impulses which are transmitted to the brain. In general, the inner ear is not involved in what we ordinarily think of as an earache.

As complicated and as delicate as all of the mechanisms of

the ear are, we can still distinguish six general causes for an earache.

An injury or infection of the pinna should be treated as you would treat an injury or infection anywhere on the body. The pinna is very sensitive to pain. A small infection in it is likely to hurt because the skin is tight and there is not much room for expansion of the pus underneath the skin. A common infection of the pinna is related to pierced ears. If pierced ears get infected, you should keep the earring out until the infection is thoroughly healed. Assume that you will have to get the ear pierced again at some future time. Keep the earlobes meticulously clean with soap and water and keep the hair combed behind the ear; you probably won't get the infection resolved if hair covers your ear. You may have to apply an antibiotic ointment like Neosporin ointment, and if things get difficult, an oral antibiotic may prove necessary.

External otitis refers to an infection in the external canal. It is usually caused by enthusiastic poking around in the canal with some kind of weapon temporarily adapted to the purpose of cleaning out the wax. The external otitis is sometimes caused by getting contaminated water into the ear. The infection usually causes pain, a sense of fullness in the canal, and a sensation of decreased hearing on the affected side. The pain may be felt elsewhere on the side of the head (e.g., into the back of the jaw) and sometimes there is pus or blood draining from the ear. The treatment usually requires the instillation of appropriate antibiotic drops into the external canal. Sometimes the infection can be controlled with diluted Burrow's solution (dilute it 1 to 10 with water), which you should be able to get at a drugstore. The pain can be treated as you would any pain; a hot pack can be very helpful and aspirins can be taken if necessary.

Wax in the external canal. Ear wax, technically called cerumen, keeps the canal lubricated, and the wax flows outward normally and eventually falls out by itself. The amount of ear wax has nothing to do with your personal hygiene or your bathing habits. Some people naturally form more wax than others, and in some people the composition of the wax or the anatomy of the canal is such that the wax does not flow out very easily. It accumulates and may start causing pain because of its location, or it may block the canal and decrease the hearing on that side. The pain from too much wax is usually caused, not from the wax, but sometimes from the pressure it puts on the eardrum and usually from the heroic efforts to get it out. This is almost inevitably associated with development of an external otitis. The best way to get excess wax out is with a generous but gentle irrigation of the external canal with warm water delivered through a rubber ear syringe (provided that you don't have a perforated eardrum). Hot water will be very painful and cold water will probably make you very dizzy. If the wax is dry and firm, it may be useful to soften it with a few drops of hydrogen peroxide or mineral oil. Either of these should be left in the canal with the head tilted for ten to fifteen minutes before washing the ear with water.

It is risky to poke around your ear with most random instruments. Hairpins, toothpicks, paper clips, pencils, and match sticks are not useful for getting the wax out of your ear and may scratch the canal or perforate the eardrum. If you must go after the wax, gently use a cotton-tipped applicator with plenty of cotton on the tip and don't poke the applicator in any farther than necessary.

Foreign bodies. Most unusual things can get into children's ears, but adults occasionally get something bizarre wedged in that doesn't come out. Getting foreign bodies out of the ear can be a delicate business. First, try to find out what you are dealing with. You can get into a lot of trouble if you are fumbling around with something of unknown size and shape and with unknown pointed edges. Second, get some good light on the object. You can also make trouble if you are fumbling around with something you can't see. Third, get some reasonably acceptable equipment. You might try with a flashlight and a pair of eyebrow tweezers, but this may not be very successful. Good equipment probably means medical tools and a trip to a doctor or an emergency room. A number of things can be removed from the canal with simple irrigation with water from an ear syringe. Irrigation is probably not a prudent thing to do with sharp objects where you have to be particularly careful of the point(s). If a child has put a bean in his little brother's ear, warm water may make the bean swell and make it much more difficult to remove.

Insects get into ears; if they continue to walk around it is both painful and noisy. Insects can be removed in two ways. If the insect is still alive, try a bright light next to the ear. He may walk out to see what is going on and you can quickly grab him. If the insect is dead or does not respond to light, a few drops of water or alcohol will usually drown him and at least relieve the pain of his feet walking all over your eardrum. The dead insect can then usually be washed out with water from an ear syringe.

Otitis media is an infection on the inside of the eardrum within the chamber of the middle ear. Most cases of otitis media occur in children but the problem may be seen in adults as well. Otitis media usually is coincidental with an upper respiratory infection. The middle ear is connected to the back of the nose by a channel called the Eustachian tube; it is through this tube that infecting organisms enter the middle ear from an infected nose. Rarely, the middle ear infection is caused by trauma to the eardrum or through a perforation of the drum. An otitis media is always associated with a severe earache and usually with a sensation of fullness and decreased hearing in the ear. If you could see inside the ear, you would see a red eardrum frequently bulging with the pressure from the middle ear. The treatment requires antibiotics. In children it may require the creation of a small window in the eardrum to drain out the pus from the middle ear. The use of nasal decongestants to shrink the membrane in the nose will often open up the clogged Eustachian tube and permit some drainage. This relieves the pressure (and pain) and facilitates the healing of the infection. You can usually get a nasal decongestant like Neo-Synephrine nasal spray (⅛ per cent or ¼ per cent) in a drugstore without a prescription.

Toothaches can sometimes be felt primarily as pain in the ear. This is particularly true for wisdom teeth that are coming in wrong. See the following section on toothaches.

Toothaches and Dental Problems

It is surely unscientific and it is likely that careful scrutiny will refute our observation, but we are certain that virtually all dental emergencies occur at night or on weekends or at least at times and in places when and where no dentist is available. (This is similar to our non-scientific observation that most babies, certainly more than half, are born between 2 A.M. and 5 A.M.)

Almost all toothaches are due to an inflammation within the tooth, sometimes with an obvious infection. Usually the toothache originates just beneath a cavity and the cavity has eroded deep enough to produce pain. Occasionally a toothache can be caused by an injury to the tooth or the jaw. An unusual kind of toothache may occur in some people in their late teens and twenties who may have trouble which is the result of impacted wisdom teeth. (The wisdom teeth or third molars erupt in the back of the mouth between the ages of seventeen and twenty-five. They often come in crooked, and the pressure on the adjacent teeth or the infections which result can be quite uncomfortable. The wisdom teeth often have to be extracted, and they won't be missed.)

A toothache can be simply irritating with a noticeable but trivial amount of pain or it can be an incapacitating affliction with severe pain to the point of total distraction. As if the pain itself weren't bad enough, it is often accompanied by a headache, an earache (particularly associated with impacted wisdom teeth), or a swollen face, all of which may add to the discomfort.

The treatment of a toothache will almost always require the services of a dentist. Every effort should be made to salvage a tooth rather than to simply extract every bad aching tooth. It's much easier to pull teeth, but it is well worth the effort keeping as many as possible. Fake teeth are not as good as even the damaged and repaired real ones.

While waiting for a dentist there are a few things you can do that should ease the distress.

> Start by taking two aspirins. This can be repeated in three to four hours if necessary.
>
> Put a few drops of oil of cloves on the painful tooth and on the surrounding gums. This has a pleasant taste and provides some relief of the pain. It is a mild anesthetic and if it works, stick with it.
>
> Early in the process the pain is often accentuated with cold, and anything cold on the tooth is very uncomfortable. Rinsing your mouth with warm water and putting a hot water bottle or heating pad on your face near the tooth may offer some relief. Later, as the damage to the tooth increases, the toothache may become heat sensitive. Our profound suggestion in this case would be to rinse with cold water or apply an ice pack or to suck on some ice chips.
>
> Rinsing your mouth with salt water (one or two teaspoons of salt in a glass of water) will often help to relieve the pain. If there is an infection, the salt water may relieve some of the swelling of the gums and decrease some of the inflammation.
>
> These manipulations may not be successful, but any stronger medication, such as codeine (30 to 60 mg with two aspirins), will require a doctor's prescription.

Not all pain in the teeth or in the gums or mouth is the result of a cavity (caries) or an infection in a tooth. An abscess can develop and extend beneath the tooth and into the gums and surrounding tissues. This too requires treatment by a dentist, but if there is none available you may have to start treatment yourself and get the abscess drained at a later time. An abscess will be accompanied by a tender area of swelling in the gums and usually by a fever. It should be treated with penicillin (250 to 500 mg four times a day) or, if you are allergic to penicillin, you should take erythromycin or tetracycline (250 to 500 mg four times a day for either).

Broken teeth are not usually painful unless the injury exposes the sensitive nerve roots on the inside of the tooth. In this case you should treat it as you would any ordinary toothache. If the tooth is broken out of its socket, it will probably be accompanied by brisk bleeding. Part of the bleeding may be coming from a laceration of the cheek or tongue. These can bleed profusely but, unless the laceration is extensive or goes through the tongue or cheek, it heals rapidly without specific treatment. If the bleeding is not too heavy, it may be controlled by rinsing your mouth with warm salt water. Bleeding from the tooth socket can be controlled by packing it with a pad of gauze or a small handkerchief and biting down. If you have some epinephrine (1:1000 solution) available, soak the gauze in it and bite down. The bleeding cheek and tongue may be more difficult to control, but try pressing a gauze pad (soaked in epinephrine if possible) against the bleeding area. A deep laceration may have to be sutured to control the bleeding (see Chapter 4).

As with any trauma, do not neglect more subtle injuries to the head simply because of the more obvious broken tooth or bleeding mouth. Chapter 4 discusses head injuries. Special care must be taken in an unconscious or stuporous person to prevent him from choking or aspirating the tooth fragments or clots of blood. If you are looking after someone who is bleeding from the mouth, have him lie quietly on his side and have him spit out the blood or clots rather than allow it to drip down his throat or back into his lungs.

Fractured jaws require special treatment. See Chapter 4.

Acne

Acne is the great plague of the adolescent. The Madison Avenue and TV picture of America portrays handsome and beautiful people with creamy, soft, and unblemished skin; the kid with pimples is physically, mentally, or socially inferior. No one dies of acne, people rarely lose time from work or school because of it, there are no crash federal programs to cure it, and the average physician does not take it seriously. For the sufferer it can be a serious and devastating problem. The effects can be crippling psychologically as well as physically, and although the vast majority of people who have acne receive no permanent scars to either their psyche or appearance, a tough time is had by all.

About 90 per cent of all adolescents have some acne; if you are one of them you needn't feel alone. Although its intensity may fluctuate in virtually every case, you can take some solace in the realistic expectation that acne ultimately gets better, regardless of what you do to treat it or neglect it. This is philosophical solace, however; the support it offers you depends upon your capacity to take a long-range view of the world. It offers little to the immediacy of this Saturday night.

A rational approach to acne depends on an understanding of its cause and the factors which contribute to it. For generations parents have incorrectly ascribed the onset of acne or an increase in its severity to a wide variety of teenage forms of disobedience or misconduct such as staying out too late, eating the wrong foods, or masturbation. The bewildered teenager will soon begin to feel guilty for what is perfectly normal behavior. Acne is not the result of masturbation, is not due to any sexual fantasies, activities, or desires, and is possibly only remotely related to diet. Unfortunately, it may be related to staying out too late, but this only insofar as late hours represent a sort of stress. Emotional or physical excesses from the big game or a big exam or a big date or having an argument with your parents may cause the acne to flare up.

Acne usually occurs at a time in life when there is a normal physiologic increase in the sex hormones; about the time of puberty and for a number of years thereafter. One hormone, called androgen, which is normally present in both men and women, with higher concentrations in men, appears to be the most potent acne stimulus. In addition to maturing the sexual processes, these hormones also indirectly cause an enlargement and an increased activity of some glands of the skin, the sebaceous glands. These glands, which secrete a waxy substance called sebum, are most productive in the skin of the scalp, the forehead, the face, chest, and back. Acne is probably related to (1) the imbalance of sebum production relative to (2) the increasing size of the glands, (3) other factors which tend to plug the glands and prevent their normal flow, and (4) local skin infections caused by normal skin bacterial organisms thriving on the plugged, non-flowing sebum. Ideally, if a person's growth and maturation is a fully orderly process there is no imbalance and no acne. The problem emerges if any one part of the complex system is out of phase. Tension and stress add to the intensity of the problem and, as usual, the nature of the relationship of the emotions to acne is not at all understood.

There probably are a few specific individuals with a specific food intolerance, but dietary indiscretions and the consumption of specific foods are probably grossly exaggerated culprits. It is obvious that most of the forbidden foods which have established a reputation as offenders in acne are those which are favored by young people and an anathema to their parents. It suggests that their proscription may have been based on ulterior motives since their alleged role in acne fulfills the puritanical concepts of parents and physicians: "If it is enjoyable, it can't be good for you."

No presently known treatment can prevent acne. At best we can make it a little more tolerable when it is present. It would seem that all one would have to do would be to unplug the pores and cut down on sebum production. Not so simple. Only the principles of treatment are simple, and we can separate them as follows:

Local treatment: what to do with the skin.

The skin should be washed frequently and the liberal use of any ordinary soap will substantially decrease the oiliness of the skin. This will dry the skin and the outer layer will tend to flake off, opening some of the plugged-up glands. An antibacterial agent such as hexachlorophene added to the soap probably has no significant additional value.

Steam or hot and wet towels on the skin for ten to fifteen minutes two or three times a day will help open the glands and allow better deeper cleaning. Vigorous rubbing with a rough towel is effective in removing some of the superficial skin and plugs.

Sunlight or an ultraviolet lamp has the same effect by increasing the scaling of the skin. Be careful with the UV light. It can be dangerous if it isn't used properly, so follow the instructions on the lamp and make sure the eyes, the eyelids, and the lips are protected from too much UV light.

A variety of over-the-counter skin creams, ointments, pastes, lotions, soaps, powders, and impregnated towelettes are available. Some are tinted and some are supplied in various shades to cover up acne blemishes as well as to help to clear them. The important ingredients are: any form of sulfur (between 2 and 8 per cent), which helps both to peel off the superficial layers of the skin and to decrease the sebum formation; resorcinol (between 1 and 4 per cent); and salicylic acid (1 to 2 percent). The manufacturers have included a variety of other agents including antibiotics, antibacterial agents, anti-inflammatory agents, corticosteroids, and vitamin A, all of which have no significant benefit and substantially increase the price. The sulfur, resorcinol, and salicylic acid are the useful basic ingredients. They act as irritants to the skin and produce a continuous drying and peeling without causing discomfort or too much skin irritation.

A shampoo once or twice a week is usually very helpful in

decreasing the oiliness of the scalp and the problems this may cause on adjacent parts of the face and head.

Diet: If you can convince yourself that a specific food plays a role in your acne, you obviously would do well to avoid that food if you can. Unfortunately, the concept that certain foods produce acne has been accepted by most people and sometimes intentionally or inadvertently eating what you might think of as the wrong foods produces a sense of anxiety and guilt. This is regrettable, since for most people it isn't that important. If you can't identify any kind of food as the culprit, a whole set of restrictions would appear to be a lot of trouble for a very limited possible return. The foods usually implicated in causing acne include sweets, starchy or fatty foods, and some specific foods such as nuts, chocolate, cheeses, shellfish, and pork products. Some studies seem to suggest that food or medications containing iodine or bromides are bad for acne and suggest you avoid iodized salt. We don't have much faith in any of these dietary suggestions.

Antibiotics: If the acne pimples persist despite a reasonable attempt at the simpler methods, a trial of antibiotics may be useful. Tetracycline is most widely used, and some people can keep the pimples under control with as little as one pill (250 mg) every two days. Antibiotics in skin creams or lotions probably have little value.

Stress: Stress or anxiety or tension probably aggravate acne in some people. No one really knows why, but it is quite predictable in those people who are susceptible. It's easy to suggest that you avoid stress and play it cool, but that doesn't help much. If stress makes the acne worse and this leads to embarrassment and to further stress, you are entering a deteriorating cycle and you have to get off somewhere.

Hormones: Some women notice a flare-up of their acne before or during their menstrual periods. You may find that a small dose of a diuretic (a water pill like Diuril, 500 mg a day) at the time of your period may help prevent this flare-up. Better still, it has been shown that an anovulatory menstrual cycle, that is, a menstrual period without ovulation, which can be produced medically with birth control pills, will help to substantially reduce acne in some young women. This treatment is not routine, and should be tried only in resistant or severe cases, but if a girl is taking the pill for other reasons, here is another benefit to be derived. You may notice an initial flare-up of the acne in the first few menstrual cycles, but it should get better in three or four months.

Squeezing: The case for squeezing the pimples out is a matter for judgment. If a pimple is deep with a tight plug, you'll do more harm than good by squeezing because you'll probably only break the tissues within the skin to create local irritation and infection. It will look worse than if you had left it alone. If the pimple is superficial, just under the skin, you might soften the plug with a hot towel (give it at least five to ten minutes) after a thorough face washing and gently get your fingers underneath it to squeeze it out. Scars and pock marks can be caused by local infections and these should be avoided. We do not subscribe to the view that the pimples ought never to be squeezed out, but they should be selectively squeezed. If it doesn't pop easily, don't force it and leave it alone.

There are lots of simple things not to do for acne.

> Don't use greasy or occlusive facial creams to clean your face. These plug up the pores. Soap and water are much more effective.

> You don't need any vaccines or toxoids. They are of no benefit.

> You don't need any creams or lotions with any hormones or corticosteroids added. They don't help. You might benefit from an injection of cortisone into a severe or deep lesion, but you'll need a doctor to do this.

> You don't need huge doses of vitamin A. Controlled studies show this doesn't help, and too much vitamin A can produce serious side effects.

You don't need any x-ray treatments for your skin. It's much too dangerous for a disease like acne.

You don't need any antibiotics in any lotion or cream. It doesn't help and can cause further trouble if your skin is sensitive to it.

Acne decreases with aging—reassurance for all concerned. Those who note acne flaring up periodically in their thirties and forties can look upon it as a sign of their youth, virility, and continuing adolescence.

Bad Breath

Halitosis was created when the American advertising industry teamed up with, and created, the American mouthwash industry. The word probably comes from the Latin *halitus,* which means breath, which we all have. Halitosis, or bad breath, is a medical rarity. The power of advertising has created an amazing state of self-consciousness and almost paranoia among the public who are so fearful of being unpopular or of offending one another that they spend untold millions for a variety of toothpastes, mouthwashes, dentifrices, chewing gum, breath fresheners, candy mints, sprays, drops, and chlorophyll, and still they talk to each other behind cupped hands, hoping to catch the offending vapors en route. What a fantastic con job has been perpetrated on the public!

It is probably important to differentiate between *bad breath,* or unpleasant odors coming from the lungs or the nasopharynx (the back of the nose, mouth, and throat) and *bad taste,* which is generally imperceptible to anyone except to the sufferer.

Bad breath is almost always the result of smoking or eating foods which have strong odors, like garlic and onions. The odors don't come from the stomach unless you are belching up the remains of your last meal, but rather from the lungs which are exhaling the end-product vapors of the garlic, onions, alcohol or cigarettes which you ate, drank, or smoked hours before. If you have an abscessed tooth or badly infected gums or infected sinuses or severe and persistent postnasal drip, you may have bad breath as a result of the odors created by the decaying material in the infection. But most people who have any of these infections or discharges know about them because they cause a serious amount of discomfort themselves and the approach to these problems is not to fuss about the bad breath, but to treat the tooth or the gums or the sinuses which are causing the foul odor. All the mouthwash and toothpaste you can use will not help much.

It should be apparent that bad breath should not in any way be affected by anything you slosh around in the mouth. For a few minutes your supposedly offended friends smell, not your breath but the perfumes and the alcohol in the deodorant. After you naturally swallow or spit out the deodorant, the odors of the breath reappear.

There is also *bad taste* in the mouth, which is very common in people who smoke too much. Most people have a foul-tasting mouth when they wake up in the morning, particularly if they sleep in a dry room. The saliva in your mouth dries out, the bacteria between the teeth have a chance to work relatively umolested, and if you sleep soundly you probably don't swallow or chew or talk too much. In this case a gargle or rinse will get rid of most of the foul taste and odor, and you can gargle or rinse with plain tap water as well as with a fancy, colorful, commercial product. Tooth brushing is usually quite satisfactory. The alcohol in most mouth deodorants has a tendency to dry out the mucous membranes if used too frequently. Most of these mouthwash products contain some antibacterial agents to kill the mouth bacteria, but the effect is transient at best, and more likely of no consequence whatsoever. There are mint tablets and chewing gums which supposedly contain ingredients such as activated charcoal which absorb foul odors. Unfortunately, you could not possibly chew enough charcoal or gum to absorb a significant amount of odor.

The best and easiest way to deal with bad breath or bad taste is (1) avoid foods which have truly strong persistent odors such as garlic, onions, and any others which you can personally identify, (2) keep your teeth and gums in good health by brushing or massaging frequently with anything which makes you happy, (3) get sinus infections or postnasal drip checked out to make sure this is not responsible for the odors, (4) stop smoking, and (5) stop worrying about offending everyone else.

Thrombophlebitis

Thrombophlebitis is an inflammation with a blood clot in a vein. It is most commonly present in veins of the legs. It has achieved some notoriety and an increase in public concern since it recently became known that thrombophlebitis is occasionally associated with the use of birth control pills.

Human blood is a moderately thick and viscous fluid. Various forces tend to keep it flowing in the blood vessels, but many other factors tend to slow its flow or stop it altogether. Impaired flow (stasis) ultimately causes the blood to clot in the vein and thrombophlebitis is likely to develop. Man's two-legged posture has, in part, created the problem, since the erect position places an unusually large strain on the blood vessels in the legs. In the upright position the back pressure within the legs is substantial. This pressure creates difficulty in getting the blood back uphill to the heart.

Blood clots alone in the legs are fairly common, particularly in older people. Usually they go unnoticed; they produce no symptoms and are of little consequence. The body's normal protective mechanisms clear out the clot with time and there are no complications. Occasionally the problem may be more complex and serious and the innocuous clot results in some inflammation in the vein and thrombophlebitis.

There are four common factors which predispose to thrombophlebitis in young people:

Birth control pills cause what amounts to an increase in the coagulability of the blood and a slightly increased tendency for the blood to clot.

Pregnancy produces the same effect as the pills, but the situation is complicated by the weight of the pregnant uterus partially obstructing the flow of blood from the veins in the legs and producing some stasis in the veins.

Prolonged bed rest or inactivity, such as after an operation or during a long plane or bus trip, results in a decreased blood flow and predisposes to clot formation.

An injury to a blood vessel, or a damaged, weakened blood vessel, such as in varicose veins, can decrease the blood flow and, in addition, the injury serves as a site of inflammation of the vessel.

The primary concern of thrombophlebitis relates to the possibility that part of the associated blood clot may break loose and float upstream in the vein to cause problems elsewhere in the body. This broken fragment of blood clot, called an embolus, can end up in the lungs or, rarely, in the heart or the brain. When it lodges in one of these sites, an embolus can sometimes be fatal. Fortunately, emboli are not too common, and they usually float to a site where they produce little trouble or discomfort and are not serious or significant.

If you have any of the things which predispose to the development of thrombophlebitis (if you are pregnant, if you are taking birth control pills, if you have had thrombophlebitis before, if you have varicose veins, if you are overweight), you are in a relatively vulnerable situation, and you should be a little careful and try to use some common sense to avoid the development of serious thrombophlebitis.

If you have to stand for long periods of time, you will probably benefit from elastic or support stockings. Ideally, they should be high enough to reach above the knee. They decrease the stasis and pooling of blood which result from prolonged standing. If you stand for a while, but are inactive, it helps to stamp your feet or flex your toes and ankles to increase the blood flow.

Try to avoid sitting for a long time in one position, particularly with your legs crossed or in an awkward position. A long plane or bus trip can be disastrous unless you make a conscious effort to get up and walk around every few hours, or to flex the toes and ankles while you are sitting.

If you are bedridden, or convalescing in bed, it helps to massage the calves and thighs and move your legs around to flex the leg and foot muscles.

The characteristic symptoms of thrombophlebitis usually make the diagnosis fairly obvious, particularly if you have any of the predisposing factors going against you. A cramping, dragging sensation with aching in the calf is usually present. The leg is tender to pressure and often is swollen with red streaks extending up the leg along one of the superficial veins. Remember, though, that thrombophlebitis can exist with no symptoms whatsoever.

The treatment depends on how severe the inflammation is and how uncomfortable you are. A conservative, cautious approach is often all that is necessary. Rest in bed, with the legs in a comfortable position, slightly elevated on a pillow, is the best initial treatment. Warm compresses, either dry or moist, around the calf are useful. Aspirin decreases the inflammation and is effective in relieving the pain.

If the pain and tenderness don't get substantially better in about twenty-four hours, you may need more vigorous treatment and possibly hospitalization. You may need stronger antiinflammatory drugs or anticoagulants which act to prevent further blood clotting. These measures require competent medical supervision.

We do not think that the problem of thrombophlebitis and the development of emboli should elicit panic in the minds of those who are using birth control pills. The increased incidence of blood clots in women on the pill is real and statistically significant, albeit very small. It represents a very rare, unpredictable complication of this contraceptive method. The use of these pills must be weighed against other factors that are important in birth control techniques (see Chapter 6), and the recognition that pregnancy itself carries a significantly greater risk to the well-being of the mother than does the use of birth control pills.

Motion and Seasickness

If you have never been seasick or carsick, you probably can't appreciate why everyone makes so much fuss about it. If you have had the unpleasant experience of being seasick, you understand. Anyone who is seasick is about as miserable and uncomfortable as one can get without being seriously ill; fortunately, the problem is rarely serious.

There is no real difference between carsickness, seasickness, airsickness or any form of motion sickness. There are people who are sensitive to vertical movements, and they get nauseated in elevators, during a bumpy trip on an airplane, on a ship in rough weather, or in cars or buses. Some people are particularly sensitive to changes in linear movement—anything going forward or backward, as in stop-and-go traffic; they get uncomfortable on carnival rides, and children get sick on the swing in the playground. Most people are sensitive to a greater or lesser degree to any changes in angular acceleration, the normal pitch and sway of any moving vehicle or boat.

Everyone will get motion sickness if the stimulus is severe enough or prolonged enough. Some people are obviously more sensitive than others, and your ability to eat huge meals while everyone else aboard ship is vomiting up his entire intestinal tract is no indication of how tough you are, but rather a sign of how insensitive your semicircular canals are. There are three semicircular bony canals which are tiny and deep inside your ears. They contain an extremely delicate mechanism which can detect the slightest changes in your position. They help control your sense of balance and do other interesting things like telling you whether you are going forward or backward, if you are upside down or right side up, or if you are falling down. If these canals get shaken too vigorously, you get motion sickness.

The pattern of motion sickness is fairly reproducible. Its severity ranges from the slight queasy feeling you may get when an elevator starts or stops too fast, to the fatigue, malaise, lassitude, and yawning you get on a long car ride (which you don't even appreciate until you get out to walk around), to the severe nausea, vomiting, and dizziness you may experience if you have ever been fishing at sea in a small boat. Some people notice sweating and a sense of suffocation or difficulty breathing when they have motion sickness. In extreme cases, particularly if prolonged, the motion sickness ultimately may result in prostration, dehydration, and even depression and apathy.

The sensation of motion sickness is produced by movement or, more particularly, changes in position, acceleration, or deceleration in any direction. This is necessary, but the symptoms can be accentuated by a variety of other sensory stimuli, such as the sight or smell or taste of food, the sound of waves, or the vibration of a motor. Of course, your reaction to the discomfort is predicated on, or mediated by, your psychological attitudes or emotional state at that time.

The symptoms usually rapidly decrease when the motion stops. You can almost feel the relief experienced by a seasick man as he steps off the boat onto the dock. Sometimes, however, the symptoms may persist for hours or days, and then you have to determine if the symptoms are due to the motion or some other concomitant illness.

The treatment sometimes is the uniquely simple process of getting off the boat, but this is often impossible and not much consolation when you are out at sea or on a cross-country flight. There are some precautionary measures if you have a tendency to get sick.

> Don't eat or drink anything for at least four hours before the trip starts. An empty stomach is less likely to get upset, and the vomiting will be less of a problem. Pick as large a vehicle as possible or practical. A large boat bobs less than a small one. A large jet is more stable than a smaller plane and it doesn't get tossed around as much in turbulent air currents.
>
> Use a little care in choosing your seat or location. Sit in the middle of the bus, because if you sit over the rear axle you will maximize the vertical bouncing. On a boat, sit or stay as close to the center as possible. The pitching and rolling of the boat tends to occur around some central point; when one side goes up, the other goes down, but the center stays relatively fixed.
>
> Try to hold your head as fixed as possible. If your head nods or tilts with each wave, it shakes the semicircular canals around all the more. Lean your head against a post or a firm pillow.
>
> Focus your eyes on some distant or fixed object, a cloud or a hilltop.
>
> Stay in bed if you can on a ship.

There are a number of medications which are variably effective in preventing or treating motion sickness. Some of these may be obtained without a doctor's prescription. They all have some side effects, as do virtually all medications. These will make you sleepy. They work much better if you can take them thirty to sixty minutes before you anticipate trouble, but they can be taken when you are sick if you can keep them down. They are available by injection and even by rectal suppositories for people who are too nauseated to take pills, but if you have the foresight to take along the fixings for a shot of Dramamine or a suppository of Compazine, you should have had the foresight and experience to take the pills before you left.

Meclizine (Bonine) in a 25–50 mg dose lasts for about ten to twelve hours. Cyclizine (Marezine) in a 50 mg dose, dimenhydrinate (Dramamine) 50 mg, and prochlorperazine (Compazine) 10 mg are effective for about four to six hours. None is superior to any of the others as far as we can determine, but these are probably better than most other drugs or combinations on the market. When you get anything at the drugstore, look on the label to see what is in it and how much. These are recommended doses for adults. Children need much less and you should be guided by the label. Meclizine and cyclizine are teratogenic in animals (cause fetal abnormalities) and should not be taken during pregnancy.

For chronic and recurrent motion sickness, for the poor guy who always gets sick and has to make the trip, one or two sleeping pills before you step on board may help. They won't do much for the nausea, vomiting, and dizziness, but maybe you can sleep through it all.

As a very last resort, you can contemplate (when you are seasick) the possibility of having the semicircular canals destroyed by surgery. You will have trouble walking up and down stairs, won't be able to drive or change positions too rapidly, won't be able to walk around in a dark room, but you won't get seasick any more. Anyone so desperate should stay home.

Insects, Rabies, and Snakebites

Man has gained dominance over the world around him and almost everything that lives is subdued by him. However, some of the non-microscopic things living on earth still persist in being medical problems: unpleasant, annoying, or dangerous. We have selected only a few groups of these creatures for discussion here. Not all of man's biologic enemies are included. There are a number which we don't discuss because they inflict wounds which are not unique and are no different from any other wound (e.g., the tearing gash of a grizzly bear). We don't discuss the many insects which transmit diseases to man (e.g., the mosquito and malaria), nor do we discuss a group of worms and parasites which find their way to man's intestinal tract to establish a new home. At the risk of appearing unreasonably restrictive, we have tried to limit our discussion to some of the biologic adversaries in the United States which are potentially more applicable to our readers. We don't discuss the dangerous animals which are found in the seas and the large number which are not encountered in the United States. Our selection is incomplete and entirely arbitrary, and our organization defies the ritual of biological classification. Our main concerns are practical.

We have split the discussion into three categories: 1) the insects that live on people; 2) animal bites and rabies; and 3) snakes, or the problems that arise from animals with a poisonous venom.

THE INSECTS THAT LIVE ON PEOPLE

Any of a number of friendly animals might find that you will make a comfortable home if conditions are right. Let us assume that they have a right to a pleasant environment, and that their selection of you is a reflection of their good taste and judgment. You don't want to appear an ungracious host, but you would rather not have them around since they are not very gracious guests.

There are a number of types of lice, scabies, mites, nits, chiggers, fleas, maggots, and a few other things which can settle in your hair and skin and clothes. They are not all the same. Their elimination can sometimes be troublesome and you may have to be persistent.

Lice. The adult of the species is a louse. The eggs are called nits. Nit-picking, then, is the process of removing the louse eggs, a very laborious task since there are many nits and they are very small. The process is well suited for a nit-picking personality. There are three kinds of lice that live on man: the head lice, the body lice, and the crab lice (crabs). The crab lice live in the hairs around the pubic area, near the genitalia. The nits of the crab and head lice live on the hairs; the body nits live in clothing. All of them suck blood, although not very much. It is their saliva and their excreta which makes them unpleasant, since this is what causes the itch. They are all transmitted by close personal contact.

If you have lice you should be able to see the nits. They adhere to a hair shaft and can be slid up and down. The lice and nits can be very effectively eliminated by treatment with various kinds of lotions and shampoos. You can get these without a prescription. A particularly effective skin medication known as Kwell does require a prescription, however. It is well worth the trouble of getting one or hustling some Kwell somewhere since it is so effective. Your clothing and bedding should be sterilized; an easy way to accomplish this is to dip them into some boiling water. You can also get rid of the lice by dusting yourself, your clothing, your bedding, and your friends with DDT powder. DDT is quite innocuous in these small doses, and unless you have a large number of friends, the environmental consequences will be small. It is something you'll have to settle with your own conscience. For those of you who are unhappy about killing the lice (or anything), try to understand that you are just putting the lice to sleep and washing them off.

Scabies. A minor epidemic of scabies is sweeping the country. The outcry over the scabies epidemic reflects the puritanical attitude of the worried health officials (since scabies is often a problem of counter-culture people living in a loosely structured way) rather than more appropriate official concern for the comfort and well-being of those who are affected.

Scabies (or mange, as it is sometimes called) is caused by a type of mite. Mites are tiny (1/100th of an inch) insects which burrow into the skin, laying eggs and depositing small amounts of excreta en route. The itching starts about a month after infestation (it takes about this long for you to get sensitized). The itching disappears promptly when the mites are removed. Kwell (see above) can get rid of the mites, but you may need two or three treatments. Mites are common in situations of close contact, overcrowding, and poor sanitation.

Bedbugs are not serious but their disagreeable odor can be annoying and their puncture bite can cause wheals or hives on the skin. They are not known to be involved in the transmission of any human disease. They can be disposed of with DDT (5 per cent solution in kerosene) spread on beds (not on bedding), furniture, crevices, etc.

Chiggers, redbugs, or mites (not all mites cause scabies) cause an intense itching when the insect larvae attack the skin. The symptoms can be relieved with cold packs or a towel dipped in ice water. Kwell (see above) on your skin is very effective. You need an insecticide to get them out of your backyard and your privy or wherever they are coming from.

Fleas are not a serious problem or threat. When they get on your skin they tend to migrate to a tight area (along the belt line or the top of your boot) and they suck a bit of blood which causes a mild burning or itching sensation. If they are driving you mad you can try a little insecticide powder, but you will have to powder your environment and all the local cats, dogs, chickens, rats, and mice who carry the fleas. These animal fleas tend to migrate when the going gets rough and they will leave your pet and settle on you. If you are a persistent target for fleas (some people seem to be selectively desirable), try taking thiamine (vitamin B_1, 100 mg a day). It's excreted in your skin and makes you less tasty to the fleas.

Ticks should technically be classified with the snakes since they inject a venom when they bite, but we have decided not to be too technical here. When they feed on human blood, a small drop of a toxin from their saliva is deposited under the skin. They can hang on for a few days and can get buried among long hairs. The venom can cause a slowly developing paralysis in small adults and children in addition to an itch. The paralysis is rapidly reversible if the tick can be removed. It is better to remove the tick rather than to kill it. If you can get your fingers or a pair of tweezers on it, you can remove the tick with a slow steady pull. You can sometimes encourage it to come out of the skin with a glowing cigarette, a drop of oil or freezing with an ice cube. If it comes out voluntarily you won't have any of its parts left behind.

Maggots are extremely unpleasant but fortunately relatively uncommon. They feed on feces, garbage, and dead or dying tissue. If you are careless and let an open wound get dirty, maggots can get in to feed on the dead or devitalized tissue. If maggots are present in a wound, you can assume that it is grossly contaminated and needs irrigation, antibiotics, and proper dressing. Rarely, food contaminated with maggots can cause intestinal maggots, but most of them are killed by the acid in your stomach.

ANIMAL BITES AND RABIES

Rabies is caused by a virus which is carried in the saliva of rabid animals. Although rabies is rarely seen in humans in the United States, it is not infrequently found in wild animals. Contrary to common belief, rabid dogs are not the major problem; transmission occurs more commonly from other animals: wolves, foxes, skunks, bears, squirrels, bobcats, and particularly bats (partly because they can fly and attack without warning). Rats and mice do not appear to carry rabies. The disease kills the infected animals rapidly, but in the wild, they transmit it to one another and maintain a reservoir of infection which defies elimination.

Although the symptoms of rabies in humans can appear anywhere from ten days to as long as two years after the bite, there is, on the average, a two-month incubation period between the exposure to the infected animal and the time of first onset of symptoms. This incubation period is shorter when the wound is on the head or neck and is roughly related to the distance from the wound to the brain.

Rabies always has to be considered if there has been an animal bite, particularly if the attack appears to have been unprovoked. If at all possible, the attacking animal should be captured, but not killed, since the diagnosis of rabies is much easier to confirm in a live animal. If you must kill the animal or if it dies, save as much of the carcass as you can. If you can't carry it all back to town, save at least the head; keep it on ice if at all possible, to preserve the tissue as best as possible for the important pathologic study. The live captured animal should be observed for about a week. If the animal remains well, it doesn't have rabies and you don't have to worry about the bite in any way other than ordinary concern over an ordinary wound. If the animal dies during the observation for no obvious reason (e.g., a bullet wound), you have to assume that it died of rabies. You should arrange to send the carcass to the State Health Department Laboratory for their confirmation. Rabies immunization should be started as soon as possible after the bite, or as soon as the animal appears sick or dies (see below). It is obvious that not every animal that dies has rabies and it is also true that not every bite from a rabid animal will transmit rabies. However, we recommend that you don't take the risk. Once the symptoms of rabies appear in man, death is inevitable and the vaccine will do no good. There have been some extremely rare reported cases of recoveries from rabies but, retrospectively, the diagnosis in all these cases but one was never firmly established.

Any animal bite should be thoroughly washed with copious amounts of soapy water and any dead tissue should be cut away. Rabies vaccine should be given for:

Any unprovoked attack by an animal which escapes;

Any attack by an animal that appears rabid (is acting strangely in any way);

Any attack which results in multiple bites or head, neck, or hand wounds; and,

Any bat bite.

Administering the vaccine is not a pleasant procedure for it requires multiple injections which often have to be given in the skin of the abdominal wall. The reluctance to administer the vaccine has been related to its discomfort, but this is not a good enough reason considering the consequences and the risk. The danger of side effects and possible serious complications from the vaccine has been substantially reduced by the development of newer vaccines. There should be no reason to delay rabies immunization when it is necessary.

The following table summarizes the normal immunization recommendations suggested by the United States Public Health Service:

Animal	Apparent Health of Animal	Treatment for		
		Contact but no injury	Scratches, licks, single bites	Multiple bites or any head, neck, hand bite
Dog, Cat	Healthy	None	Maybe*	Vaccine
	Questionable	None	Vaccine	Vaccine
	Escaped, unknown or rabid	None	Vaccine	Vaccine
Wild animals	Provoked attack, captured animal, appears healthy	None	Maybe*	Vaccine
	Any unprovoked attack	None	Vaccine	Vaccine
Bats		None	Vaccine	Vaccine

* Depending on the circumstances, vaccine may be started and discontinued if the animal remains healthy for seven days, or vaccine may be delayed and started immediately if the animal develops any symptoms within the time (seven days) it remains under observation.

Note: Where vaccine is recommended, if the animal is captured and remains healthy while under observation, the vaccine can be discontinued.

Veterinarians, spelunkers, who may get bitten by bats, and those who have frequent exposure to wild animals should give serious consideration to immunization as a routine procedure even if they haven't been bitten.

SNAKES, AND THE PROBLEMS THAT ARISE FROM ANIMALS WITH A POISONOUS VENOM

Snakes. There is an astonishing amount of local folklore about local snakes and an amazing inability of local experts to identify what snake just bit you. You will frequently find that, short of a real expert or a good snake atlas, you will have a difficult time with certain identification.

There are two principal types of poisonous snakes in the United States: the coral snakes and the pit vipers. Coral snakes are found across the southern part of the country. Pit vipers are found everywhere; rattlesnakes, which are a type of pit viper, are found in every state except Maine, Delaware, Hawaii, and Alaska.

The coral snakes will not attack unless provoked. Their bite may leave small or inconspicuous fang marks, but despite its small, relatively benign appearance, the coral snake bite produces an immediate, intense burning. The symptoms may progress to somnolence, nausea, vomiting, incontinence, paralysis, coma, and sometimes, but not always, death.

The pit vipers are so named because of the presence of an indented "pit" which is located between the nostrils and the eyes. The vipers often attack without any apparent provocation and will leave obvious fang marks. The bite causes intense pain which may be excruciating. The symptoms progress to weakness, a tingling and/or numbness of the extremity, a developing sense of suffocation, severe itching (from hives), and problems with bleeding, internally or in the lips and eyes. Untreated, a severe bite will cause circulatory collapse and death.

There is much first aid that you can do without any specific drugs while you are getting the victim to the hospital. First, determine if the snake really has bitten. If there are no fang marks, no pain, and no swelling within twenty minutes, you can assume that there has been no bite. If there has been a bite on an arm or leg, place a tourniquet between the bite and the body. The tourniquet can be made of anything that you can wrap and tightly tie around an arm or leg; a belt, necktie, rope or torn-up shirt. Tie the tourniquet as tight as you can and release it only about one minute every half hour. If you can, put some ice on the limb (but don't immerse the limb in ice) and then immobilize the limb with a splint. These three procedures, tourniquet, ice, and immobilization, slow down the transport of the venom to the rest of the body.

With a knife or razor blade make some straight cuts about ¼ inch deep and ½ inch long directly over the fang marks and suck out the venom. Don't worry about getting poisoned yourself, unless you have an open wound on your lips or in your mouth, since you can spit the venom out, and the venom which you may accidentally swallow is quickly destroyed by the acid in your stomach. This suction procedure is well worth the effort and well worth not being squeamish about; it can remove most of the venom if done properly and quickly enough.

Keep the victim calm and quiet. It's probably not a good idea to use alcohol for sedation. Some people are not calmed by alcohol, and since alcohol dilates the blood vessels, it may increase the absorption and transport of the venom. Almost anything else which may calm an uncomfortable and anxious snakebite victim is preferable to whiskey.

Kill or capture the snake if at all possible and take it with the victim to a hospital as quickly as you can. Antivenins are substances which neutralize the venom, and are now commercially available. Most hospitals in areas where snakebites are a problem have various and appropriate antivenins available. It obviously helps if you have the snake for identification since the antivenins are relatively species-specific.

There are a number of interesting and pertinent features about snakebites.

Bites sustained by children are more serious than those by adults. The snake injects the same amount of venom in any bite and the lethal dose is smaller in children.

Bites on the trunk, face, and neck are more serious than those on the extremities. They are more difficult to treat and tourniquets are not feasible.

Large snakes have more venom and are more dangerous than small snakes of the same species.

Exercise after a bite increases the undesirable absorption of the venom. Rest and immobilization are crucial.

Sometimes poisonous snakes bite but do not inject any venom.

Vigorous snake control campaigns frequently eliminate the beneficial varieties of snakes which help to control rodents.

No diseases are transmitted by the non-poisonous snakes.

It is important to make an effort to remove the fangs which are sometimes left in the skin in non-poisonous bites.

Lizards. In the United States the lizard problem is the gila monster problem, and the gila monster problem is mostly the problem of people who won't leave them alone. These orange and black lizards, found mostly in Arizona and New Mexico, will only attack if you really provoke or tease them. The venom is not as serious as snake venom but it can be fatal. It should be treated as you would treat a snakebite. Hospitalization is probably a good idea, even though antivenins are not available.

Spiders. There are many poisonous spiders in the world, but only a few potentially dangerous spiders in the United States. The most dangerous is the black widow. The female black widow spider can occasionally cause death, mostly in small adults and children. The black widow is easy to identify; it has a black body with a red-orange hourglass mark on its underside. Its bite produces two small puncture points which cause a sharp sting. The sting lasts briefly but there is a rapid emergence of weakness, tremor, and severe abdominal cramps and muscle spasms. The general treatment is similar to that for a snakebite. An antivenin is available. The best treatment is prevention, and if black widows are found in your area it may be worthwhile spraying with DDT any area where they might be, such as lumber piles, junkpiles, basements, privies, or similar dark areas. You should weigh the potential benefits against the possible risks with the use of anything like DDT.

Scorpions. These are present in most of the United States, but only a few varieties, which are found in the Southwest, are dangerous. Their bite is rarely fatal to adults but they can be serious, or even fatal, in small children. The symptoms of a bite are like those of a bee sting. The treatment is the same as for a snakebite (but suction probably isn't worth the effort). An antivenin is available but it may have to be obtained from the Mexican government. Scorpions don't attack unless there is an accidental contact with them. They may climb into your shoe and object to the insertion of your foot. Experienced campers shake out their boots and clothes in the morning. DDT helps to get rid of them, but you have to make your own compromise between the scorpions, the potential danger to you and to the environment.

Bees, wasps, hornets, and ants. Some people are exquisitely sensitive to these insects and may develop a rapid, severe, or even fatal allergic reaction when stung. If you know you are sensitive, you can be desensitized to the venom. You should avoid bees and avoid places where bees are likely to be. In case you are bitten, you should keep drugs like epinephrine or Isuprel on hand to treat the allergic reaction. You and your family should know how to use these drugs. People not extremely sensitive to insect stings can use cold packs and household ammonia to decrease the pain and stinging. Remove the stinger if it is still in the skin. Mud packs are of no value.

Blister beetles are interesting only because one of the beetles, Spanish fly, is a notorious aphrodisiac. The Spanish fly secretes a blister-producing substance called cantharidin. The cantharidin will irritate the skin, and when the dried, powdered flies are ingested, the cantharidin causes an inflammation and irritation of the penis or clitoris. The sensation is reported to be unpleasant rather than stimulating. Since sexual stimulation is primarily, if not entirely, a psychic reaction, the fabled aphrodisiac qualities of Spanish fly will add nothing but discomfort to your otherwise valiant efforts.

Centipedes have a reputation which far exceeds their capacity to make trouble. Only one variety in the southern United States is toxic to man and that one is probably not fatal. It makes two puncture wounds and injects its venom through two hollow fangs. There is a burning, aching, and swelling sensation which decreases in about four to five hours. Cold packs are useful.

Sunstroke and Frostbite

The human body generates heat, disposes of the excess, and maintains its temperature within very narrow limits despite wide variations in the temperature of the external environment.

Circumstances associated with extremes of temperature may cause serious injuries, but considering the magnitude and frequency of the exposure, the injuries are surprisingly uncommon.

HEAT

Heat problems don't necessarily require a tropical climate. We have seen serious problems with heat exhaustion and the potential for heat injuries of epidemic proportions (prevented only by the provision of salt along with the drinking water) in Washington, D.C., during a hot summer day when 250,000 people gathered for a demonstration and marched and sat unprotected in the blazing sun.

Much of the problem with heat relates to the controlling role of sweat. Sweat rids you of the excess body heat; the evaporation of sweat cools your skin and thereby cools your body. Under extreme conditions of heat and physical activity a person can lose two to three quarts of sweat an hour. Sweat is a salt water solution and both water and salt have to be replaced when the sweating is profuse. Under normal conditions the salt in food and usual seasoning will replace the salt lost in your sweat.

There are three kinds of problems associated with the body's failure to adjust to excess heat. The differentiation of these problems is more than just academic since their treatment is different.

Heat cramps (muscle cramps): This is the problem of people working hard on a hot day, sweating profusely, and drinking only water. The development of heat cramps does not necessarily require excess heat or exposure to a hot sun, but rather only profuse sweating and the concomitant consumption of large quantities of water without salt. The onset of muscle cramps is the typical first sign (other than thirst) that something is wrong. Treatment is primarily with salt and secondarily with water, rest, and a cool environment. This whole problem can be thought of as water intoxication; an affected person has diluted himself with too much water at a time when he is deficient in both salt and water.

Heat exhaustion: This is the most frequent problem with heat. The symptoms can develop within a few hours but can develop slowly over a period of a few days. Most commonly there will be weakness, dizziness, headache, nausea, vomiting, loss of appetite, fainting, and possibly the development of more severe forms of shock due to dehydration. This patient will be sweating profusely, his temperature may be normal, slightly elevated, or even low. He has lost too much salt and too much water. He needs replacement of both. It is possible to overdo one or the other in the treatment, but unless the situation is extreme, the kidneys will compensate for an imbalance if both salt and water are given. The patient also needs rest and a cool environment.

Heat stroke: This is a serious emergency and it can be fatal if untreated. By a number of mechanisms, including a prolongation of heat exhaustion, the patient becomes dehydrated with a profound loss of body fluids and he stops sweating entirely. The heat regulating machinery fails; the patient has lost his ability to dissipate the heat which he is constantly generating through his normal metabolism. The symptoms may at first be similar to those of heat exhaustion. Surprisingly rapidly, though, the patient may become confused, delirious, and go into shock. His skin is hot and very dry. He is not sweating at all. His body temperature will be high, frequently over 105°. The temperature will continue to rise and will soon destroy brain tissue at high enough levels. The patient must be treated immediately. If possible, it is best to place him in a tub of ice water. In the absence of a tub, ice packs should be used, particularly in places like the armpits and in the groin. In the absence of ice, ordinary water or a sponge bath will do, but none of these will do as well as an ice bath. The patient's temperature must be brought to less than 103° and the best way to do it is with ice water. The patient will need hospitalization for fluid replacement.

COLD

Cold injuries occur in three types of people: (1) soldiers and people who are required to stand or play in the snow; (2) skiers and mountain climbers or people who choose to stand or play in the snow, and (3) the poor, lost souls who fall asleep in the street whether it's snowing or not. The basic injuries caused by excessive cold are those due to actual freezing of the fluids within the cells of the skin or underlying tissues (a process which destroys the cell) or those due to constriction of the blood vessels and compromise of the blood supply to a cold part.

There are two major types of cold injuries:

Trench foot or *immersion foot:* This is almost invariably a disease of war and exposure. Soldiers are probably the only people who are required to stand in cold water for a long time. If your feet get cold and wet from prolonged standing in a trench or dugout and you add to this the local trauma due to immobility or prolonged marching, and add the malnutrition and dehydration often seen in soldiers, the development of trench foot is likely. Shipwreck survivors or those with actual immersion of limbs in water for prolonged periods of time, particularly cold water, will develop immersion foot. The pathological process is the same; interference with the blood supply to the feet. There is swelling of the feet and pain and breakdown of the skin. The feet need tender, loving care and a dry, warm supportive environment. Rewarming of the feet should be slow; if the feet are reheated too rapidly, particularly before the blood supply can be reestablished, there is a good chance of injuring the macerated tissues.

Frostbite: The skin in frostbite is actually frozen, and tiny crystals of ice forming within the skin destroy the cells. Frostbite occurs most commonly in the hands and feet, the tip of the nose and ears, in areas of the body where the circulation is diminished when exposed to cold. It can often be prevented with proper clothing, the avoidance of wet shoes or gloves, and, most important, the buddy system to watch the nose and ears of your companions. If the tip of the nose or ears gets cold, painful, pale or white, that part can be warmed and the circulation restored to normal with a warm hand. If frostbite is extensive, the treatment must be more careful and elaborate. The frozen part should be rewarmed slowly, preferably with a bath of circulating water at about body temperature (100° F). Try to avoid any unnecessary trauma to the tissues and don't massage too vigorously. Everything must be gentle. Immersion of the frozen part in too hot water will create two new problems. First, the frozen extremity, with a poor blood supply, will be easily burned by hot water. Second, when the blood supply does get reestablished to the frozen area, the blood will suddenly be rapidly cooled as it passes through the thawed limb and the cooled blood returning to the body's central core will cause a precipitous cooling of the rest of the body, an event that may have serious consequences itself.

6 Social and Political Medicine

Psychotropic Drugs

There are too many people who have never taken or used any psychotropic drugs advising people who are taking or using drugs regularly. It is interesting but discouraging to observe what is being said and written by so many self-appointed experts and ill-informed authorities. There has been a deluge of nonsense, myth, superstition, hearsay, anecdotes, and pseudo-scientific observations made by everyone from Spiro Agnew to Timothy Leary, all trying to outdo each other with tales of horror and bliss. We will make no attempt to enter this competition.

It is not our intent to condone or condemn the use of drugs. That they are used widely, indiscriminately, and sometimes carelessly, is obvious. That the best benefit of these drugs can be achieved when they are taken "properly" is perhaps less well appreciated. We will assume that our readers have had some experience either directly or indirectly with drugs, and therefore we will not dwell too long on those aspects which we assume are common knowledge. Although there is much confusion and misunderstanding and some commercially self-serving dishonesty about alcohol and cigarettes, we have not included any specific discussion of these agents, the most abused psychotropic drugs of twentieth-century America.

It is useful and important to understand the difference between addiction, habituation, and tolerance. Many drugs are habituating (habit forming) but not all of these are addicting. The addictive drugs are those which produce some kind of symptoms if the drug is suddenly withdrawn; the withdrawal reaction is somewhat characteristic of the particular drug. The addictive potential of drugs varies widely; the intensity of the withdrawal symptoms with a particular drug depends on the individual using the drug, the dose being taken, and the duration of its use. The opiates and their derivatives (including heroin) are very addictive. Less addictive are drugs like alcohol, barbiturates and the nicotine in cigarettes. Although it is not as easy to become addicted to these latter drugs, once addicted their discontinuance will yield a typical withdrawal reaction in susceptible individuals.

Habituation is less of a problem than addiction. A drug habit, like any habit, may be difficult to break, simply because of gratification received by the use of the drug. No characteristic withdrawal symptoms are present when a habituating, nonaddictive drug is discontinued. Marihuana is not addictive (no withdrawal symptoms) but for some it has slight habituation potential. When an addictive drug is taken, habituation always precedes addiction, since true addiction, and the need to take a drug to avoid withdrawal symptoms, takes time to develop, even with heroin. Tolerance to a drug refers to the need for continually increased doses to produce a similar effect. Cocaine, for example, has a high habituation potential, but tolerance does not develop; the dose requirements are fairly constant regardless of how long or frequently it is used. Tolerance to alcohol and cigarettes (nicotine) is not a significant problem; habituation varies but can be intense; withdrawal (addiction) can be substantial (alcohol) or simply uncomfortable (cigarettes). The opiates, barbiturates, and speed develop tolerance rapidly and have a high habituation potential.

Many "experts" would put all psychotropic drugs in one category and condemn them all (except alcohol and nicotine, of course) as guilty by association. Not true, no matter how the facts are distorted. You cannot confuse marihuana with heroin or acid with speed. Marihuana does not lead to heroin and LSD is not addicting. These drugs have entirely different effects, chemical structures, toxicity, tolerance, habituation, and addictive potential. Much of the panic, confusion, and anxiety of the American public has been the result of a poorly informed or misinformed or malicious press, a vicious, punitive, and puritanical attitude on the part of the police and demagogic public officials, and an inaccurate and anachronistic attitude of the Federal Bureau of Narcotics. The forces of repression can be held directly responsible for muddling and confusing everything in 1914 with pressure for bad legislation (and again in 1937 when marihuana was added to the list of controlled substances) and for stubbornly refusing to recognize its own absurd mistakes even today.

A simple and convenient classification would put the psychotropic drugs currently in vogue into five distinct categories.

- Marihuana (grass, pot, etc.) has the same effect and is the same substance as hashish (hash). The grass is less potent, the hash is more concentrated.
- All varieties of barbiturates, sedatives, and tranquilizers are similar except for differences in time of onset and duration of effect. They are all downers with varying degrees of potency.
- The stimulants include the amphetamines and cocaine. The amphetamines (speed) are prepared commercially in a number of different forms but the effect of each is similar to all the others.
- The hallucinogens, LSD, mescaline, peyote, are roughly similar with small variations which are noted below. The person using these drugs is more dependent on "the set and setting" than which of the drugs is being utilized.
- The "hard-core" drugs (morphine, heroin, opium) are similar chemically and physiologically and all have high addictive potential.

There are laboratory tests which can identify three of these five categories of drugs in the urine or the blood: the barbiturates, the amphetamines, and the opium alkaloids. The tests for amphetamines and opiates are not generally available to doctors in most hospitals, are expensive to perform and take time to complete. For practical purposes they are unavailable generally and, unless you are a captive patient as you would be if you were in the Army, you needn't delay or avoid necessary medical treatment because of your fear of having the drug detected in your urine. There are no satisfactory methods for detecting any of the drugs in the LSD group or for marihuana or hashish.

If you overdo the drugs or if you don't do them right, you may run into some of the medical problems which are directly or indirectly related to using the drugs. Many users take these medical problems for granted and assume that they are inescapable risks or even part of the price to be paid. Many of the less compassionate, less perceptive public feel that the medical complications "serve you right" and are just punishment for your defiance of the rules and your indifference to established authority. Unfortunately, this attitude extends to a significant part of the medical community, the Hippocratic oath notwithstanding; you will sense the condemnation in most medical offices, clinics, and hospitals.

Even if you don't overdo the drugs and even if you do use them carefully and correctly, you still are far from safe and you get no guarantee that you will avoid medical problems. Shooting anything into a vein is dangerous; once you start meddling with syringes and needles you can soon expect problems.

The most notorious and common but not necessarily the most serious complication of intravenous injections (shooting) is hepatitis. Hepatitis is an inflammation in the liver which is caused by injecting some of the hepatitis virus into your blood. The virus comes from the blood of someone else who has or had hepatitis and who used the same needle or syringe. You can also transmit malaria and syphilis this way if you are selective and choose friends with special or exotic diseases to share your outfit. You can possibly sterilize the needle and syringe after each use, but it's hard to be sure it's clean, the hepatitis virus is very resistant to even careful cleaning and sterilizing, and most people don't bother to be careful when they are busy getting stoned. Realistically, unless you are obsessively compulsive and stingy (features which are not too common in heroin users), you can expect to get a dose of the hepatitis virus sooner or later. What it will do to you and your liver depends on many other factors. Chapter 5 discusses the medical problems of hepatitis.

If you use your veins regularly, even if you are good at it and if you are careful, you will ultimately clot up your favorite vein and you can expect an occasional abscess to appear under the skin at the injection site. Abscesses are usually due to contaminants and debris in the junk you are injecting. These will be present even if you filter it first. Sometimes the contaminants are in the dirt on the needle or on your skin and they are pushed under the skin with the needle. Swabbing the skin with alcohol first may clean the skin somewhat, but it certainly will not sterilize it. The abscess is an area under or within the skin which is swollen, tender, and usually hot and painful. The best treatment is to rest both the arm and the vein, and apply heat with a warm towel, hot water bottle, heating pad, or anything similar. If the swelling, pain, and tenderness get worse, if you have a fever, you should get some antibiotics like penicillin to help in the battle against those rapidly multiplying and spreading bacteria.

A special kind of abscess and infection is tetanus, which is discussed in Chapter 4. Tetanus is particularly dangerous; it releases a toxin which causes lockjaw and paralysis. The toxin isn't controlled simply with a shot of penicillin. Tetanus is rare but increasingly frequent in addicts.

Since most of the junk you shoot is contaminated in one way or another, consider yourself lucky that you don't get a fever, chill, and infection each time you shoot anything. Hope that your dealer is benevolent and is cutting your junk with something relatively harmless like sugar or lactose and is not adding talcum or Ajax. Sometimes the junk or the speed is so contaminated and is so irritating to the vein that it clots the vein, causing painful thrombophlebitis (Chapter 5) all the way up the arm. If the damage to the vein and adjacent tissues is severe and extensive, you may be lucky to get only thrombophlebitis with the resulting infection.

Sometimes the bacteria and debris get carried into the bloodstream to get destroyed by the white blood cells, or filtered out by the lymph glands. If you are less lucky, or if your dose of bacteria and miscellaneous other material is large and frequent enough, or if you have anything wrong with your heart beforehand, some of the bacteria may settle and colonize on your heart valves to produce bacterial endocarditis. Without treatment, this is almost always fatal. Even with the best treatment over an extended period of time, the disease carries with it a significant risk, a high mortality and a good chance of permanent damage to your heart. The chances of survival depend, in part, on which bacteria or fungi are contaminating your smack or speed.

These are the more common serious medical problems you may encounter if you inject your tranquilizer or pacifier instead of drinking it, smoking it, or dropping it like the rest of the world. Remember that most addicts shooting speed have little or no appetite, and those using smack have little or no money, so malnutrition ultimately gets to be a problem. Malnutrition sets you up for a whole variety of other medical problems from pneumonia to tuberculosis. If you should fall prey by natural means to virtually any other illness or ailment, your experience with overusing drugs will complicate the disease and treatment tremendously and undoubtedly slow the normal recovery process.

Swallowing or smoking or sniffing your drugs is a lot safer and more predictable than shooting them, but whenever there is a profit to be made in any dealing, you have to be very careful of what else you are getting to dilute your efforts. Pure anything is virtually impossible to get on the street or from normal sources. Virtually all pharmacologic studies of drugs obtained from the usual and common street sources have shown them to be only occasionally as advertised, frequently mixed in with a variety of substances as benign as milk sugar and oregano to drugs as powerful and potentially deadly as strychnine and scopolamine. Some samples are absolutely inert with no active ingredients and some contain such weird compounds as tranquilizers used for horses and cows. Probably the worst that will happen from a pill or a joint will be a bum trip, some nausea or vomiting or a bad headache, but no hepatitis, no abscesses, no endocarditis or tetanus to worry about.

You should have some information about a wide variety of drugs which are commonly used. The emphasis is on the short-term and long-term effects of the drugs and on the best and most appropriate treatment at this time for the ill effects and overdose of the drugs. If you are taking care of someone who has had a bad trip or an overdose or just a bad side effect, don't panic. Gentle and firm reassurance will help tremendously until you can get whatever help is needed.

The psychiatric aspects of drug abuse or the long-term psychiatric problems which are seen in addicts are not discussed here. The focus is on the medical problems, both immediate and long term, with which we have more experience; without meaning to ignore or minimize the problems, we leave the enormous field of psychiatric rehabilitation to others more expert in these matters.

MARIHUANA AND HASHISH

These drugs are the same except that hash is about five to eight times (maybe more or less, depending on the product, where it is from, and how much it has been cut) as potent as grass. The tetrahydrocannabinol is the active ingredient in both. Comparing the two is like discussing the relative alcohol content in whiskey and beer. There is a wide spectrum of other substances similar to marihuana with exotic names such as charas, bhang and ghanja, What it is called depends on where it is from. For practical purposes what you will be dealing with in the U.S. is grass usually and hash occasionally.

Duration of action: The effect of the drug lasts about one to six hours depending on the amount inhaled or ingested. More important for the question of duration is the nature of the grass, which varies greatly, partly in the intrinsic quality of the original product and partly in how much it has been diluted on its way to the user. The inhaled drug is usually shorter acting than the ingested form but its onset of action is noted more rapidly.

Short-term effects cannot be summarized briefly since the effects are so much dependent on the experience of the user and the circumstances of their use. An oversimplified list would include mild drowsiness, euphoria, heightened sensory awareness, and distorted perception of time and space. Increased appetite, dryness and irritation of the eyes, and thirst probably due to dryness of the mouth are often noted.

Hallucinations or an acute psychosis is very rare.

The "spaced out" phenomenon seen with pot is probably related to an impairment of immediate memory formation. We don't know much about the neurophysiology of memory, and the obscure explanation we have had from experts thus far leads us to believe that no one else knows much more. Spaced out is when you are stoned and start to say something but forget what you started to say, and when the end of your sentence has nothing to do with its beginning. It is why a stoned driver will stop carefully for a red light but forget why he stopped. Remote memory relates to what you recall from long ago and recent memory reminds you of what you had for breakfast. These aspects of memory are apparently unimpaired by marihuana. Immediate memory is related to the formulation of memory, the recall of things which you are doing right now. It seems that pot retards or restricts the formulation of immediate memory and all the thousands or millions of bits of information entering your brain each second when you are stoned are lost, never to become recent or remote memory. Some small part must be retained however, or no one would remember what spaced out is like.

Long-term effects: The most commonly seen long-term effect is a bronchitis manifested by a dry hacking cough. Less well defined and very infrequent is the "amotivational syndrome" sometimes seen in heavy and regular users of the drug. This is manifested by listlessness, loss of ambition and drive, and loss of interest in the external environment. It is not clear whether the excessive use of marihuana is responsible for the decrease in drive and motivation, or whether some of the people who are dropping out anyway became intense potheads. We tend to favor the latter view, but recognize that we have no rigorous evidence to support our prejudice. Some authorities suggest that psychological, albeit not physical, dependence can occur after continued use, and that psychoses do occur and marihuana and hashish can precipitate acute schizophrenic reactions in susceptible individuals. Again we have the problem of which comes first, marihuana precipitating psychosis or a psychotic or pre-psychotic individual who happens to fall apart while using marihuana. Problems with psychosis may occur more frequently with hashish excess than with marihuana, but if they do occur they must be extremely rare; many experienced observers question the occurrence of any psychotic reactions even with large doses for long periods.

Treatment: Generally no treatment is necessary. The bronchitis responds to discontinuation of the drug and a decrease in the dose subsequently. The rare patient with an acute anxiety psychosis will probably respond to reassurance and only rarely is hospitalization necessary.

BARBITURATES

The barbiturates are the prototype of a large number of central nervous system depressants. We include in this group most of the common tranquilizers such as Miltown, Equanil, Librium, and Valium; all of the common sleeping pills such as Doriden, Noludar, Placidy, and chloral hydrate; and of course all of the common barbiturates (which are usually used as sleeping pills) which come in a variety of preparations, but most commonly, Seconal, Nembutal, Amytal, Tuinal, and phenobarbital. All of these products, which have achieved widespread use and distribution in the underground marketplace, have been given local descriptive "code names" such as reds (Seconal), rainbows (Tuinal), and yellow jackets (Nembutal), and the original knock-out drops (chloral hydrate) popularized in 1930 movies.

All of these depressants have the same basic effect with varying side effects and duration of action. There are some subtle differences which may be important to regular users and connoisseurs of the various pills. These differences are also important for the doctor if you've taken an overdose and he has to figure out how to get it out of your system to save your life. The differences are of no real relevance for the casual user.

Duration of action: This depends on what you have taken, how much, and whether you were drinking any alcohol at the same time. Alcohol markedly and dangerously increases the effect of any of the barbiturates. If you take the pure natural uncontaminated downer, it is best to figure an effect lasting four to eight hours; much longer if you've taken a whole handful of pills, or any combination of different ones.

Short-term effects: The sleeping pills and tranquilizers are legal. When parents criticize your pot smoking and flush your stash down the toilet, you may want to retaliate by emptying out the medicine cabinet and throwing away their supply. Just as pot has a way of relieving anxiety and producing a mild euphoric state, the barbiturates and tranquilizers have short-term effects in lessening tensions, relieving anxiety, and "taking the edge off," although they don't characteristically produce the same or similar sense of euphoria as pot. When taken in larger doses, the barbiturates and tranquilizers have a substantial sedative effect, probably more so with barbiturates than the tranquilizers. However, the tranquilizers can produce just as much sedation, particularly when they are taken in slightly larger than usual doses.

Associated with the relaxation produced by these drugs is a degree of impairment of memory, a variable amount of physical incoordination, and probably some defect in the higher intellectual functions such as judgment, intellect, and imagination.

In some ways, these drugs are like alcohol, which is also a sedative. Because the most sophisticated and highest centers of the brain (involving such things as imagination, coordination, judgment, etc.) are depressed earliest, with the lowest doses of either barbiturates or alcohol, the more primitive or the more instinctive centers of the brain take over, resulting in a transient high (often very brief or absent with the central nervous system depressants) with a decrease in inhibition, some excitement, slurred speech, garrulous behavior, stumbling, and all the features characteristic of someone high on alcohol. As the dose increases you rapidly pass through the high on your way to increasing sedation, somnolence, and ultimately coma.

Long-term effects: The more often you take the barbiturates and some of the tranquilizers, the more you need to achieve the same effect. For the guy who takes a sleeping pill every night, the problem is simple; after a while one pill doesn't seem to work and he needs two or more to get his "good night's sleep." This development of tolerance is not as marked as with speed or the opiates, but it is a definite and reproducible phenomenon. Chronic users get to be dependent on the barbiturates both physically and psychologically. Regular and heavy users may get to be irritable, a little dulled and apathetic, and sometimes confused. There is an unusual accident proneness, probably due to impaired judgment, as well as poor muscle coordination just as in an alcoholic. The impairment in intellect and mental function is probably reversible; when you stop the drugs your thinking becomes clearer and more lucid and alert, but no one has scientifically measured what happens to the intellect after prolonged regular and heavy use of barbiturates.

The diagnosis of an overdose of barbiturates may be difficult, but you should be alerted when you see someone who behaves as if he was drunk but you can't detect the odor of alcohol on his breath. The pattern of drowsiness, slurred speech, a stumbling gait and clumsy movements, confusion, and irritability in a non-alcoholic is suggestive of barbiturate overdose. You shouldn't cold-turkey the barbiturates and don't expect a chronic user to stop abruptly without suffering serious ill effects. It's not the addiction and the psychic craving that creates the problem. The user who has taken a large amount for a short time or the heavy, regular addict develops a pattern resembling alcoholic delirium tremens (d.t.'s) and convulsions (which are sometimes fatal) when the drug is abruptly withdrawn. An overdose of barbiturates almost always requires hospitalization and may require the gradual tapering of the drug or substitution with other similar drugs to prevent the convulsions and their complications.

THE STIMULANT DRUGS

For years, at the suggestion and urging of the pharmaceutical industry, doctors have written millions of prescriptions for billions of amephetamines for hundreds of thousands of patients for the alleged weight-reducing effects with which the pills were endowed. It is likely that most of those involved in this grotesque fraud, the doctor, the patient and the drug company, suspected that the pills weren't worth a damn for weight reduction; the effects are temporary, the determined fat person can easily out-eat the pills, and the side effects of the pills are substantial. What most people didn't suspect, or didn't want to admit, was that it was precisely the side stimulant effects that made the pills so sought after. Weight reduction was the excuse or trivial bonus to justify the prescription ethically.

Other drugs in the same category, similar to the amphetamines with similar effects (Preludin and Ritalin), are no better and no safer than speed. There are dozens of varieties, trade names, and slang expressions for the drugs which fall into the same stimulant category.

A typical starting dose of amphetamine (speed) may be 5 mg. This is usually enough to keep the first-time user alert and tense and to produce a feeling of energy and excitement for about three to four hours. Continued use requires progressively larger doses to produce the same effect. Shooting speed to produce the euphoric rush sensation in an experienced user can require enormous doses, up to 1,000 times as much as the starting 5 mg dose and as often as four or five times a day. When you get up to the larger doses, the amphetamines will (as the drug companies advertise to the doctors) suppress the appetite and produce a weight loss. The speed freak has no appetite; if he sticks with it long enough he will get malnourished, and a variety of nutritional deficiencies will become serious. The speed run is a demanding one and it is hard to get off. The freak incorrectly figures that the best treatment for the fatigue is another shot of the same. If he keeps at this for a while he isn't worth much after a few days. It can go on for weeks but both the supply of speed as well as the speed freak become exhausted. His judgment is impaired and a behavior pattern resembling paranoid schizophrenia develops. The speed freak often becomes suspicious, frightened, and then depressed and suicidal.

Sometimes a ping-pong pattern is established when a barbiturate or some other downer is taken to come down from a speed run and then another shot of speed is taken to get out of the depression of the downer, until you need a downer again so you can get some rest. It's similar to a pharmacologic manic-depressive psychosis.

Shooting speed, like shooting anything, carries with it the danger of hepatitis, abscesses, endocarditis and thrombophlebitis. If you use it long enough, often enough, and in large enough doses, it will produce what some people call a toxic psychosis and some people call an acute brain syndrome.

Amphetamine tolerance is a problem but it does not produce a classical addiction. Abrupt withdrawal may be associated with ravenous hunger, prolonged sleep, muscle aches, depression, and apathy.

Cocaine has been around for centuries. The Peruvian Indians knew very well about the stimulant effects of cocoa leaves many hundreds of years ago. Peruvian miners today still depend on the cocoa leaf. Cocaine became quite fashionable in nineteenth-century Europe and was widely accepted as a cure for alcoholism, morphine addiction, and as treatment for a vast selection of poorly understood phenomena from syphilis to impotence. The cocaine user today will surely find some reassurance in the fact that some outstanding men of the nineteenth century (the portrayal of Sherlock Holmes and the reality of Sigmund Freud) were among its devotees. Freud's description based on experiments made on himself and among friends is of interest. "The psychic effect of cocaine consists of exhilaration and lasting euphoria, which does not differ in any way from the normal euphoria of a healthy person . . . I have tested this effect of coca, which wards off hunger, sleep and fatigue and steels one to intellectual effort some dozen times on myself . . . opinion is unanimous that the euphoria induced by coca is not followed by any feeling of lassitude or other state of depression . . . It seems probable . . . that coca, if used protractedly, but in moderation, is not detrimental to the body."

When Freud compared cocaine with morphine, he wrote, "To be sure, the instantaneous effect of a dose of coca cannot be compared with that of a morphine injection; but on the good side of the ledger, there is no danger of general damage to the body as is the case with the chronic use of morphine."

It should be noted that Holmes (who was created by the physician Sir Arthur Conan Doyle) gave up the cocaine in his later years and Freud was obliged to retract much of his endorsement for cocaine for medical use, particularly for curing morphine addiction, although he continued to maintain that it was an effective stimulant and not addictive.

In 1914, the Federal Government classified cocaine as a narcotic.

Cocaine may be sniffed, injected, or ingested. It is difficult to add to Dr. Freud's description of its effects. Later writers describe the aggressive behavior of the cocaine user, the hallucinations, the garrulousness, the feeling of great mental and muscular strength. The euphoria is relatively brief; it lasts fifteen to thirty minutes.

The chronic usage does not produce any physical dependence or tolerance, but contrary to Freud's observations it does produce a marked psychic dependence. There is an intense craving for the euphoric effects produced by cocaine and often an associated personality change manifested by indifference to usual interests, and a fairly consistent paranoia, characteristics which were often obvious in Sherlock Holmes.

Too much cocaine, too often and too frequent, will produce an intoxication which is characteristic; muscle twitching and quivering, shuddering, and ultimately convulsions and coma. The acute intoxication is often followed by a state of profound depression, and suicide is a serious risk.

For those of you who may be intrigued by the stimulating potential of cocaine and the enthusiasm of Freud, remember that the euphoria is very brief but the depression is very profound and prolonged and the sensation of great muscular and mental powers is nothing more than a sensation.

HALLUCINOGENS

For generations many Indian and South and Central American cultures have used a variety of hallucinogens regularly with no apparent drug problem and no discernible ill effect. The advanced and scientific Western society discovered the hallucinogens in the 1950's; they were popularized among an extremely small group in the early 1960's, illegalized shortly thereafter, and then the hallucinogens became a drug problem.

It is worthwhile making distinctions among the various hallucinogenic compounds, but more for academic purposes than because there is any practical difference. The prototype drug is LSD, lysergic acid diethylamide. It is semi-synthetic, that is, it is made by chemically treating naturally available purified ergot alkaloids. Psilocybine, sometimes known as mushrooms, is a natural product which is produced by a fungus found on a type of mushroom. Mescaline is the purified product of the buttons of the peyote cactus and the words peyote and mescaline are used interchangeably. DMT (dimethyltryptamine) and DOM (or STP) are entirely synthetic and made in the chemical laboratory.

It is very doubtful that any psilocybine is now available on the streets, and we suspect that most of the stuff peddled as mescaline is probably LSD, but this type of claim is hard to document unless one obtains samples from a variety of sources around the country. The point is that it is extremely difficult for a casual or even experienced user to distinguish reliably between the different hallucinogens because their effects are basically so similar; because purity is a problem and the dose administered is not easy to measure; because the effects are so much related to the set and setting as well as the previous experience of the user; because there is little to compare the drug against except what you had last time (but you can't really be sure what that was either); and despite the fact that your dealer swears that this is good and legitimate stuff, he really doesn't know either unless he has made it or harvested it himself. The two commonly used synthetics, DMT and DOM, can sometimes be identified by the duration of action. DMT is relatively brief and the DOM effect can last for days (see below), hardly a reliable sign in either instance.

Duration of action: This is very variable and is related among other things to 1) the dose taken and 2) the state of the head of the user, neither of which can be accurately quantified. LSD effects last about ten to twelve hours, but there is no abrupt onset or cessation of the effect. It's very difficult to say precisely when the drug effect has worn off. Some of the effects are not related to the drug primarily but are secondary effects related to the suggestible state the user is in during the acid experience.

Psilocybine probably has a shorter duration of action, maybe six to eight hours. DMT, one of the synthetic hallucinogens, has an unusually brief duration of action, and the trip is over in about an hour. DOM (or STP) is an unusual synthetic hallucinogen because the duration of action depends on the dose more than with the other drugs in this category. In small standard doses, the effect probably lasts ten to twelve hours. Larger doses, in addition to intensifying the effect, seems to prolong it, and the trip may last up to two or three days.

Short-term effects: Many literate and imaginative people have had difficulty describing the effects of the hallucinogens. Nevertheless, "authoritative and scientific" technical descriptions of the effects of LSD appear regularly in a variety of scientific and medical journals with unquestioned credentials such as *The Los Angeles Times* and the *Reader's Digest*. These descriptions have probably been written by people who have never been near an acid pill or acid trip.

An important feature of LSD which makes a description so difficult is that the experience varies with each trip, and the same person taking the same pill on two different occasions under differing circumstances might justifiably think that he took two different pills.

Some useful generalizations can be made, however, which are more in the realm of objective physiology and medicine; we will avoid those which deal in the dramatic excitement of literary excesses. There is usually some agitation, anxiety, and hypomania. Most people get restless and hyperactive. These sensations are almost incidental but may be a result of what would appear to be the primary effect of the acid, which can be described as a distortion of sensory perception. There are illusions, hallucinations, and delusions, and these are not just auditory or visual, but tactile as well. Sometimes these are pleasant, beautiful, and exciting. Sometimes they are frightening and horrible distortions. It is these changes in your sensory perception which are so much mediated by your previous experiences, by the circumstances of the trip, by your surroundings, the people you are with, and the sensory input which you are subject to during the trip. Many people on acid are very suggestible although some get quite paranoid and a gentle suggestion may be interpreted as a threat. Sometimes there is what has been called a "breakdown in personality," but we aren't sure what this means and it must be rare. Occasional unusual and bizarre behavior may be noted, but these are probably related to the distortion in sensory perception and the interpretation by the user of the distorted input.

Some people become nauseated and will occasionally vomit. We suspect that some of this may be due to contaminants in the drug. Mescaline fairly regularly produces some nausea and this appears to be a primary effect of the drug itself. Mescaline may have more of a stimulant effect than other drugs in this group.

DMT, the short-acting hallucinogen, produces intense excitement and exhilaration when injected intravenously rather than swallowed, and less intense of an effect when smoked. DOM (STP) in large doses can produce marked disorientation, trembling, and confusion and, most alarming, it can provoke marked psychotic reactions in some susceptible people.

Long-term effects are even less well documented, and less well understood. Some people don't really come back from the acid trip and sometime later they are still involved in the perceptual distortions the LSD produces. No one knows whether the drug itself produces the psychosis or the acid is the vehicle through which an underlying psychosis is unmasked. There is no doubt that some people with a well-compensated psychosis can function effectively and happily under normal circumstances but when subject to stress, whatever the cause, the psychosis becomes more manifest, and flagrant and persistent. LSD may represent this stress for these people.

The flashback phenomenon is a recurrence of the drug experience at a later date without further exposure to the drug. This is a well-documented phenomenon and not too infrequent. We do not understand how or why this happens, and the explanation lies in the realm of science fiction.

There was a lot of unfortunate and hysterical publicity a few years ago about the possibility of chromosome damage and birth defects in people taking acid during their pregnancy. The cases reported were very poorly documented. Many things, including the common cold virus and the caffeine in coffee, can produce the type of defects which were noted. There is no convincing evidence that LSD is a cause of birth defects. However, before we get accused of sanctioning acid and credited with the theory that LSD is no different from a cold, we would remind you that we emphatically urge that no drugs be taken during pregnancy. Too much about the effect of any drugs on pregnancy is unknown. To take a drug with as potent an effect as LSD during pregnancy is foolish.

There is no reason at this time to believe that the long-term effects of psilocybine or mescaline are any different from LSD. They may be, but no one knows. Experience with DMT and DOM is even less extensive, and with these drugs we can safely draw a large question mark to describe the long-term effects.

Treatment: For the uneventful good trip nothing need be done, nothing should be done, and almost anything that is done will mess things up.

For the bad trip, for the frightened, agitated, and upset patient, the most satisfactory, although not necessarily the simplest treatment is often a quiet room with a minimum of external stimuli, the gentle and firm reassurance of a friend, and gentle suggestion and orientation toward more pleasant stimuli and experiences. This "talking down," first utilized at the Haight-Ashbury Free Medical Clinic in San Francisco, proved to be enormously successful in treating the many bad acid trips who were brought in during the early days when people knew even less about acid than we do now. It's a novel and exciting approach to the bad trip and much more satisfactory than the use of sedatives or tranquilizers. It is true that sedatives or tranquilizers are sometimes necessary if the patient cannot be managed by talking down, but we would like to urge that they not be used initially if at all possible. If a bad trip can be turned into a good trip with friendly reassurances, you have accomplished more than by just putting the agitated or frightened patient to sleep with a large shot of Thorazine; all of the implications and side effects of the unpleasant experience can be avoided if the trip can be turned around.

Extreme caution is necessary in treating anyone on a bad trip with DOM (STP). Thorazine can be very effective with standard bad acid trips, but it may prolong and intensify the effect of DOM. Sometimes it is impossible to know what drug a person has taken, and the agitated patient is the last person to give you an accurate description of what he took. If you suspect DOM and the trip continues for more than twelve hours, you have to assume that DOM is involved. No Thorazine should be used to terminate or decrease a prolonged bad trip. Valium, 10 or 20 mg (intravenous or intramuscular) is probably safer and better.

We have no recommendations on the wisdom of the use of any hallucinogen. These are extremely potent drugs with bizarre and confusing effects about which very little is known. However, if you can't resist the urge or temptation to satisfy your curiosity, we would like to offer some suggestions to protect you and to help maximize the possibility of a good trip.

- Make sure that you have your head together before you start. The acid will not help get you together; it is bad therapy if you are anxious, upset, or depressed. You stand a good chance of a bad trip if you've just broken your engagement or flunked out of school.
- Don't take acid if you are going to be by yourself. You should have someone sensible and responsible who is not going to take anything, stay with you just to make sure you

don't try to fly out of the window, and so you don't have to think about the telephone or the neighbors.
 • Pick a place where you are comfortable, someplace with which you are familiar, and a spot where you are surrounded by beautiful and pleasant stimuli. Don't expect a good trip if all the input is ugly and unpleasant.
 • Everyone is different, but most people find they enjoy the experience more if it is shared with friends they know and love.
 • Choose a time which is open-ended. No sense in taking acid and worrying about getting your head together to be at work in the morning.
 • Don't drive and don't plan on doing anything which requires mechanical ability. Don't do anything which can't be undone and redone later if you change your mind.
 Bon voyage.

OPIATES

These are the hard-core drugs which are supposed to be at the end of the line. These are the drugs which marihuana is supposed to lead to. We can speak lightly and nonchalantly about pot and hash, we can caution about acid, we can worry about speed or the barbiturates, but when anyone talks about hard-core and dangerous drugs, these are the drugs which he should be talking about.
 The natural alkaloids derived from the unripe seed capsules of the opium poppy (*Papaver somniferum*) are morphine, codeine, and, of course, opium. Heroin is made by chemically treating either the opium alkaloids or the morphine itself.
 The opiates are extremely effective drugs in the treatment of pain. *Morphine* is the standard drug for the treatment of severe pain. Although a number of other drugs may be used, they all are compared to morphine to determine their effectiveness. *Heroin* (smack) is a simple chemical derivative of morphine. *Codeine* is similar although less potent and is the result of another simple change in the morphine molecular

structure. *Demerol* and *methadone* are not derivatives of morphine or opium, but are synthetic opiates with morphine-like action. There are dozens of other natural, semi-synthetic, and synthetic opiates and there are dozens of other preparations containing variable amounts of the opiates. Many cough syrups have codeine (e.g., elixir terpin hydrate with codeine), and most of the drugs used to control diarrhea are opium derivatives (paregoric is a 4 per cent solution of tincture of opium).

The primary differences among the various opiate derivatives are their addictive potential, the dose required to produce an equivalent amount of pain relief, and the amount of euphoria which is produced. The medical effects, which must be considered by some addicts to be the side effects and not the primary purpose of the drugs, are extremely potent. They are pain killers of course, but they also are effective sedatives. They elevate the mood to produce a gentle euphoria and tranquillity, particularly in depressed people. They suppress cough and are constipating. They usually produce dizziness, nausea, and sometimes vomiting, even in small doses.

Notwithstanding the acknowledged medical benefits of this group of drugs, their major disadvantage is unquestionably the high potential for both physical and psychologic dependence, not only in susceptible addictive personalities, but in well-adjusted individuals with high self-esteem who are subjected to repeated doses of these drugs. Both heroin and Dilaudid have a greater addictive potential than morphine itself.

A standard dose of virtually all the opiates has an effect which lasts about four to six hours. There are some differences depending on the drug, the dose, and how it is taken (by mouth or by vein). Some of the effects are more prolonged than others. Methadone has a pain relieving effect for about four to six hours, but it can block the euphoria of heroin for about twenty-four hours.

The initial effects of shooting smack are usually what everyone thinks all the fuss is about. It produces an intense euphoria and what has been described as a total body orgasm. None of the other opiates duplicates the intense effect which is produced by heroin, although most of them produce the drowsiness, the sense of tranquillity, and the peaceful relaxation which follows the initial "up" effect. Many long-time users prefer the lost intensity of the secondary "down" effect. The effect depends on the user, his state of mind when he takes the drug, his experience with the drug, and his poetic ability to re-create it to others.

The long-term effects of these drugs are more often situational and societal rather than pharmacologic. The addict is almost always preoccupied with obtaining money for his next fix or making contact with his dealer or getting his outfit together. The proclivity to produce criminal behavior in opiate addicts, said to be greatest in heroin addicts, is probably a myth created intentionally or out of stupidity by the Federal Bureau of Narcotics, and unfortunately reinforced by the criminal behavior of opiate addicts. The cause and effect relationship is more obscure, but most intelligent observers agree that the criminal behavior is a result of artificially inflated costs of addiction and not a direct result of the opiates or the addiction itself.

Poor appetite, weight loss and poor nutrition, loss of sexual drive, and chronic constipation are part of the penalty for the euphoria of smack, but apparently for some people this is a small price to pay.

Heroin is the prototype drug for producing addiction. Repeated usage produces a high degree of tolerance; increasing doses are needed to produce the same effect, and abstinence is associated with characteristic withdrawal symptoms. The severity of the abstinence syndrome depends on the daily dose of the drug administered and the regularity and the duration of use. It is impossible for the addict using heroin purchased in normal street conditions to judge doses, but anyone using a small dose for less than a month may, if he goes cold turkey, get by with no symptoms of withdrawal at all. Moderate doses produce moderate abstinence symptoms, and only for about three or four days. If you have worked your way up to high doses for a long time, the symptoms produced by abstinence may be severe and may last up to seven or ten days.

Nothing happens for the first eight to sixteen hours of abstinence except possibly some slight drowsiness. In twenty-four hours this is followed by restlessness, yawning, sweating, nasal congestion, and tearing of the eyes. After a day or more the restlessness becomes more severe, the characteristic goose flesh appears (similar to what might appear in a "cold turkey") and uncomfortable muscle twitching is a problem. The full-blown pattern develops with loss of appetite, vomiting, diarrhea, insomnia, and severe aching muscles in the arms and legs. The symptoms reach the maximum intensity about forty-eight hours after withdrawal, persist at peak severity for another day or so, and then gradually wane in the next week. The severe acute symptoms are gone in ten days, but persistent weakness, irritability, nervousness, and insomnia may be present for months. All of these physical symptoms are complicated by anxiety and sometimes extraordinary tension and nervousness. Convulsions are rarely if ever seen as a result of opiate withdrawal; if they do occur, it may be due to concomitant withdrawal of barbiturates which often produces convulsions when abruptly stopped in a heavy user. If an addict has no access to a methadone withdrawal program, the symptoms of abstinence should be treated sympathetically and patiently with aspirin, fluids, mild sedatives or tranquilizers, and firm but friendly reassurance. Hospitalization is often necessary in severe cases.

There is a lot of confusion about morphine and heroin. Most doctors don't understand or appreciate the differences between them, and the confusion filters to the press and then to the public. As we noted before, heroin is a simple chemical derivative of morphine. Heroin is illegal for any purpose in the U.S. and in most other countries as well. It is not available even for medical purposes under any circumstances, whereas morphine, although extremely restricted, is medically available and is frequently used to kill pain and alleviate anxiety. The distinction between the two drugs relates to the addiction potential, and this is probably related to the euphoria produced by the drug. Heroin, it has been claimed, has more addictive potential than morphine and is said to be the most addictive drug available. (Although we have no reason to doubt this assertion, it appears to be another medical phenomenon which is accepted *prima facie*. We have never seen any scientific evidence to substantiate this statement, but we accept it as true since it probably is so.)

Accidental heroin overdoses occur frequently and probably account for the majority of heroin deaths. The overdose phenomenon, another side benefit of the unenlightened attitude of the Narcotics Bureau toward the control of narcotics, sometimes occurs in the form of small epidemics. When some relatively uncontaminated heroin hits the streets, the addict, having no way to judge its purity, takes his usual dose. This may be substantially stronger than the adulterated junk he is used to. Overdoses also occur in heroin novices using inappropriate amounts of the drug when they have not established high tolerance to it. The pattern is repeated frequently with minor variation in the emergency room of most large city hospitals: two men arrive with a comatose friend but strangely disappear when the confusion settles. This addict is lucky to be brought into the hospital for treatment; many are left alone, to be found dead of an accidental overdose days later.

The treatment for heroin (or any of the opiate narcotics) overdose is relatively simple and extremely effective. The primary effect of an overdose is respiratory depression; the victim has shallow and slow breathing or simply stops breathing entirely. Nalorphine (Nalline) specifically reverses the sedative effects of the opiates and frequently awakens a comatose addict within minutes. Nalline is a semi-synthetic opiate and can produce all of the undesirable effects of morphine but has very little of its beneficial effects. It has some side effects of its own, such as a tendency to produce hallucinations and confusion, but when it is given to counteract an opiate overdose, it can be lifesaving. It rapidly blocks the effect of the heroin or other opiates. It is very specific in reversing the coma. If Nalline is not effective in fifteen or twenty minutes, you can assume that the respiratory depression is not due to morphine or heroin.

Nalline can be used to treat an overdose of methadone but more care is required. Methadone, which is discussed below, has a duration of action which may last twenty-four hours or more. Since Nalline lasts about as long as an ordinary dose of heroin (four to six hours), it may be necessary to use repeat doses of Nalline to prevent a person with a methadone overdose from lapsing back into coma four to six hours later and the Nalline, but not the methadone overdose, has worn off.

Methadone is the drug which is employed most extensively now in detoxification programs for heroin addicts. There are many good reasons to try it and some problems with it, but it is no panacea by any means. (The major problems with methadone, aside from the problems of the effectiveness of substituting one drug for another, appear to be related to the failure of many methadone programs to provide the supportive ancillary and rehabilitative services which are necessary if an addict is likely to be cured. An addiction which has roots in intense social disorganization is not likely to be resolved simply by getting a person off one drug on to another.) Methadone has less of a euphoric effect than heroin, it has a longer duration of action, and it can be given by mouth. In many ways methadone is similar to morphine. It is potent as a pain killer and produces the same drowsiness, nausea and constipation which make it difficult to take on a regular basis. Methadone produces tolerance and dependence just like all the opiates, but the experts seem to feel that being addicted to methadone is better than being addicted to heroin. Apparently the methadone addicts can function more satisfactorily in the community than heroin addicts, but it is not known how much of this change in social adaptation is due to the social services provided in good methadone programs; how much is due to the different drug; and how much is due to the fact that the methadone addict takes his pills and doesn't have to hustle twenty hours a day worrying about his next fix or stealing two or three television sets to finance the whole operation. The withdrawal symptoms of methadone addiction are probably less intense and more prolonged than those with heroin. A man can skip methadone a day every so often and probably get away without feeling too sick. Note that heroin can be differentiated from methadone in a urine specimen, so if you cheat and get some smack when on methadone, the urine may give you away.

Medical Draft Counseling

Although the Selective Service System is likely to be eliminated within the next few years, we do not think it wise to base your draft deferral hopes entirely on the expectation that you can wait the system out. Hopefully, some day young men who will not fight will not have to resist, refuse, or emigrate. However, the termination of the draft may still be a long way off and, should the Vietnam War get more elaborate or any other new war develop, you can be confident that the draft, like the poor, will always be with us.

If you choose not to serve as a warrior for the U.S. Government, you owe yourself the careful examination of all of the legal and ethical methods of having yourself declared unsuitable for this service. Remember that it is much easier to stay out than to get out. Once you are in, the process of changing your mind, and theirs, is substantially more complex. It is worth your while to make your serious draft deferral effort as soon as possible.

We would like to offer some suggestions about medical and psychiatric military deferments. These should not be your only approach to the problem, but they should be high on your list if you ever consider the possibility of trying to get deferred. We urge you to talk to a competent draft counselor. If none is available, check with the standard handbooks which will provide some details on draft resistance ("Handbook for Conscientious Objectors," CCCO, 2016 Walnut Street, Philadelphia, Pennsylvania 19103, $1.00; or "Manual for Draft Age Immigrants to Canada," Toronto Anti-Draft Programme, Suite 15, 2279 Yonge Street, Toronto 12, Canada; $2.00).

Despite the fact that all draft boards are supposed to adhere to rigorously defined common standards, there is a tremendous variability in their interpretation and their attitudes toward some kinds of medical problems. It has been our experience that what is accepted unquestioned at one draft board or pre-induction physical, may be highly suspect and rejected at another. We cannot say that there is any detectable or predictable pattern. This variability may be the personal idiosyncrasy of the examining doctor more than a policy of the draft board itself.

There are specific Selective Service regulations which spell out in elaborate detail what medical conditions and physical defects are causes for rejection from military service in peacetime. (We have included these regulations in their entirety in Appendix 3.) If you are threatened by the draft, it is probably worth your while to go through the regulations carefully to see if there is anything which may be even remotely applicable to your personal history. Most of it is in technical language and may not mean too much to you, but something in it might ring a bell. A detailed manual of procedures related to 4-F classification, prepared by CCCO is reproduced in part in Appendix 4.

It is very desirable to have a doctor examine you, document the abnormality, and then write a letter for you to the draft board. It is sometimes difficult to find the right doctor who is qualified, sympathetic, and willing to help you. Keep the following considerations in mind:

- Your own family doctor, if you have one, who presumably has known you for years, is often best qualified to document a serious or recurrent illness. Specific documentation is very helpful and this is the major reason to try your own physician. The Selective Service System is impressed by exact dates of illness, enumeration of lab tests, hospitalizations, etc., and your own doctor can do this best. Unfortunately, "old family doc" may not be totally sympathetic to your interests, particularly if you've taken to growing your hair a little long or if he feels that anyone who does not want to fight for his country is unpatriotic. It is not easy to force him to write a letter even if you only want the facts without embellishment, elaboration, or opinion. Moreover, he may feel that the Army is just what you need to get that bad knee into shape or to get rid of that funny heart murmur you have had for years. You could do well without his help. You may not know how he feels about these things, so it may be necessary to see him before he writes a letter and seals your doom. If he sounds like a pamphlet from the John Birch Society, seek help elsewhere.

• Most draft counseling services know which doctors in town are sympathetic and realistic about draft problems. Have a draft counselor give you these names.

Sympathetic doctors are often well known among people who need their help, but they have limited time and their reputation sometimes gets to the local draft board as well (although not to your draft board back home). In some large cities there are medical draft referral services who put potential draftees in contact with appropriate doctors. You may be able to get in touch with these people through the local chapter of the Medical Committee for Human Rights (see Appendix 1).

• If your family doctor will not or cannot do, or if you are 3,000 miles away and you need to get your medical problem documented, it is best to try to see someone who has a particular interest in your type of problem; that is, a "specialist." If it involves your knee or your back, you are better off seeing an orthopedist, and if you have a heart murmur, a letter from a cardiologist will be a lot more valuable than one from a general practitioner. This is not essential, but the doctor at the draft board will be a little more cautious about ignoring or rejecting an impression of a specialist with fancy credentials.

- Don't expect the doctor to lie on your behalf. He can bend over backward, perhaps elaborate a bit, and be generous in his assessment. He can help you with a particular interpretation of the regulations and can possibly elevate a possible diagnosis to a probable one. But it would be unreasonable to expect him to commit perjury on your behalf.

Don't expect the Selective Service doctors to find and document any abnormality at the time of your draft physical. Their examination is perfunctory at best and often borders on malpractice. You are run through the system quickly and efficiently, but usually not very carefully. The system is not set up to detect any subtle abnormalities or anything but the most obvious defects. They are very paranoid about malingerers, they are worried about getting tricked, and they are often unimpressed with your problems unless you can document them. Don't assume that they will detect or make any effort to note even a serious hearing loss, for example, and there are well-documented instances of men being drafted with missing limbs, unnoticed at the time of their physical.

You should have a number of copies of your doctor's letter with you, since the system has a way of losing things and letters get misfiled. Your records sometimes don't follow you around at the time of the physical. Don't give your letter to anyone except to the doctor who has the final authority to make the decision on your status, unless you have a copy. This sometimes requires some persistence on your part, since the sergeant will want to have the letter for your files and the doctor somehow won't have it in the end. You can outwit and placate the sergeant by having an extra copy of the letter to give him.

The letter from your doctor should spell out as precisely as possible what your problem is, and should include the results of laboratory tests, x-ray reports and whatever documentation he has. It should give dates of hospitalization, if pertinent, since this contributes to the impression of severity and authenticity.

It is probably useful for your doctor to state specifically, in whatever appropriate fashion, how military service will make your defect worse or how the presence of the defect will make you unable to contribute to the military and carry out your assigned duties. There are many chronic problems which plague the patient but are not particularly serious; for example, low back pain, or a whiplash injury. These defects would not in themselves be any great problem in civilian life when the patient can voluntarily temper his activities according to his own experience and tolerance. But when confronted by the necessity of carrying a fifty pound pack for fifteen miles or jumping from the back of a truck, the patient may find that the minor problem has become a major disability. It is useful for your doctor to point out how a defect may be increased at times of stress, such as on patrol or in combat, when a recurrence could endanger the lives or safety of the group. Of course, the military knows the risks of inducting a man with a bad knee or bad back who washes out after a few days or a few weeks of basic training and then may be entitled to a disability pension for life.

Your doctor's letter should also refer to the specific Army Regulations which disqualify you (for example: ". . . therefore this man is not a suitable candidate for induction into the Armed Forces according to AR 40-501, section____, part____, paragraph____"). This may be a two-edged sword and may irritate the examining doctor, but it alerts him to the fact that you have done your homework, and more important, it puts the burden of proof on him to demonstrate that you do not have what it is you claim. When confronted by this, it usually is not worth his time, and he often doesn't pursue it any further.

The Selective Service System is not enthusiastic about homosexuals, alcoholics, or drug addicts. It is not our intent to lump these three into the same category, but the regulations put them together under Section XVI, 2-34, "Personality Disorders," (a) "character and behavior disorders." If you fall into one of these categories and are willing to have it documented and go into your records, then the Army would probably rather not have you and the problems they think you are likely to cause them. This is not to say that there are no homosexuals, alcoholics, or drug addicts in the service.

It is relatively easy to document your homosexuality if you should desire, but a letter from a psychiatrist will help. You really have to do a lot of heavy and serious drinking to be an alcoholic in the eyes of the Army, but if you "use drugs frequently" (and the word "use" is ill defined as is the word "frequently"), including the non-addicting drugs like marihuana or LSD, you probably qualify as an addict. The Army is equally concerned with the bad habits you might bring with you or the bad influence you might exert on the clean-cut Scotch and beer drinkers of which they are so proud, as they are with the possible psychological and physical dependence they believe to be associated with the use of these agents. If you are qualified to be disqualified on any of these grounds, you expose yourself to the risk of future embarrassment or possible difficulty getting a job or various kinds of credentials (teacher's license, bar exam, medical license, etc.). Your records are supposed to be confidential and available only to you or your representative, but have no illusions about the privacy of these records if the Civil Service Commission or any federal agency wants to check out your background. If you are concerned about jeopardizing your future career, you might think twice before putting any of these "problems" into the record, but if you are anxious not to spend a few years of involuntary servitude, you might find that these "personality disorders" will serve you well.

Keep in mind the fact that the military has no use for, and

little patience with, troublemakers. If they have reason to believe that you will be a troublemaker or a nuisance in the Army, they would generally rather not allow you anywhere near the rest of the troops who are training to be good soldiers. They call it "frequent encounters with law enforcement agencies or antisocial attitudes or behavior." If you have had difficulty dealing with authority figures or have a habit of provoking your boss or your teachers, you may qualify as a troublemaker. You will probably need a letter from a psychiatrist to document this as a legitimate behavior pattern. The Army used to pride itself on being able to take these troublemakers and discipline them into shape, but they have discovered that troublemakers thrive on provoking authority, encourage punishment, and spend too much time in the stockade to make it worth their while, so they would rather not have you.

There is one final aspect of medical deferments which causes us some discomfort and concern. Although we know the draft is unfair and discriminatory, medical deferments are even more so. In a subtle but definite fashion this pattern of deferment tends to discriminate, as usual, against the black, the poor, the less sophisticated, and the less well educated. Those who had little or no previous exposure to good medical care are often unaware of deferrable defects. Documentation of illnesses costs money, sometimes a lot of money. For every man who gets his legitimate medical deferment, someone else serves in his place, and it usually seems to be the black, the poor, the less sophisticated and the less well educated.

Tear Gas and Chemical Warfare

The use of chemical warfare agents has become so frequent during police and military operations, that we must expect the use of them in virtually any confrontation, regardless of how peaceful or legitimate it may be. To be unprepared or uninformed about these agents is naïve and foolish. When used properly, these weapons are extremely effective in crowd control and dispersal and can be relatively harmless. Despite the disclaimers of the police and the generals, all of the chemical warfare agents, even tear gas, can be extremely dangerous when used improperly or in the wrong circumstances.

Individuals who are exposed to any chemical agents should be alerted to the possibility of increased danger if any of the following conditions or circumstances exist. Risks of serious injury are substantially increased if the agents are:

> used indoors or in any enclosed area such as a car, bus, or classroom;
>
> used under circumstances in which the victims are trapped, cordoned, or denied an escape route from the contaminated area;
>
> used against individuals who are particularly sensitive to respiratory irritants or who have precedent heart or lung diseases (such as asthma);
>
> used against victims who may be taking certain medications such as Tedral or Isuprel or certain kinds of related drugs;
>
> used in improper or excessive dosages;
>
> administered directly into someone's eye or into his mouth (as can be done with mace);
>
> used when wind conditions prevent the dissemination of the vapors;
>
> used so as to affect unsuspecting bystanders, particularly the very old, the very young, and pregnant women.

PRECAUTIONARY MEASURES

The likelihood of suffering serious ill effects may be diminished by attention to some simple precautionary measures. Obviously, the circumstances of the encounter may limit the applicability of some of these suggestions.

- If you have any significant heart or lung disease (particularly asthma) and the use of gases is likely, you would do well to stay away. If your participation is necessary for whatever reason, stay near the periphery of a crowd where your rapid departure can be facilitated if gas is used.
- If you use any medications with Isuprel, Ephedrine, or similar drugs such as might be contained in any asthma pills or in an inhaler for asthma, do not take any medication on the day that you anticipate that you might be exposed to any of the war gases.
- Ski goggles are very effective in protecting your eyes. A clear plastic or yellow lens is advised and will not decrease normal visibility, although your peripheral vision will be hampered.
- Elastic bands at the wrists and ankles are helpful in decreasing the skin exposure. An elastic band is not recommended for the neck, but a tighter rather than a looser collar may be helpful (e.g., a turtle neck). Some people recommend adhesive tape for the collars, sleeves and ankles to minimize skin exposure. This should be balanced against the discomfort and delay when removing contaminated clothing.
- If you see gaseous agents being used, don't wait around to get a whiff before you start to move. Many agents are odorless and invisible and the first sign you get is the toxic effect itself. Although this crowd dispersal is precisely what the police want, you can function a lot more effectively later if you haven't previously suffered the ill effects of the gas. The dose you get is related to many factors, but chief among them are the duration of exposure, and how deeply you breathe. Holding your breath probably helps but is difficult when you are running. Running tends to increase the depth of breathing, but it gets you away from the gas faster. A wet cloth or handkerchief over your nose or mouth helps to trap some of the larger particles in a mist (like tear gas) but is actually probably little help if the agent is a gas and not a mist.
- Try to get upwind from the agent if at all possible. Try to

get to an area where the wind blows the gas away from you and not toward you.

TYPES OF AGENTS USED

There are four types of agents which are likely to be used in crowd and riot control. These are: tear gases, incapacitating gases, vomiting gases, and mace.

Hopefully the police and the military will not resort to using some of the other toxic chemical agents, which have been stockpiled and are ready for use. These include the choking agents, the nerve gases, the blood gases, and the blister agents. If any of these is ever used on any population, be it civilian or military, you can assume that the authorities have taken leave of their senses and extreme measures are imminent. These agents are potent lethal weapons and are not intended to be used for riot control and crowd dispersal.

Tear Gases constitute the mainstay of the police and military crowd dispersal agents. They characteristically provoke a flow of tears and cause skin irritation. The Army manuals and the instruction manuals distributed by the manufacturer describe them as having "nuisance value." This concept is unfortunate, because under some circumstances they can be highly toxic and they can be more than just a nuisance. Anyone exposed to any of the tear gases should have a great deal of respect for them. They have caused serious reactions in many people including permanent eye damage and major respiratory problems, and in certain conditions they could cause fatalities.

There are five tear gas agents which could be used. Their general properties are similar except for the small, important differences which are noted. There probably is no real benefit to be derived from extensive efforts to determine which agent is being utilized.

Note that none of the tear gases is really a gas but is a fine dispersal of a mist of the toxic chemical. This has particular implications as to simple precautionary measures and in treatment. Thus, a wet handkerchief held firmly over your nose and mouth may be helpful, in this case, in filtering out some of the mist particles. The fine particles, on the other hand, will remain on the skin and clothing for many hours. Virtually anyone who has been exposed to tear gas will recall innocently touching his eye or face even hours after exposure and experiencing a fresh irritation. This is caused by rubbing a bit of tear gas particle which has probably been dislodged from the clothing to the hand and then to the face.

CN—Chloroacetophenone: This is the standard tear gas. It has an odor similar to apple blossoms if one has the presence of mind to make note of it. Its action is instantaneous. In addition to its primary action as a powerful tearing agent, it is extremely irritating to the upper respiratory passages, the nose, throat, and lungs. It causes a burning and itching sensation on the skin, particularly in the moist regions. In high concentrations on the skin for a prolonged period of time, it can produce blisters, but generally in small doses on the skin its effect is similar to a strong sunburn, and the irritation subsides in a few hours. In some sensitive people it produces nausea.

CNC—Chloroacetophenone in Chloroform: This form of tear gas is similar to CN except it has an odor of chloroform.

CS—Ortho-Chlorobenzyl-malanonitrile: This agent has the characteristics of a tear gas but carries with it far more serious additional effects. It has an odor similar to pepper and it is immediately effective even in low concentrations. The victim is incapacitated in twenty to sixty seconds after exposure, but the duration of action is short—only five to ten minutes after the victim can be removed to fresh air. Its most devastating effect occurs immediately and is manifested by the inability of exposed individuals to perform effective concerted action. Its physiologic effect is similar to standard tear gas: intense burning of the eyes, with a copious flow of tears, coughing, difficulty in breathing, and a tightness of the chest. There is an involuntary closing of the eyes, a stinging sensation of the skin, particularly in moist areas, a running nose, and dizziness or swimming of the head. If the victim is exposed to an unusually large dose, nausea and vomiting may occur. The treatment after exposure to CS is different from that for standard tear gas and you should check the section on treatment which follows.

CNS—A mixture of Chloroacetophenone (CN) and Chloroform with Chloropicrin: This has an odor which has been described as similar to flypaper, for those who are familiar with flypaper. The effects of CNS are similar to CN, except that the addition of chloropicrin provides the effects of a vomiting agent and a choking agent as well as a tearing agent. The nausea, vomiting, colic (paroxysmal abdominal pain), and diarrhea may persist for weeks after exposure to CNS and, therefore, it is not likely to be used except under unusual circumstances. Note the special comments on treatment, below.

BBC—Bromobenzylcyanide: This agent is similar to the standard tear gas, except its effect is primarily as an irritant to the eyes and respiratory passages and not as a tearing agent. It has an odor similar to soured fruit. One unusual effect is a rather severe headache and pain in the forehead. Its effect can persist up to twenty-four to forty-eight hours. This agent is distinctly lethal in enclosed spaces. Treatment is the same as for CN.

Treatment of Tear Gases: This section, and the following ones dealing with treatment of other gases, includes a general discussion of how to treat chemical warfare injuries. We have included some comments on what few home remedies are available and applicable. Since so few professional medical people have had any experience with these agents, we have also recommended prescription medications in particular cases. These professional comments appear in brackets.

> Get as far away as possible from the source of the tear gas. Do not allow your curiosity to delay your departure. If possible, get upwind from the gas. Face into a gas-free wind.

EYES

Do not rub your eyes.

Blot your tears with a clean handkerchief or gauze pad. Do not rub or brush away tears. Do not blot your eyes with the same handkerchief you have used to cover your exposed nose and mouth; it will be filled with tear gas particles which you will then rub into your eyes.

Immediate and thorough irrigation of the eyes will decrease the irritant effect of the tear gas. This can be done with plain tap water or, if available, a 1 per cent boric acid solution, a 1 per cent salt water solution (one part boric acid or salt to 100 parts water), or a 2 per cent sodium bicarbonate (baking soda) solution (2 parts baking soda to 100 parts water) may give more immediate relief than tap water. However, if these solutions are not immediately available, do not waste any time preparing or seeking them. Use an irrigating syringe or any device which can gently spray the solution into the open eye. Direct the stream into the nasal side of the eye and tilt the head so that the fluid runs down the eye toward the side of the face. Copious and continuous irrigation is necessary.

If the face and eyes are heavily contaminated, and particularly if the eyes are so affected and irritated that they cannot be opened to be irrigated, it is useful to place the victim's head under running tap water or, if available, immerse his head in a tub of cool water.

Obviously, a water supply is critical. The effectiveness of water is directly proportional to the quantity used. This may pose a severe logistical problem in field or street conditions where you may be lucky to have only a canteen of water. In any planned event, the planning should involve consideration of the sources of a generous water supply. The absence of a source of water will prolong the incapacitation of a gas victim and this should be balanced against other needs in any contemplated encounter.

Some photophobia (irritation and pain in the eyes and spasms of the eyelids when exposed to light) may persist for a variable time after exposure to tear gas. This may be relieved by staying in a darkened room or wearing dark glasses in the daylight. The eyes should not be bandaged.

Most non-prescription eye drops available in drugstores are only mild pain killers at best. In the absence of a specific eye anesthetic, these may be worth a try. [If available, an ophthalmic anesthetic such as Ophthaine or Pontocaine will be quite effective in relieving the pain and spasm. If an anesthetic is used, the eye should be patched closed for at least three to four hours.]

If eye pain persists for more than a few hours or if blurred vision persists, there is a possibility of corneal damage and you should check with an eye doctor.

SKIN

Wash the exposed skin as soon as possible. Note that perspiration tends to increase the irritant effect of the tear gas. You can use plain cool tap water but soapy water is probably better and a solution of 2 to 5 per cent baking soda (2 to 5 parts soda in 100 parts of water), or 4 per cent sodium sulfite in 50 per cent alcohol) (4 parts sodium sulfite in 100 parts of 50 per cent alcohol) are perhaps more soothing. Use copious quantities of water to flush the skin. Shower if possible.

Do not apply any creams, oils, salves, or bandages.

First- and second-degree burns can be treated effectively after the tear gas has been removed (see Chapter 4).

Exposed clothing should be removed outside or away from the treatment area. The clothing will retain particles of tear gas and will continue to exude noxious effects providing a continuing source of irritation, particularly if kept indoors. The clothing should be aerated vigorously and washed as soon as possible.

LUNGS

Avoid overbreathing or breathing too rapidly. Exhale slowly and deeply as if you were talking.

If difficulty in breathing persists and particularly if the respirations are wheezing or whistling in character, it is important to keep the victim quiet, sedated if possible, and give him plenty of fresh (uncontaminated) air. If available, a cautious dose of one of the asthma spray mists (i.e., Mistometer) may relieve the wheezing.

[Definitive therapy is the treatment of an asthmatic attack. Tedral or Quadrinal, sedation with barbiturates, fluids, and, if necessary, slowly administered intravenous or rectal ammophylline, 250 to 500 mg, or epinephrine, 0.5 to 1.0 mg subcutaneously should resolve the episode unless a continuous asthmatic stimulus persists in the environment.]

PREMISES

Maximum aeration is essential for decontamination indoors.

Tear gas is heavier than air. The lower floors may retain the fumes longer than the upper floors. Get above the gas if possible.

If persisting tear gas fumes are present, it may be necessary to wash the floors and walls. Soapy water is effective, or you may use hot washing soda (sodium carbonate), one pound added to six gallons of water.

Special Treatment of CS: Basic measures are similar to those for standard tear gas exposure. If CS can be identified as the agent used, there are some other considerations which are pertinent.

> Because of its short duration of action and because of the inability of exposed individuals to perform effective concerted action, the victims should move to fresh air, face the wind, stand well spaced apart and should be cautioned against rubbing their eyes.
>
> As with ordinary tear gas, copious flushing of the skin with tap water is effective in removing the agent, but if the CS is used as a powder or dust, exposure to water will increase the skin irritation and it may be best to wait six hours before washing. Brushing, aeration, and mechanical removal of the dust appear to be the only methods available in the interim.

Special Treatment of CNS: Initial treatment is the same as for CN.

> [The nausea and vomiting can be controlled with something like 10 mg of Compazine. If this cannot be given by mouth because of the nausea and vomiting, it can be administered intramuscularly or in the form of a rectal suppository. This latter route may not be satisfactory in the presence of persistent diarrhea. The Compazine may be repeated in four to six hours.] Generally, nothing should be given by mouth until the symptoms of nausea and vomiting subside, and then start with small sips of water—a teaspoon every five minutes—or have the victim suck on ice chips.
>
> Colic is paroxysmal or spasmodic abdominal cramps which may be quite intense. [When the nausea and vomiting subside and the symptoms of colic are clearly related to the gas inhalation, one or two tablets of Donnatal may give some relief.]

Diarrhea may itself be associated with abdominal cramps. Bloody diarrhea carries many other implications and may not be just the effect of gas exposure (refer to the section on diarrhea, Chapter 3). If the diarrhea is clearly related to the gas, it can be treated with Kaopectate, one or two tablespoons every three to four hours.

[More definitive control will be obtained with an opium preparation like paregoric, one to two teaspoons every four hours, or with Lomotil, one or two tablets after each bowel movement but not to exceed eight tablets in a twenty-four hour period.]

Incapacitating Gases: These agents are capable of producing physiologic or mental effects that prevent the exposed victims from performing their normal activities for a significant length of time. Two general groups have been developed: those which produce primarily temporary physical disability manifested by paralysis, blindness, or deafness; and those agents whose action is to produce temporary mental aberrations.

These agents are different from the lethal nerve gases, choking agents, blood gases, or blister agents since the incapacitating agents produce only a temporary effect without evident permanent damage. They are therefore available for riot control.

Army chemical agent manuals suggest use of this type of agent "where military necessity requires control of a situation but where there is good reason for not harming the surrounding population or even the troops." It is also suggested for use to "confuse defense or retaliatory forces" and, most foreboding and ominous, "to affect the rationality of an important leadership group at some particularly crucial point."

Only one of the incapacitating agents appears to be generally available. It is identified only as "BZ." It is a potent psychoactive agent and it is capable of producing both mental and physical incapacitation. It is dispersed as an aerosol and is inhaled. The effect begins thirty to sixty minutes after exposure, becomes maximal in four to eight hours and may persist for two to four days in untreated victims.

[Its effects appear to be similar to a large dose of drugs such as atropine or scopolamine, but the effects persist for a longer duration.] Early signs of toxicity in the first one to four hours after exposure to BZ include rapid heart rate, dryness of the skin and mouth, increase in body and skin temperature, dilated pupils with blurred vision, dizziness, stumbling and loss of balance, vomiting, disorientation, confusion and sedation progressing to stupor. If a small dose is received, the victim may note only sleepiness and decreased alertness.

If the victim has received a large inhaled dose, there is increasing inability to respond effectively or appropriately to ordinary stimuli for a period up to about twelve hours. Following this and for periods up to four days, the victim demonstrates increased activity and random unpredictable behavior.

No treatment for the direct toxic effects of the drug are described. We have not had any experience with this unknown drug, and we are reluctant to advise anyone on how to deal with it definitively. [If presented with a patient demonstrating the symptoms of BZ toxicity, treatment with a drug such as neostigmine (0.5 to 1.0 mg) or esterase inhibitor such as Tensilon (10 mg or 25 mg) intramuscularly would be reasonable, but we do not know how effective, or possibly dangerous, such treatment might be.]

Contaminated parts of the skin should be washed with soap and water. The eyes should be irrigated with large amounts of tap water. Clothing should be removed, shaken or brushed, and then washed.

One should be cautioned that very little is as yet known about this agent, or similar agents which have undoubtedly been developed but not yet publicized. The unique effects of this type of drug would appear to make its use possible when military personnel are faced with a desperate situation, or with the tempting possibility of gassing an isolated leadership group of demonstrators at a crucial time.

Vomiting Gases: These gases can cause great discomfort to

their victims under normal circumstances. When released indoors, they can cause serious illness or even death. There are three types of vomiting agents which may be used.

DA—Diphenylchloroarsine: This is an odorless gas which is irritating to the eyes and skin. It has a rapid rate of action and the effects can be noted within two to three minutes after a one-minute exposure. The victim first notices an irritation of the eyes and a thick viscous nasal discharge similar to that caused by a cold. This is usually followed by sneezing, coughing, severe headache, acute pain and tightness in the chest, and finally intense nausea and vomiting.

The effect can last for thirty minutes after the victim has left the contaminated area, but at high concentrations with high dosage, the effects may last for hours.

DM—Adamsite: This has the same effect as DA.

DC—Diphenylcyanoarsine: This agent is similar to the ones described above. It may be recognized perhaps by its odor suggesting a bitter almond-garlic mixture, but the specific identification is not important for practical purposes, and no unnecessary risk should be undertaken to identify the gas.

Specific treatment methods are roughly the same as those outlined in the section on tear gases, specifically for CN and CNS.

Mace: Although this is a variant of ordinary tear gas, the unique properties of mace, its widespread availability, its indiscriminate and frequently inappropriate use, warrant a separate section on the subject.

Mace is tear gas (CN or Chloroacetophenone) marketed in a special solvent which permits its adherence to skin and prolongs its local irritating action. The solvent may also facilitate penetration of the irritant into the skin, thus causing greater discomfort. It is distributed in a container designed to disperse it in the form of a stream rather than as a vapor or mist.

When mace is sprayed directly onto the skin it causes extreme pain. Some protection is offered by covering the skin with Vaseline before exposure, but this must be wiped off immediately after contact since the mace will dissolve in the Vaseline and increase skin irritation. Experience suggests that the benefits of Vaseline are small and not worth the increased and potential danger; it is best avoided entirely. After exposure, copious irrigation of the burned area with plain tap water is advised.

If mace is sprayed directly into the eyes, it can cause permanent eye damage or blindness. Unfortunately, although it should not be sprayed into the face, many policemen do just that to achieve maximum effectiveness, and the incidence of facial and eye burns appears to be disproportionately high. Ski goggles are effective protection here.

The best and fastest treatment for eye exposure is continuous irrigation of the eye with large quantities of tap water. If pain and spasm of the eyelids prevent proper irrigation, it is useful to place the victim's head in a bucket or sink full of cool water (don't forget to allow him to breathe). Some authorities suggest dilute boric acid or dilute sodium bicarbonate solution (baking soda). These probably offer little advantage over plain tap water, and if time or facilities are a crucial factor, don't delay by preparing or seeking special solutions. Eye anesthetics, as discussed in the treatment of tear gas, are similarly applicable here. If blurred vision or pain persist for more than a few hours, there is a possibility of corneal damage and you should check with an eye doctor.

Mental confusion is noted frequently after exposure to mace. It is not clear whether this is due to the intense pain on exposure or from inhalation of the toxic solvents which accompany the tear gas. The confusion and irrational behavior may last for a few hours and require no treatment except reassurance and friendly supervision.

Venereal Disease

The method of catching syphilis or gonorrhea is almost always fun. Since both usually can be easily and, in general, successfully treated, and neither is particularly unpleasant, they should be freed of the hysteria that surrounds them. In certain segments of our society, syphilis and gonorrhea represent a standard of some accomplishment—a reverse status symbol of sorts.

But for the sake of perspective: syphilis and gonorrhea are highly contagious infectious diseases. Treatment can be difficult and is too often neglected. In these cases the diseases are potentially quite serious. Syphilis may be fatal if untreated. Although syphilis may appear to go away by itself, untreated it may develop complications years later which may be very unpleasant, uncomfortable, and can lead to an untimely death. Infected people who have not been treated may retain their ability to transmit their disease unsuspectingly to spouses, friends, and children (during childbirth). We recommend that you try to avoid syphilis and gonorrhea; failing that, we urge their prompt and vigorous treatment.

Public health officials express alarm over the increased evidence of venereal disease and proclaim an epidemic in progress. From a statistical viewpoint, they are right. Gonorrhea is now the second most common reported infectious disease in the U.S. after the common cold. There are, however, many public health "menaces" which are far more serious than syphilis and gonorrhea, and we would like to see public health officials adopt a more dispassionate approach. Were it not for the sexual connotations associated with venereal diseases, the official posture would be about as enthusiastic as with an epidemic of measles or malnutrition.

Why we have still not been able to eradicate entirely these two easily treated diseases in the 1970's is a continuing problem for the epidemiologists. Why an epidemic now? There are many good reasons: the sexual revolution, the availability of good contraceptive methods, the increased access to abortions, and the increased sophistication of the public, who, knowing the ease and effectiveness of treatment, are less cautious and more nonchalant about possible exposure.

Why the anxiety about epidemics of syphilis and gonorrhea? Aside from the purely intellectual and academic concern that it isn't right to have an epidemic of anything, particularly something that is so easy to treat, there are some problems which are potentially serious. First, there is increasing evidence that the bacteria which causes gonorrhea (and possibly the organism which causes syphilis also) is becoming resistant to penicillin and perhaps to some other antibiotics as well. This is cause for alarm since the easy and successful treatment which we have been relying on for the past 30 years may not be so useful in the future and stronger antibiotics with increased toxicity and side effects may be necessary. Secondly, many people do not know they have syphilis or gonorrhea; there are frequently no obvious manifestations of gonorrhea in women. (About half the women who have gonorrhea never know it.) Untreated, syphilis is severe and devastating and has long-range effects on the brain and the heart. Untreated, it is ultimately fatal. Gonorrhea, if untreated, produces a chronic infection in women, and almost always leads to sterility. Chronic untreated gonorrhea infections in men are unusual since they almost always cause burning on urination and a penile discharge and one would have to be very stoic or very stupid to put up with this for very long. If a man does ignore gonorrhea, there is a reasonable possibility of a stricture developing in the urethra (the canal passing through the penis), and the resolution of this problem is a most unpleasant experience.

One interesting aspect of venereal diseases which should not be ignored is the varied forms they may take in people who are more imaginative and vigorous in their lovemaking. Syphilis and gonorrhea are not confined to the genitalia, and the manifestations can be seen in less expected and more unusual places. Doctors not uncommonly see venereal disease in the mouth or the rectum.

As we have indicated, *the main danger from syphilis and gonorrhea is not in getting it, but in not knowing about it or in ignoring it.* We will discuss how to recognize it and how to check when you suspect you have it. Remember, venereal disease specifically refers to a "disease of love" and is invariably the result of sexual contact with someone who has it. It has been said that the only people who get venereal disease from toilet seats are wives of officers in the Army and clergymen. The rest of us acquire the disease by natural means.

Syphilis and gonorrhea are the venereal diseases which we are concerned about. There are other venereal diseases, but they are unusual in the United States and are medical curiosities only. The section on vaginal discharges (Chapter 5) discusses some of the other non-venereal vaginal problems and the section on urinary tract infections (Chapter 5) discusses cystitis (bladder infection) and some of the non-venereal diseases which may cause a discharge from the penis.

Gonorrhea is an infection caused by the bacteria *Neisseria gonorrhoeae*. You get it very simply by having physical contact, either genital or anal or oral, with someone who has the infection. It is the same for men and women. Occasionally an infant is born to a mother who has gonorrhea and the baby gets an infection in the eyes. If not treated, it can result in blindness. These infants are the only "innocent victims" of gonorrhea.

The symptoms in men are distinctive. It starts with some burning and pain on urination two days to two weeks, but almost always within five days, after exposure. When a thick mucous discharge from the penis is present, there are very few other things it can be. If treatment is not or cannot be obtained shortly, some patients will notice an increasing difficulty in urinating, probably due to infection spreading to the prostate, a gland located near the base of the penis. There may be fever, pain, and tenderness with swelling of the testes and scrotum.

In women, the symptoms are not quite so obvious and, as we indicated, about 50 per cent of women and maybe more have no symptoms at all. When there are symptoms, they are initially generally mild and rather nonspecific. There may be a slight burning on urination and there may be a vaginal discharge. Some women note lower abdominal pain later in the course of the disease. If not treated, gonorrhea can progress to a severe and serious inflammation of all the pelvic organs, leading to scarring, possible sterility, abscess formation, and generalized infection. If the extent of the infection is very severe, surgery may be necessary to drain the abscesses.

There are no generally available blood tests at this time to confirm the presence of gonorrhea. The only way to be certain of the diagnosis is to obtain a specimen from the penile discharge in men or from inside the vagina at the cervix in women. If the symptoms appear elsewhere, a specimen has to be obtained from inside the anal canal, the mouth, or whereever else the symptoms may be.

Treatment is direct but not as simple as it used to be. When penicillin was first used successfully for treating gonorrhea thirty years ago, 75,000 units was plenty. Now the recommended dose is 4,800,000 units for women and 2,400,000 units for men and even then the cure rate is not 100 per cent.

The bacteria are getting tougher and we can anticipate that penicillin will be less successful or even useless in the near future. For people who are allergic to penicillin, other antibiotics can be used satisfactorily but should be given in appropriate dosage schedules by a doctor.

Since the bacteria are getting tougher and wiser, this treatment schedule is not always effective, particularly in the Vietnamese varieties. In men, the symptoms may be diminished with treatment, but if urinary burning or a discharge persists after three days, it may be necessary to get an additional shot of penicillin. For women, particularly those who were asymptomatic initially, a repeat check-up and a repeat test should be done routinely after a week or ten days. Remember that only 75 to 95 per cent of patients are cured with the first shot, and this means that as many as one in four people with gonorrhea will need further treatment. Some men will note a slight mucus-like penile discharge for weeks or months even after an infection has been successfully treated. It is probably a manifestation of subsiding inflammation, but you can't be sure without getting an additional check-up. There are a few other important aspects of gonorrhea that you should know about.

- Gonorrhea infection confers no immunity on the patient.
- Gonorrhea and syphilis travel together very often, and if you have gonorrhea, you had better get a test for syphilis as well (see below).
- It's your obligation to tell your sexual contacts that you have gonorrhea, so they can get treated. This is particularly important for the women who often don't know they have it. If you can't or won't tell your contacts, tell the doctor and he can usually arrange for a professional and confidential follow-up of your contacts by the local health department. Your sexual contacts will have to get in touch with their recent partners and they too will have to get treated. A very awkward situation develops when a man gets gonorrhea in an extramarital contact and then gives it to his wife before he knows of his infection (or vice versa). Someone has to tell his wife something; she too will need treatment. Honesty may be the only way out, but consider all the implications and you may find that an elaborate fabrication is necessary.
- Gonorrhea involves people of all ages. While no attempt is made to initiate an international contest for the youngest and oldest patients with gonorrhea, one hospital in Paris reported gonorrhea in a twelve-year-old boy whose father took him to a brothel (the father paid), and in an eighty-four-year-old man whose son took him to a brothel (the son paid). No mention was made if it was the same brothel.
- It is probably wisest to practice abstinence until you are certain the infection is cured. (A poster issued by the San Francisco VD clinic summed up the warning succinctly: "If you dig your lovers enough to ball them then you dig them enough to not give them the clap. Help keep our neighborhood

clean.") This means sexual abstinence until a repeat pelvic exam is made and a negative cervical smear is obtained for women at least one week after treatment and all symptoms in men have disappeared at least three days after treatment.

- The best, although still unsatisfactory, way to prevent gonorrhea for both men and women is using a condom. (See the discussion of birth control in this chapter.) It helps a little but it is far from foolproof and should not be relied upon. Some people with little ingenuity and imagination manage to get infected despite it.
- Some authorities in the Army, worried about frequent gonorrhea in servicemen patronizing local prostitutes while on leave, have distributed penicillin beforehand. This treatment system probably is of very little benefit and it encourages the development of resistant strains of the organism. It treats a lot of people unnecessarily, it probably provides an inadequate dose for the vast majority of gonorrhea now seen in Vietnam, and it is likely to cause significant penicillin reactions in about 5 per cent of those treated. It certainly cannot be recommended as a routine measure for civilian or casual sexual activities.

Syphilis is a fascinating and extremely complex disease. It is an infectious disease caused by the organism *treponema pallidum*. There are three phases of the disease.

- Primary syphilis is manifested by a small and painless sore, called an ulcer or chancre, usually on the genitalia. It may be located anywhere, however, and is sometimes absent or not visible at all (50 per cent of women and 30 percent of men have no primary chancre). The chancre usually appears between ten days and three months after infection. It is usually solitary, but multiple ulcers may occur. There are no associated symptoms except sometimes a mild headache; certainly nothing to alert you that anything is wrong. The chancre if untreated will gradually heal in about four to six weeks. During this time, the infected patient is highly contagious.

- Secondary syphilis occurs at the same time or shortly after the primary chancre appears. It is usually manifested by a rash, with no particular distinguishing characteristics. It may be fairly widespread but the patient still does not feel particularly sick and the rash also may go unnoticed. The skin rash and any chancre associated with syphilis are literally teeming with syphilis microorganisms, and the likelihood of spread if not treated is very high.
- Tertiary syphilis occurs usually many years after manifestations of primary and secondary syphilis have receded. It may take twenty or thirty years for tertiary syphilis to appear (it may never appear), but when it does the results are severe with brain and/or heart damage frequently producing a fatal result.

Diagnosis of syphilis:

1) The discovery of any ulcer on the genitalia, no matter how benign or nondescript, should arouse your suspicion, particularly if the ulcer is painless.
- Any generalized rash or eruption, when there are no systemic or generalized symptoms and if you feel good, should arouse your suspicion of syphilis.
- Aside from obtaining a specimen from the chancre for microscopic examination, the best way to diagnose syphilis is with a blood test. The blood test usually becomes positive between the third and sixth week after the disease has been contracted, but it may not become positive for up to three months and repeated testing is necessary if your suspicion is high. It does no good to get a blood test the day after the night before. Unless you've had syphilis from a previous exposure, the test will be negative this early. The appearance of a chancre in primary syphilis is usually, but not always, associated with a positive blood test. A scraping from the chancre may be negative, so repeat blood tests will have to be taken at intervals for up to three months to rule out syphilis. If you have the rash of secondary syphilis, the blood test will almost invariably be positive and if the test is not positive, you almost certainly don't have syphilis.

- Most hospitals routinely check a blood test for syphilis on every admitted patient. Most states require a blood test for syphilis before getting married. These two measures detect a small but significant number of people who have previously undiagnosed syphilis.
- The presence of a positive blood test is suggestive, but by no means absolutely diagnostic of syphilis. A significant number of people will have what is called a biologically false positive test for syphilis; that is, a positive blood test but no other evidence of syphilis. Your doctor will have to determine the likelihood of infection, but if he doesn't treat it he will have to get additional blood tests to monitor how strongly positive the test is or to determine if it was a temporary abnormality. More specific tests have been developed recently which can give an answer with a high degree of accuracy.

How do you get syphilis? Probably the best way is by sexual intercourse, but any sort of physical contact involving moist surfaces of the body like the mouth, lips, eyes, or anus with someone who has syphilis will spread the disease. An infected pregnant woman can give it to her newborn baby. There are no other ways to get syphilis. You can't get it from toilet seats or dirty linen. The organism is particularly fastidious and delicate and will not survive outside the body for very long. Of course, indirect transmission can occur under unusual circumstances, such as cutting yourself with a knife which has just cut someone who has secondary syphilis, or using a needle which has just been used by your friend with syphilis. These are relatively uncommon methods of transmission and usually not as satisfying as nature's way.

Treatment: Treatment is relatively simple but must be adhered to compulsively and followed up carefully. Penicillin is given, preferably by injection; the dose depends on what stage of the disease and what complications, if any, are present. For people allergic to penicillin, other antibiotics are equally effective, but make sure you tell the doctor that you have an allergy to penicillin.

The future of venereal diseases. It seems odd that we

haven't been able to eradicate these two diseases, since we have plenty of adequate antibiotics and the diseases have no place else to go and no one else to infect except man. Surely part of the explanation is related to the large group of untreated and unsuspecting women who carry gonorrhea in an asymptomatic state. The social stigma which our society has placed on people with VD has, until recently, hampered adequate treatment and follow-up of contacts. The epidemic will probably get worse for the next few years, and you may find it easier to catch syphilis or gonorrhea than ever before. The public health officials anticipate that the epidemic which is now upon us will evolve into a plague very soon if we don't take elaborate measures. Two hopeful possibilities are being studied. A vaccine against syphilis is almost ready and a vaccination sometime early in life will protect you, hopefully for years. Some people want to put anti-VD medicines into birth control pills to give you double-barreled protection. We personally favor the vaccine.

Sex and Pre-Marital Counseling

If we assume that not all men and women are as accomplished and as experienced as *Playboy* and *The Berkeley Barb* would like us to believe, then it is reasonable to assume that most people, even those with some experience, could use some advice about sex, particularly before getting married. Unfortunately, there is virtually nowhere to turn. The family doctor is among those least qualified to help. He has had no training (until recently) while in medical school in dealing with these questions, and his advice is tempered by his own experience or lack of it, his own moral and religious background, his personal hang-ups and problems, and what little he may have read in the general and medical literature. Doctors graduating from medical school today usually are much better trained to advise patients on sexual problems, but while the specifics of their training may be better, they have their own particular view of sex, and these may not be consistent with your views. They are no less human than anyone else. Clergymen are unusually poorly qualified to give advice on sexual problems: their intelligence, compassion, and insight are often profound, but may be distorted by a failing sense of reality, lack of experience, inhibited religious and moral views toward sex, and, frequently, major personal hang-ups. Your mother, father, and friends are not authoritative sources of information. They may be fun to talk to, but they probably learned it all from their mom, dad, and friends and, likely, in a less permissive era than today. You might get some more authoritative information from newspaper columnists, but their views of sexual problems seem remarkably distorted and are often more intent on amusing the readers than disseminating information.

The problems of sex are complex and depend, at the very least, on a reasonable familiarity with the anatomy and physiology of sexual functions; an understanding, or at least a perception, of the infinite variety of emotional and psychological reactions to sexual experiences; and the evolution of individual attitudes about sex which make each person comfortable, make it an enriching experience, and enable him to enjoy it without fear, confusion, anxiety, or guilt. We make no pretenses about our own capacity to be helpful in a short section in a general book such as this, and we are going to refer you to a number of good marriage manuals and guides to sexual practice which are commonly available. The best among these will take enough time and provide enough detail to accommodate the needs of most readers. You will have to select among them with consideration of your own attitudes, experiences, and personal philosophy and find one that makes you most comfortable. It is worth careful browsing. In general, we have found that those that deal with sex in a more direct and forthright way are preferable to those that substitute nice words for reality or those that suffuse platitudes about love and marriage. We recognize, though, that this represents our own individual views and may not be consistent with the views of some of our readers.

Even though your doctor (or any doctor) may not be the man to ask about your sexual problems (as if you could or would anyway), you should see a doctor before you get married. Most states require a blood test for syphilis before getting married, so you'll have to get it somewhere. It's a good chance and a sensible time for women to get a routine pelvic examination to make sure everything is in order inside. Some girls who have had no sexual experience before are surprised to discover that they have an imperforate or very tight hymen, a rigid membrane at the opening of the vagina. This can be stretched or cut without much trouble. If it isn't cut or dilated, it can be an unusual impediment to progress later and quite painful during sexual intercourse.

Young women should be alerted to the possibility of a bladder infection which occurs fairly often shortly after marriage and is euphemistically called "honeymoon cystitis" (cystitis refers to an infection in the bladder). Honeymoon cystitis is the result of frequent sexual intercourse in the first few weeks of marriage. The trauma, the stretching, and the frequency of intercourse result in some bacteria getting into the bladder. This warm, moist, and dark area is an ideal place for bacteria to multiply, and an infection, producing burning and frequent urination, often results. Once you have cystitis you'll probably need a sulfa drug to get rid of it (see Chapter 5, Urinary Tract Infections). One good way to prevent it from recurring is to urinate soon after intercourse. It gets most of the bacteria out of the bladder and is usually all that is needed.

Although the sexual activities and problems of youth, of newlyweds and of those during the reproductive years are what we mean when we talk about sex, we would like to emphasize the importance of the sexual needs of middle-aged and elderly people. Once the family is completed, or once the menopause sets in, the fires of passion and desire are not extinguished and buried forever. If we avoid equating sexual intimacy and sexual responsiveness solely with sexual intercourse, it becomes obvious that sexual needs in older years are often the same as those of younger people. True, there is a variable decrease in sexual activity as one gets older, both in men and in women, but it is not predictable or quantifiable and there is no value in keeping count, enumerating successes or initiating competition for the most frequent, the oldest or the best. What is much more important is the realization that middle-aged and older people have a continuing need for, and derive considerable satisfaction from, warm, close physical and emotional contact with other responsive human beings which transcends their overt sexual needs and does not diminish in intensity with age. Sexual activity takes the natural form its participants desire, and you may be reassured if it is different at age sixty from what it was at age twenty. A couple may get more real pleasure and satisfaction from just holding hands at age seventy-five than they did when they were fifteen and may enjoy each other sexually as much as whatever they were doing at age twenty-five.

Birth Control

The separation of sex from reproduction is now reliably possible. The factors which you must consider when deciding on which form of birth control you will use include: (1) the effectiveness of the method, (2) its convenience or inconvenience, (3) the esthetic aspects, (4) the potential side effects, (5) the dangers and problems, (6) what other benefits can be expected, if any, and (7) the relative cost.

There are five recommended forms of contraception: birth control pills, an intrauterine device (IUD), a diaphragm, a condom, or jellies, cream, foam, etc. There are many other forms of contraception which have been utilized, some for centuries, but which we cannot recommend primarily because they are not reliable. Cross off your list: the rhythm method, coitus interruptus or withdrawal, and abstinence, none of which is much more reliable than maybe chance alone.

Birth Control Pills: These pills act by preventing ovulation. If ovulation (which normally occurs monthly about halfway between the menstrual periods) does not occur, there cannot be any conception, since the sperm will have no ovum (egg) to fertilize. There are two types of birth control pills: the combination pill, which is much more commonly used, and the sequential pill, which will probably be withdrawn from utilization in the near future. There are no significant differences between the two in effectiveness or side effects.

Taking the pill requires a moderate amount of motivation, a fairly disciplined life style and the absolutely compulsive requirement that your pill be taken every day with religious devotion. Although it cannot be established with certainty, it is assumed that the vast majority of the very few "pill failures" are the result of skipping or forgetting a pill once too often. There are good instructions and advice included in the pill package and it is well worth your while to read them. Briefly, the pill is taken every day for twenty-one days. Two or three days after the last pill is taken, a normal menstrual period should begin. The next cycle of pills should be started on the fifth day of the period or the seventh day after the last pill from the previous cycle was taken, even if the bleeding persists or if the menstrual period is missed.

About 20 per cent of women taking the pill will have some undesirable side effects. These include a wide variety of problems such as nausea, swelling of the legs, weight gain, headaches, fatigue, mental depression, breast tenderness, and nervousness. Fortunately, the side effects generally are mild, almost always occur in the first one or two menstrual cycles after starting the pill, and tend to disappear subsequently. If these side effects persist or are severe, it may require discontinuation of the pills. More often, the troublesome side effects will diminish or disappear if a different pill formulation is used, particularly if you take a pill which has a lower dose of active constituents.

So much (maybe too much) has been said and written about the dangers of birth control pills. Let us try to offer some reassurance. The dangers of the pill are less than the dangers of pregnancy, particularly an unwanted or poorly timed pregnancy. The number of women who die during or as a result of their pregnancy is greater than the number of deaths among women who are taking the pill to prevent pregnancy. The pill is probably no more dangerous than tobacco or alcohol and, as a rough estimate, the risk of driving a car in the U.S. today is about equal to the risk of taking the pill. However, women who have certain medical problems, such as a history of thrombophlebitis (see Chapter 5), pulmonary embolism, hepatitis (Chapter 5), or cancer of the reproductive organs should not take the pill; nor should the pill be taken if you are already pregnant. These warnings suggest the importance of medical evaluation prior to starting the pills and regularly every six to twelve months as long as you continue to take them. There doesn't seem to be any reason why you can't take the pills indefinitely and some women have been using them for up to ten years with no serious consequences. Some doctors have suggested that you stop for a month or two every two or three years, during which time you can either get pregnant or use some other contraceptive technique.

The pill is extremely effective in preventing pregnancy. For every one hundred women taking the pill for a whole year, less than one pregnancy will result, and as we noted, this probably is not a failure of the pill, but of the pill taker.

There are additional benefits for some women taking the pill. There is a regularization of the menstrual cycle, usually a decrease in painful menses, and a decrease in the menstrual flow. Even if you are not concerned about getting pregnant, these might be good reasons to take the pill anyway.

Intrauterine Device (IUD): This is a small coil-like device that has been used for forty years and has only recently been widely accepted now that it can be made out of satisfactory and inert materials which don't produce any irritation. When the loop or the coil is inserted into the uterus, pregnancy only rarely occurs.

The IUD has to be inserted by a doctor. It is best put in during the last days of a menstrual period to make sure it isn't interfering with a preexisting pregnancy, but it can be inserted during the first week of the menstrual cycle as well. The IUD is less uncomfortable in women who have had a previous pregnancy. Women who have never been pregnant have a higher frequency of cramps from the IUD but it can be used nevertheless. There is a high incidence (about 30 per cent) of menstrual irregularities in women with an IUD and about 10 to 20 per cent of women have cramps. Like the pill, these side effects generally sort out and settle down after the first few menstrual cycles. For the 60 or 75 per cent of women who have the IUD and have no cramps or menstrual irregularities, the device is ideal. It is convenient, inexpensive, and requires no effort except an occasional check to see if it is still in place. Occasionally, the loop or coil will be spontaneously expelled but this can often be noticed by the patient herself. It can easily be reinserted by a doctor.

Pregnancy does occasionally occur with an IUD that is properly in place. It doesn't happen very often, but slightly more so than with the pill. The best estimates now are in the range of two pregnancies occurring in one hundred women using an IUD for a year; about twice as often as the pill.

The Diaphragm or cervical cap is a rubber cup on a flexible metal spring. It is inserted into the vagina and placed so as to close off the cervix, the opening of the uterus, and mechanically prevent the passage of sperm up into the uterus. It is best used with a sperm-killing cream placed inside and around the edge of the diaphragm before inserting it. It must be carefully fitted by a gynecologist and its size adjusted from time to time, particularly after a pregnancy. It will not do to borrow your friend's, even if you know precisely how to insert it.

The main problem with a diaphragm is its inconvenience. It has to be inserted before intercourse and left in place for at least eight hours afterward. It requires a conscious, deliberate act, it requires some manipulation of the genitalia, and in those circumstances where intercourse is not anticipated it retards the spontaneity of the process. In some people, these features make the process esthetically unacceptable; in others, these factors are incorporated into the foreplay with beneficial effect. Most of the problems can be obviated, though, by leaving the diaphragm in place for prolonged periods of time —days or even weeks if you care to, although you cannot have it in place during a menstrual period. Its presence, by the way, is not felt by either partner.

It certainly is a satisfactory method if the pills or an IUD cannot be used.

Pregnancy rates with a diaphragm are higher than the rates in those using the pill or an IUD. Estimates run in the range of five to ten pregnancies in one hundred women using a diaphragm for a year.

Condoms: These are named after the French physician Condom, who first thought of the idea, but it is likely that primitive variations were used for centuries before. A condom is a thin rubber sheath which is placed on the penis and acts as a simple mechanical barrier to the passage of sperm. It is probably best used in combination with a sperm-killing cream or jelly which is placed inside the vagina in case the condom should break or tear. It seems that while some women find the diaphragm inconvenient and unesthetic, some men find the condom as inconvenient and unesthetic and they also find that it interferes with the tactile sensation of intercourse. Other couples utilize the condom as part of the foreplay and prefer this method for that reason. Condom companies now manufacture thinner and stronger products to overcome some of the problems of sensory impairment.

One major advantage of the condom is that it decreases slightly, but does not entirely eliminate, the possibility of venereal disease. The condom is about as effective as the diaphragm in preventing pregnancy and about five to ten pregnancies occur in one hundred couples using this method for one year.

Jellies, creams, and foams: These materials contain a variety of sperm-killing agents. If any of these preparations is inserted into the vagina prior to intercourse, they do a fair job in killing sperm and preventing pregnancy. The protection is not as good as the other methods and the pregnancy rate goes up to twenty to twenty-five per one hundred women per year. This is almost in the range of being unreliable. However, the jellies, foams, and creams are simple, relatively safe, and fairly inexpensive. One major disadvantage has been the mess and sloppiness of it all, but some enterprising manufacturer is now producing a series of flavored products, a novelty which should compensate for some of these difficulties.

Non-Recommended Methods: The rhythm method is complicated, requires a high degree of motivation, periods of abstinence, and even when done correctly produces about thirty-five pregnancies in one hundred couples using this method for one year. That comes to about one chance in three of a pregnancy for each year of use, and statistically, you can count on a pregnancy about every three years if you use this method exclusively. This is not good enough by present standards.

The technique of withdrawal may have been admirable and satisfactory in 1850 when little else was available. It may be acceptable today in an emergency situation, but is not recommended for routine use.

Abstinence, of course, is 100 per cent effective if practiced regularly. It may be perfectly suitable during short periods, for example, the month or two when you stop the birth control pills every few years or during short periods when other methods must be discontinued or changed. Abstinence is an all-or-nothing phenomenon; it must be total or else forget it.

A COMPARISON OF BIRTH CONTROL METHODS

It is simple to compare the objective considerations with different methods. But people's personal preferences and habits, wide variations in normal sex practices and frequency, and many other subjective aspects can't be evaluated.

Effectiveness: When used properly, the pills are far and away most effective for birth control. In a semi-quantitative fashion the pills rate about 0.5–1.0, the IUD rates 2, the diaphragm and condom between 5 and 10, and jellies, foams, etc. get 20 to 25. The ratings represent the number of pregnancies resulting in 100 women who use this method for one year. The pill is 40 to 50 times more effective than foam.

Convenience: This is best measured in terms of how much or how little effort has to be expended to use the method. Far and away, the most convenient method is the IUD, which requires zero effort once it's in and settled. All the others are inconvenient to a varying degree. If you set up a pattern, the pills are not too inconvenient. The other three methods, the diaphragm, the condom and foam, are inconvenient at the very least because they interrupt the spontaneity and naturalness of coitus. The diaphragm has to be left in place for at least six to eight hours but can remain in place continually between menstrual periods.

Esthetic Aspects: The IUD and birth control pills do not in any way interfere with the enjoyment of coitus; some women, however, note a decrease in libido with the pill, while other women feel less constrained and inhibited on the pill and libido is increased. The diaphragm, if properly fitted, should not be felt by either partner, so it cannot be considered esthetically unacceptable except possibly in that it interrupts coitus. However, with a little foresight, the diaphragm can be inserted beforehand. The condom may decrease tactile sensation in some men, but its use, as with the diaphragm, can be incorporated in the foreplay and increase the enjoyment in some others. As we have noted, the foams are now favored

	Effectiveness	Convenience	Esthetics	Side Effects
	(Pregnancies per 100 women per year)			
BIRTH CONTROL PILLS	0.5	+	++++	Short term and Long term
IUD	2	++++	++++	Early and Transient
DIAPHRAGM	5–10	±	+++	None
CONDOM	5–10	±	+++	None
FOAM	20–25	±	++	None

and in fact act as a lubricant, so esthetically they can be quite acceptable.

Potential Side Effects: These are minimal with the diaphragm, the condom, or the foams. The side effects with the IUD are usually evident early, and if they are too troublesome, it can be removed. For a significant number of women with the IUD such effects are too severe and it can't be used. Most others have no trouble and for them the IUD is ideal. The side effects for the pill users are relatively frequent, annoying, but generally transient.

The Dangers: The diaphragm, condom, and foam carry with them no significant risk to the user. The IUD rarely can get into the wrong place, can perforate the uterus and can cause trouble. The dangers of the pills are notorious, probably greatly overstated considering the vast number of people taking them with no problems whatsoever, but can't be ignored. It is likely that other dangers will become more evident in the future.

Other Benefits: Besides preventing babies the pills tend to make menstrual periods more regular, frequently decrease or eliminate cramping pains during periods, tend to decrease the amount of bleeding and thereby decrease the problem with anemia. The foam or jellies can act as an effective lubricant.

	Dangers	Other Benefits	Cost
BIRTH CONTROL PILLS	++++	Substantial	Fixed and moderate
IUD	++	None	Once and moderate
DIAPHRAGM	None	None	Once and moderate
CONDOM	None	Prevents VD	Variable—Small
FOAM	None	Lubricant	Variable—Small

The condom may help prevent venereal disease. It probably decreases the likelihood of VD but it won't eliminate it completely and don't rely on it alone. As best as we can determine, the IUD and the diaphragm have no conceivable use other than preventing pregnancy.

Cost: The IUD and the diaphragm have one initial cost, and this includes the doctor's fee to insert the IUD or to fit the diaphragm. With reasonable care the diaphragm should last about two years, but it will have to be refitted after each pregnancy. The IUD can be left in place for years if desired. The cost of the foam or the condom depends on the frequency of coitus. It is relatively small, even for the most active couple. The pills represent a continuous expense regardless of frequency of coitus and a once or twice yearly doctor fee has to be considered.

The Future: The possibilities for the future are the once-a-month shots instead of the daily pill, pills to be taken after coitus to prevent pregnancy, and oral contraceptive pills for males. Post-coital pills or shots are available now to prevent pregnancy in unusual circumstances like rape. They have major side effects, however, and must be administered by a physician. (See the section on rape below.) These and many others are in varying stages of development. They may be years away, so don't postpone your plans.

Pregnancy

ARE YOU PREGNANT?

The most common cause of a missed menstrual period in a woman of childbearing age is childbearing. Simply stated, if you are between the ages of about eighteen to thirty-five, if you are not using any contraceptive device or technique, if you have had intercourse in the past two to four weeks and if you miss your period, the best bet is that you are pregnant. The age bracket could well be extended to about fourteen to forty-five. However, the likelihood of pregnancy is less after a missed period in the lower age level since so many girls normally have irregular or missed periods during their teens anyway. There is less of a likelihood of pregnancy in the upper age group because ovulation is less frequent. A significant number of older women start having irregular menstrual periods with the onset of the menopause.

If you are in a hurry to find out if you are pregnant, and can't wait until the pregnancy is obvious, a test for pregnancy can be positive as soon as three to four weeks after conception or about ten days after the missed menstrual period was to have begun. To be absolutely certain, it may be wise to wait for another week or two before getting the pregnancy test. All that is needed is a urine specimen. A concentrated urine is best, so bring in the first specimen obtained in the morning on arising. The results of the pregnancy test are accurate but not absolute. About 5 per cent of women who are really pregnant will have a negative test initially and about 2 per cent of women who are not pregnant will have a positive test. These results can disturb you, so if the test doesn't seem to fit with what you suspect, have the test repeated after a few weeks' delay. If the pregnancy test is done too early the results may be in error and may be very misleading. Better be patient than confused.

Many women, particularly those who have been pregnant before, can tell they are pregnant simply by how they feel, and the pregnancy test is really not necessary. However, it is probably wise to get your impression confirmed.

DO YOU WANT TO HAVE A BABY?

Once the pregnancy is confirmed, a few details may come to mind. You have only two months or so to decide if you want to have a baby. Having a baby is not like getting a kitten or buying a house, or even getting married. It's a major responsibility and an irrevocable decision. For some people, considering their life style, having a baby is a major disaster, a grotesque error and a tragic source of unhappiness for both the parents and the baby. For most others a baby is a source of enormous pleasure and brings a great deal of happiness and love into one's life. Don't have a baby to save a dying marriage or love affair, and don't have a baby to encourage a reluctant boyfriend. It is probably best to postpone a baby until you can swing the added financial burden, and until after you have done all those things you always dreamed of, or you may resent the baby. Some people aren't ready for the responsibilities and restrictions a baby brings. Some are never ready. For many, age is no factor and having a baby is the greatest thing in their lives. Having a baby is not simply a nine-month commitment but a full-time responsibility for years.

Think about it carefully before you make any definite decisions. Now for the first time in many states you have the right, the privilege, and the obligation to make that decision and it is a responsibility you should not ignore or assume lightly.

For the vast majority of women who happily look forward to having a baby, there are a few old wives' tales that should be buried, some advice you may need, and some questions we can answer.

DO YOU NEED A DOCTOR?

Why should a woman have to tolerate the impersonality, the sterile, aseptic, routinized pattern of obstetricians, hospitals, and delivery wards, with anesthetics, medications, masks, rules and regulations? Simply answered, you don't have to put up with this type of twentieth-century efficiency. If you were the only person involved, you would be free to make the simple decision and do it your own way. However, the baby is at least a 50 per cent partner in pregnancy and it is entitled to the best that medicine and science can manage.

Billions of women for thousands of years have had billions of babies all over the world without benefit of hospitals, episiotomies, saddle block anesthesia, visiting hours, or isolation. The world has managed to survive and those children who lived don't seem to be at any great disadvantage. Those babies who died or didn't make it through the first few months of life might not agree. Although we are doctors and are probably biased, we have no stake in trying to enrich the coffers of obstetricians. There are, however, so many good reasons for not having your baby at home and so many reasons for having your baby with the assistance of a competent doctor or midwife, particularly the first baby, that we are extremely reluctant to advise unattended home delivery under any circumstances.

If you live in a remote area, on a farm or on a rural commune, you may have no choice and may have to have your baby without medical assistance. In any case you should have a competent doctor or midwife check you periodically during the pregnancy to make sure none of the serious but potentially treatable and reversible complications is developing. We would like to stress the necessity for medical care during pregnancy by calling your attention to some statistics. In sections of rural Southeastern U.S. where about 50 per cent of women have their babies without a doctor's care, about five to ten times as many mothers will die during delivery as in urban, affluent America. On American Indian reservations, about three times as many mothers will die. It is obviously not as simple as all this, because other health and environmental factors are very much involved, but it is still reasonable to say that good medical care during pregnancy and delivery increases your chances of surviving your pregnancy and delivery about five- to eight-fold. The statistics are also impressive for the infants. The infant mortality in sections of the rural Southern U.S. is about 60 per 1,000. On Indian reservations about 38 of every 1,000 infants born will die. In affluent America it is reduced to about 20 per 1,000 babies. Your baby has a three-fold better chance if you get good and early medical care, twentieth-century style.

Don't confuse home delivery with natural childbirth. Natural childbirth techniques teach and prepare women to have their babies as naturally as possible, but under the care of a doctor, with modern medical facilities available if an unusual complication should develop. Natural childbirth requires a great deal of training and preparation of the mother during pregnancy so that a child may be born without pain medications and anesthesia and without the associated problems and complications sometimes seen with these medications. This can only be done if the mother is highly motivated and willing and able to prepare for her delivery. For those who stick with it and succeed, natural childbirth is a gratifying and joyful experience. Some women, despite adequate preparation and training, are not able to go through labor and delivery as naturally as planned and are sometimes left with a sense of failure, inadequacy, grief, and guilt. The alternative, if natural childbirth is unsuccessful, is a delivery which utilizes the normal medications available to medical science to make the delivery a less painful and safer process. The methods of natural childbirth are certainly not applicable to all women in all circumstances.

MEDICAL PROBLEMS OF PREGNANCY

It is a rare woman who is pregnant who doesn't have some medical problem of pregnancy. Most are only annoying, trivial, and transient. Some of these problems can make you miserable, and some can be devastating, threatening the life of the mother and the baby.

PROBLEMS WHICH REQUIRE A MEDICAL EVALUATION

Bleeding during pregnancy. This is seen in about 20 to 25 per cent of all pregnancies. It's usually nothing serious. It can be the first sign of a miscarriage (a spontaneous abortion) and it may be a sign of something as serious as a cancer of the cervix. There is no sense in just worrying about it. Have a doctor check it out.

Headaches, swelling of the feet and ankles, and blurred vision may be the sign of toxemia of pregnancy and/or high blood pressure, two common problems of pregnancy which can complicate things substantially and which must be treated. If the headaches persist, you should get your blood pressure checked and get your urine tested for protein. Swelling of the feet is common during pregnancy, but should not be ignored. It may require nothing more than a change in your diet with some salt restriction, or the use of a mild water pill to get rid of the extra fluid. Blurred vision may suggest high blood pressure and it, too, should not be ignored.

PROBLEMS WHICH USUALLY DON'T NEED A DOCTOR

Morning sickness: Some experienced women know they are pregnant when they feel nauseated and start vomiting in the morning. Nausea is a very common problem in the first two or three months of pregnancy. It usually occurs on an empty stomach, characteristically in the morning before breakfast. The nausea discourages the woman from eating breakfast, and of course this makes it worse.

Try keeping some dry food like dry cereal or crackers at the bedside and eat a handful before getting out of bed. Some women find sucking on some ice chips or drinking ginger ale relieves the nausea. There are pills and shots to take and they do work, but it is best to avoid any medication, no matter how urgent, during pregnancy, particularly during the first few months. Don't despair, the morning sickness usually clears up in a month or two.

Heartburn occurs toward the end of pregnancy. It is that burning, belching, and uncomfortable feeling in the pit of the stomach and up under the breastbone. It's advertised on TV a lot, and oddly enough, the antacids advertised are quite effective for relief of the symptoms. Any and all of the antacids are about equally effective. You can take the one that tastes best and is least expensive. Other than taste and cost, there is no significant difference among them for short-term usage and they are generally harmless. If you want to avoid medicines, take some baking soda, about a half teaspoon in a half glass of water. It's just as good as the antacids and is much cheaper. Too much baking soda may produce some fluid retention, as would ordinary salt. If you have noted ankle swelling or puffiness in the fingers or face, go easy on the baking soda and salt.

Vaginal discharge is a frequent annoying problem during pregnancy. There usually is nothing wrong and nothing need be done. If the discharge is very heavy, very itchy, or odorous, check the section on vaginal discharge (Chapter 5) to see if you can get any ideas there about what is going on. If it isn't too bad but bothersome, you might want to try a vinegar douche (add one-half cup of white vinegar to two cups of water) to restore the normal acidity of the vagina and give you some relief.

Hemorrhoids: These may first appear during pregnancy, but if you've had trouble with hemorrhoids before, they are almost certain to get worse during pregnancy and kick up during each subsequent pregnancy. The baby in the enlarged uterus puts pressure on the veins in the pelvis and the veins around the anus tend to engorge with blood. The hemorrhoids itch, frequently bleed, and sometimes are very painful. See the section on hemorrhoids (Chapter 5) for comments on how to deal with this problem.

Varicose veins are similar to hemorrhoids but appear in the legs, usually in the veins on the back of the calves and behind the knees. Don't confuse the small and thin bluish veins seen just under the skin with varicose veins. These small visible veins are normal and of no consequence, except that most women are very sensitive about their appearance. Not much can or should be done about them. The varicose veins are enlarged, thick, and swollen veins, sometimes with a lumpy feeling, sometimes painful and tender, and often associated with a dragging, cramping sensation in the legs. The single best thing to do for varicose veins is to try to get as much rest as possible with the legs elevated. This is foolish advice if you have other kids to take care of or are working and standing all day. Support stockings may help relieve some of the discomfort. If the veins get very tender and inflamed you may have thrombophlebitis (see Chapter 5). The veins can be removed surgically if necessary, but wait until the end of pregnancy and reconsider it then, when you've taken the stress off the veins.

Urinary frequency occurs early, and in mid-pregnancy. It gets better toward the end of pregnancy as the enlarging uterus starts to lift out of the pelvis, taking the pressure off the bladder. There isn't much you can do about urinary frequency. You may cut down on the amount of water and fluids you drink, particularly in the evening, so you can get an uninterrupted night's sleep. If the frequent urination is associated with burning or pain, with flank pain or pain in the mid-abdomen or with fever, there may be an associated urinary tract infection (see Chapter 5).

GENERAL ADVICE

If it's your first pregnancy, you are sure to have many questions you often forget to ask the doctor or feel embarrassed to waste his time on such trivia. Most people turn to their family and friends and get the advice that is passed on from generation to generation as old wives' tales, a combination of superstition, myths, black magic, frustration, and fears, mixed in with a generous helping of experience. Some of the advice is sound and some is foolish. Some is dangerous. Times and attitudes change along with the accumulation of knowledge and new experience. We think the advice we offer is sound. It will undoubtedly be disputed by your mother and mother-in-law who know better.

Expected date of delivery: There are lots of methods for calculating when you are due, but the simplest is to add seven days to the first day of your last period (if you keep track of such things) and then subtract three months. For example, if your last period started October 8, add seven days to get October 15 and then subtract three months to get July 15. It's a pretty good approximation. You can work it the other way around if you want your baby to be born on a certain date. Say you pick Christmas. Add 3 months to get March 25 and then subtract a week to get March 18. If your period starts near this date, you should concentrate your efforts in the next two or three weeks to coincide with the next time of ovulation, about April 1.

Drugs or medicines: As a simple rule, no drugs at all should be taken during pregnancy, particularly in the first three months, except those given to you by your doctor. He will probably confine his medications to vitamin pills, maybe some iron pills (see comments on nutrition below), a diuretic if you are accumulating fluid, and maybe some aspirin. You should certainly avoid any psychedelics, hallucinogens, stimulants, barbiturates, or any other drugs (see the section on psychotropic drugs in Chapter 6). No one knows what kind of effect these drugs have on the very delicate and small baby trying to get a very complex human being all together in the right order and in the right place, particularly in the first two months. Some drugs (such as Thalidomide) have proven catastrophic effects and no one really knows which ones are harmless and which ones are destructive and in what dose taken for how long. It is best to assume that they are all dangerous, and we suggest a little discipline for the baby's sake.

Coitus: This old habit is one which you needn't give up once you get pregnant. Another old wives' tale shot down. Some people may notice a little mechanical problem in the last month or so, but you are free to use your imagination as necessary. If you have had previous medical difficulty with abortions or premature labor it probably would be wise to practice abstention rather than jostle things too much in the last month or two. No birth control measures are necessary during pregnancy.

Tobacco and Pot: There is some evidence that women who smoke during pregnancy have a greater likelihood of having an unsuccessful pregnancy than non-smokers. The risk is small, although definite and probably more significant in women who have had unsuccessful pregnancies in the past. Babies born to women who smoke generally weigh less at birth than those born to non-smokers, for whatever importance that may have to anyone. No one has any idea whether smoking pot has any deleterious effect on the baby if you smoke it while you are pregnant. Marihuana does not appear to have any profound effect, but don't take this as a scientific fact. We don't know, just like everyone else doesn't know.

Alcohol: Alcohol has never been shown to hurt the baby unless Mom has a habit of falling off bar stools. Too much of anything is no good for you, and too much booze can't be good for the baby.

Constipation: Before we get too involved in this, we suggest you turn to the discussion on bowel habits in Chapter 3. The uterus, which is enlarged with the growing baby, tends to put pressure on the lower intestine and some mechanical constipation may result, usually in women who have had trouble with constipation in the past. Try the simplest things first for the sluggish bowels. In the past you have been advised to try to arrange a general daily habit or pattern for bowel movements, but in some ways, for some people, this makes them obsessive and compulsive about their bowels—an objectionable feature, in most people, and probably more so in people who tend to have sluggish bowels in the first place. Drink lots of fluid, eat lots of granola, drink lots of prune juice, eat lots of roughage. If you still have no luck, an ounce of milk of magnesia every so often should do it, but don't make a habit of it. Your next best bet is some mineral oil taken at bedtime only if necessary and certainly not regularly. If you are still having problems and your diet is pretty sensible, we suggest you have a long talk with the doctor and see if he wants to look into it any further. We have avoided suggesting any enemas, since most people having babies these days have either never dealt with an enema and are completely turned off by the whole concept, or have unfortunately had to deal with them sometimes in the past and loathe using them. We don't like to make anyone unhappy when another solution may be available, so no need to resort to enemas.

Douching has been discussed above in commenting on vaginal discharge, and in Chapter 5, on vaginitis. Generally we would advise keeping it to a minimum with the simplest and mild solutions. Use a bag with low pressure and stay away from bulb syringes which may inadvertently inject some air into the uterus.

Exercise is a good idea and should continue during your pregnancy. It's probably a good idea to avoid contact sports, since a sharp blow to the abdomen may do a little damage to a very soft baby. Don't push the exercise. Fatigue, like sloth, is no good for you. Swimmers may be reassured that water does not enter the vagina to infect the baby, an observation which demolishes another old wives' tale. Regular and moderate exercise will improve your general sense of well-being.

Travel: There is no reason why you can't travel anywhere

by any means you desire. Commercial airplanes are satisfactorily pressurized and there is no risk to you or the baby. Long car trips tend to be tiring. If you have varicose veins, a long trip by any conveyance, if you have to stay put for a long time, may cause trouble with an increase in leg swelling and pain. Don't plan your trip so you end up having your baby in an airplane en route anywhere. If you have to be away for an emergency near the expected time of delivery, it may be wise to try to make some medical arrangements in advance or as soon as feasible.

Nutrition: There is nothing magical or obscure about your diet during pregnancy. Remember that you have to supplement your normal intake to allow for the enormous needs of a rapidly growing baby, and to simultaneously avoid excessive weight gain. During a normal pregnancy, you should expect to gain about sixteen to twenty pounds. Most of this will be rapidly lost at the time of delivery or shortly thereafter. If you are overweight to begin with, you have to be particularly careful about weight gain during the pregnancy and keep in mind the additional nutritional requirements of the baby. The emphasis should be on moderation of calories without unnecessary sacrifice of essential nutrients. See the discussion of food, eating, and weight reduction later in Chapter 7.

Weight maintenance during pregnancy is not just a cosmetic necessity or a convenience. Excessive weight gain will increase the risks of kidney and heart problems of pregnancy. These occur with much higher frequency in fat women. The pregnancy and delivery are more difficult and the risk to the baby is increased substantially when the mother is overweight.

Unfortunately, the eating habits of young women in America today are intemperate, eccentric, or impulsive. They represent the conglomerate of the stresses of chronic, unsuccessful weight-reduction efforts and Madison Avenue pressures. A few scattered recent attempts at more wholesome food are encouraging. The consequences of the unusual eating habits of malnutrition of young women may be quite serious during pregnancy. They certainly are poorly understood. Many women are malnourished in one way or another and some are anemic due to an iron deficiency. The effects of these deficiencies on the state of health and the well-being of a non-pregnant adult are not too clear unless the deficiency is profound or chronic. The effect of maternal malnutrition on an unborn infant is also not clearly established, but the infant is almost surely substantially more vulnerable to a slight nutritional deficiency. The evidence that malnutrition impairs optimum brain development in the fetus is now starting to accumulate, and the evidence is strong enough to warrant serious concern. Furthermore, the brain damage is likely to be permanent. A slight deficiency may result in a significant defect in the growing infant. Babies born to malnourished mothers are starting off with a handicap, and pregnant women should make a serious effort to eat sensibly and supplement their diet with vitamins and minerals if there is any question about the nutritional adequacy of their diet.

HAVING THE BABY

Most doctors and hospitals will have standard instructions for you regarding the procedures and policies which you will encounter when you are ready to deliver. Any specific advice which we may give you here may not be applicable to your own situation. If your doctor doesn't spell out what, where, and how, when you are ready, ask him.

Your first labor pains may be phony and you needn't summon the fire department when you get your first cramp. Women who have never had a baby before have a fair amount of time from the onset of labor until the baby is delivered. A great deal of haste and panic—speeding along highways with its attendant anxiety and more importantly, its dangers—is usually not necessary. The average time of labor for the first pregnancy is fourteen hours. Once you've had a baby the subsequent deliveries are usually much faster (the average duration of labor is only eight hours). If you've had a whole bunch of kids, don't dawdle around. The labor is likely to be precipitous and rapid and you may end up having your baby in the back seat of a car or in a hospital elevator en route to the delivery room.

BREAST-FEEDING

For several reasons, it seems logical that breast-feeding is better than bottle-feeding in the first few months of life. One of its primary advantages appears to be the touching, holding, and cuddling of the baby during the feeding, but this is a sensation that the baby can appreciate just as well if bottle-feeding is done properly. Some women can't breast-feed. Some women find breast-feeding impossible for social, economic, or cultural reasons. Only about 5 per cent of women in America breast-feed the baby. The other 95 per cent are not bad or inadequate mothers for taking to the bottle, particularly if the bottle is done well. For comments on how and when check with Dr. Spock.

Abortion

Attitudes, policies, and laws are rapidly changing in the world of abortions. This has largely been the result of a combination of three concepts whose time has come: (1) a new understanding and appreciation of the rights of women, (2) a much more far-sighted and informed understanding of the population problems and the need for population limitation, and (3) a reluctant realization that hundreds of thousands of women were getting criminal and dangerous abortions, often at the hands of less than competent practitioners. We shall make no effort to enter the complex emotional, ethical, religious, and moral aspects of abortions or the rights of the unborn child. We shall discuss some of the medical aspects of abortions as they are pertinent today to the many women faced with the problem of an unwanted or unplanned pregnancy.

A number of states are rapidly moving into enlightened abortion reform. In other states, the courts are dragging governmental officials into modification of legal sanctions and requiring public health agencies to make abortions available to any woman regardless of her ability to pay. The laws, which vary from state to state, are confused still further by policies and practices which frequently vary in a major way in different localities or different hospitals within a state.

Whatever advice we offer is not uniformly applicable and must be modified to your particular needs and your locality. The latest compilation of the status of abortion laws is included in Appendix 5. Regardless of these differences, some generalizations are useful.

The demand for abortion has increased so rapidly in those states with liberalized abortion laws that hospitals are often not able to keep up with the increased need. Many hospitals now arrange to do out-patient abortions without the need for hospitalization. In many communities non-profit clinics with hospital back-up arrangements can do careful abortions at a reasonable cost and provide a comfortable, sympathetic and dignified atmosphere. In these out-patient abortions you can expect to go home a few hours after a relatively simple procedure. The need for overnight hospitalization arises only if a complication develops or if an underlying medical problem is present.

An abortion should be done as soon as possible once the pregnancy has been confirmed. The state laws vary regarding the maximum duration of pregnancy permitted. Both the medical and legal problems become increasingly difficult after about the third month.

In some areas all that is needed for an abortion is the request of the mother (and sometimes the father). In others, the rules limit abortions to certain conditions or indications. These generally (but not always) include: psychiatric or medical conditions in the mother which would be made worse if the pregnancy were to be completed, rape, incest, and the probability of fetal abnormality. The psychiatric category is interpreted with a varying degree of compassion, compulsion, and caution in different localities. In some areas a non-psychiatrist can attest to the psychiatric problems associated with continuing the pregnancy.

An abortion should be done by a competent physician in a proper hospital or clinic with adequate facilities to handle any complications or problems. Hopefully and gratefully the days of the "coat hanger job" performed by the local practitioner in a small room behind a bar in the sleazy part of town are gone.

Most large cities have an abortion referral service which can advise you how to best obtain an abortion. A major consideration is the cost, and these agencies can put you on to the proper place depending on your finances. These agencies should not charge you a fee for referring you to a doctor. If they do, you had best seek advice elsewhere. If no such service exists, check with a Planned Parenthood Agency for guidance.

Rape

The legal and moral aspects of rape, the psychologic problems of the rapist or of the child molester, the problems of incest, the ethical problems of capital punishment, the paramilitary methods of avoiding rapists, or the legal methods of demonstrating and proving a rape has occurred: these profound problems are beyond the limits of this book. Although for every rape there must be a rapist and his problems, the woman who has been raped and the problems she's got to face are equally serious. (Except for pregnancy, these comments apply to male victims of rape as well.)

There are three main areas of concern for a person who has been raped. First are the sometimes severe emotional problems associated with being raped, the concern for possible venereal disease, and the possibility of pregnancy resulting from the rape.

The emotional response to being raped varies greatly. We have seen women who shrug it off as part of the risk of living in the city. At the other end of the spectrum some women are completely and permanently emotionally disabled after being raped. Probably both of these responses are unusual and extreme, although it is admittedly impossible to define a normal or appropriate response to anything as extreme as rape. The emotional response depends, at the very least, on the age and experience of the woman, the preconceived notions she has about rape, the circumstances of the rape, how well she knows the rapist, and the violence or threat of violence involved. Dozens of other factors enter into a woman's emotional response, and we should not ignore the sense of guilt she might have for allowing the circumstances to proceed to a point where a rape was inevitable or for possibly provoking or stimulating the rapist.

There are no standard or simple methods of dealing with the emotional problems of rape. The situation usually requires tact and genuine and thoughtful consideration for the woman's privacy. Sincere effort should be made to avoid increasing the victim's embarrassment, a situation one can rarely find at the front desk of most police stations. A rape victim needs to be reassured and needs the comfort and safety of friends and family, not the lonely despair and guilt she often feels by withdrawing and avoiding them. Children who are raped often suffer far more from family responses and attitudes than from the rape itself; and although the rape of a child obviously can't be taken lightly, every effort should be made to avoid making too much of a big deal about it.

Professional psychiatric counseling is probably not necessary or desirable for most women who have been raped. Some women are plagued with obsessive memories and dreams, alteration in attitudes toward sex and men, guilt and depression. If these problems persist beyond a reasonable time or are of such severity as to interfere with normal activities, professional counseling can be of some help.

Venereal disease is probably a common complication of rape. People who rape other people are not known for being considerate or for having an excessive concern about their own personal health and hygiene. In addition, an increase in sexual activity in rapists is not unusual and exposure to prostitutes may predispose to the likelihood of venereal disease. If you have been raped you should get a check-up with a gynecologist, even if you have no symptoms of venereal disease. Tell him you have been raped (or are concerned about venereal disease, if you don't want to get into the legal predicament with the rape) so he can do the appropriate tests including a blood test for syphilis. Refer to the section on venereal diseases for more details.

Many states have adapted a more enlightened attitude toward abortions in pregnancies resulting from rape, but this usually requires police documentation, and the complications of this process may well make the problem more, rather than less, difficult.

Being raped is bad enough; having an abortion because of it is another problem, but having to deal with police and legal maneuvering around the abortion is an experience that most women would not care to participate in. Substantially better and easier than an abortion is the "morning-after pill." Medications are available which can prevent pregnancy from developing if the medications are taken promptly and properly after coitus. The medications will probably make you sick for a few days but it seems like a small price to pay. The medications, pills or an injection, will have to be administered by a physician. Don't wait too long after the morning after.

If you are using a reliable method of contraception or if your next period comes on time and is normal, you are out of the woods. If your period is delayed or absent, it may be due to the fact that menstrual regularity can often be upset by severe emotional trauma like rape, but it also may be due to the fact that you are pregnant. Don't wait too long to find out.

Psychiatric Problems

There has been a flourishing of the psychiatry and the parapsychiatry business in the past decade, and it seems that almost everyone who took a semester of introductory psychology in college is now leading encounter groups or opening marriage counseling offices. This new understanding of psychiatry has dissipated many myths about psychiatric treatment. Not all psychiatry is conducted on a couch (much of it is done in group sessions) and the purpose of psychiatric hospitals is not simply confinement.

This increased sophistication and public acceptance of the role of psychiatry, however, has generated a great deal of newer confusion, misinformation, and misinterpretation.

Everyone has experienced some emotional problems at some time. Those who insist that they have no stress or problems and have never had any must surely be naïve, unaware, or dull. The vast majority of emotional problems, however, do not require the intervention of a psychiatric therapist. A specific diagnosis is rarely necessary, nor possible in most cases. Anxiety or emotional stress is often due to simple everyday problems: finances, concern about one's personal status or feelings about worth and affection. Situational factors continually reappear: job, parents, boss, in-laws, exams, girlfriends, boyfriends. Rarely do they incapacitate and very seldom are they profound or prolonged enough to require psychiatric assistance. Most of these anxiety-provoking emotional problems pass readily. Their existence and their resolution frequently serves to strengthen the ability to deal with future problems.

There are three general areas of disruption which create stress and anxiety and which may precipitate psychiatric illness.

- The most likely precipitating factor is a change in the relation to other people or objects. These are the conflicts typified by marital problems, family problems, or romantic problems. A crisis at the job, or an argument with the boss creates anxiety and stress. An unhappy marriage, an argument with unsympathetic parents or a teenage son—these are the crises in person-to-person relations which create anxiety, and if the stress is long enough or strong enough or repeated enough it results ultimately in psychiatric illness.

• A change in an individual's self-esteem or body image is a second general area of stress. Although the relationship with other people and objects is frequently more obvious, a change in one's self-esteem or body image can be just as devastating. (There is obviously much overlap since a change in your self-esteem may well be caused, for example, by a change in your relation to other people.) Stress can be precipitated by the discovery that one is not as accomplished as he thinks or by the knowledge of a serious disease such as cancer. The problems of impotence are just as real as the loss of a limb, and although the specific distortion in body image related to impotence or frigidity is entirely different from the loss of an arm, the stress it creates is very much the same.

• The third major area is the recurrent conflict, between values and the temptations of affluent society: the crisis of happiness vs. money; do what I should vs. do what I want. In recent years this has become a much misunderstood source of stress and anxiety for young people in particular.

These three categories represent an outrageous oversimplification of the complex problems of social, moral, and environmental stress. Using these generalizations, however, may provide some perspective.

The following discussion of psychiatric problems does not adhere to any precise psychiatric nomenclature. Most of the terminology is loosely used and often not defined. The discussion does not dwell on the severe or chronic psychoses which almost always require the intervention of psychiatric therapists and sometimes require medications or hospitalization. Attention is directed toward the common problems and symptoms of psychologic distress; toward what an untrained friend or family member can do to help in the early stages of an illness; and toward the signs indicating when professional psychiatric intervention is necessary.

Psychiatric emergencies are, broadly, emotional responses or behavioral patterns which seriously threaten the patient or others. They occur when an extremely stressful situation overwhelms a normal person's ability to adapt or when a mild or moderate stress overwhelms a person with impaired adaptive ability. A psychiatric emergency is not only a potential suicide or homicide. It may sometimes be an intense rage with destructive manifestations, or severe agitation. It may be a panic reaction or severe confusion of thought or intellect. The emergency is in part related to the severity and the abruptness of the problem, but more important, to its destructive potential and to its progression; a rapidly deteriorating situation constitutes more of an emergency than a stable or improving psychosis, despite the possible severity of the latter.

Among the more common psychiatric problems are the following:

DEPRESSION

Everyone will be depressed at times, since depression represents a normal reaction to an unhappy situation. Well-adjusted people have fluctuating moods of depression and elation during their day-to-day life. It isn't until the depths of depression become profound or prolonged or inappropriate that you need to get concerned. Do not confuse depression with grief. In many ways they are the same, but, as a simplification, grief is a reaction to a real external phenomenon (i.e., the death of someone you love or the dissolution of a marriage), whereas depression does not necessarily have a specific precipitating cause. A grief reaction must be measured in very individual terms, but when it becomes too prolonged, profound, or inappropriate, then you should be concerned with abnormal depression and not just reactive grief.

Some types of depression are associated with a specific

external phenomenon, but these differ from grief because they appear to be unreasonably intense. Some women develop a profound depression after the delivery of a child which may be related to a fear of the inability to perform successfully as a mother, or fear of a resentment toward the baby. Occasionally a depression results when the mother realizes that she doesn't love her baby as much as she feels she should. Menopausal or climacteric depression is common and may reflect the fear of aging or the sense of frustration of not having accomplished all that was planned in life.

There are characteristic signs of depression besides the obvious unhappiness, tearfulness, and despondency. Early signs which should alert you to a more serious depression include loss of appetite, a decrease in libido, irritability, a sense of hopelessness, a loss of interest, and general apathy. As the depression gets worse, more disabling symptoms may be noted. The loss of appetite may lead to weight loss. Insomnia, with the characteristic early-morning awakening, may lead to disturbances in the sleep-awake cycle. Bizarre physical complaints which could not have any physical basis become an obsession. There may be a paradoxical agitation and restlessness which contrasts with the apathy usually seen in severe depression.

Unless a severe depression is treated, it may get worse and more intense. The symptoms and the manifestations are unpleasant and uncomfortable for everyone, and the chronically depressed person loses his friends, alienates his family, and irritates his companions. Sometimes the best and simplest treatment is just talking about it. It is often better to discuss the problem with someone alert, intelligent, and compassionate who can remain objective, rather than a professional or a stranger. Regardless of whether the therapist is professional or not, he will be most effective if he offers empathy rather than sympathy, if he gives support and understanding, but meticulously avoids giving the depressed patient any further reason to feel sorry for himself or feel guilty. It often becomes evident that the depression is a manifestation of real guilt (i.e., "I didn't see my mother for two years before she died") or imagined guilt (i.e., "I'm not good enough for my family"). Although some of the guilt may be valid and justifiable, it serves no purpose to reinforce it and thereby the depression. Frequently the expression and the tacit admission of guilt to an empathic listener is enough to reverse the depression.

If the depressive symptoms continue, if weight loss and insomnia become severe, if the apathy and lethargy interfere with normal family or occupational obligations, if physical complaints increase in severity or if ruminations about worthlessness and suicide appear, then professional psychiatric help is needed without delay. You may find that the miserably depressed, often guilt-ridden patient greets the suggestion not with apathy, indifference, or resistance, but with relief.

SUICIDE

Suicide threats, suicide gestures, talking about and obsessions with suicide are all very much the same; they should not be ignored and must be taken seriously. Not all suicidal ruminations are the result of a severe and prolonged depression, although they frequently are. Many people who attempt suicide do so as their only way to manage, control, or avoid an acute crisis in their lives, and it may not be related to a depressive reaction. A suicide attempt is often a form of coercion; an angry wife takes a handful of sleeping pills as a gesture to her husband hoping to save a failing marriage, or a jilted boyfriend stands on the side of a bridge to rekindle a dying romance. Sometimes a suicide attempt is an extreme method of asking for help, and when someone has nowhere to go, no one to turn to and no resources and his adaptive ability is utterly exhausted, he slashes his wrists and calls an ambulance. In desperation he pleads for someone out there to acknowledge his problem and to help. Rarely is a suicide attempt a manifestation of a severe underlying psychosis, a consequence of hallucinations, or the inadvertent unfortunate result of a bad acid trip.

Suicide threats and gestures may be real or manipulative, but they should all be taken seriously. Those who threaten suicide often succeed and those who are successful have often threatened or in some way communicated their intention prior to their suicide. There are certain clues which should alert you to impending suicide.

- A deep, intense and prolonged depression sometimes terminates in a suicide. Don't ignore severe depression.
- When a chronically depressed, anxious person suddenly appears content, placid, happy, and no longer depressed, it sometimes means that he has come to terms with his problem, has decided to commit suicide, and has made his plan. It may be a great relief to him, but it should be a warning to you of possible impending suicide.
- Anyone who has made any previous suicide efforts or expressed any suicide threats in the past should be taken seriously when he starts talking about the futility of it all.
- A new pattern of alcohol excess or unusual drug abuse is sometimes a sign of depression and impending suicide.
- Beware of severe depression or anxiety in your friends or relatives who have what is called "poor impulse control" or a tendency to act out their impulses.
- An increase in interpersonal alienation or an abrupt change from a normal or outgoing, gregarious individual to an introverted and brooding loner may not have any real significance, but it may be a sign of chronic depression and impending suicide.
- If you hear expressions of utter hopelessness, which can be anything from, "I'm sure I'm going to flunk out," "No one understands or appreciates me," or "I give up on trying to work things out," you should note that a person may be trying to tell you something else besides what he is saying.
- An abrupt lowering of one's self-esteem is sometimes the precipitating event leading to suicide. Be careful when some-

one has just been humiliated in public or gets the word that he just isn't what he thought he was, particularly if he is known to be impulsive.
- If someone tells you of his plan to commit suicide, it is worthwhile taking him seriously. People don't say things like this without some reason.
- Watch out for the person who hears voices directing him to harm himself.
- Suicide is not infrequent in people with severe chronic diseases, particularly if they are associated with incapacitation, intolerable pain, or short life expectancy.

The best thing to do when you suspect an impending suicide is to ask about it. Try a little tact and discretion, but it sometimes pays to be direct rather than subtle or obscure. If you feel you can't or don't want to handle it, you should tell someone who can and should check it out before it's too late; parents, spouses, the dean or a doctor, or call Suicide Prevention if there is a branch in your city. Most people contemplating suicide are embarrassed but pleased to know that someone cares and offers to help. Perhaps, in retrospect, it may have been unwise for you to intervene in a particular situation where your assessment of a possible suicide was inaccurate, but you can't know this and it is always better to err on the side of caution.

Rarely, a suicide may be a sincere desire on the part of an intelligent, rational individual who wants to extricate himself from an intolerable and insoluble situation or from one where the only solution may appear to involve suicide. We assume that this occurs so infrequently that external manipulation and interference is justified in every case. We assume that every suicide gesture represents an error in judgment and that it is not proper to permit a suicide to proceed believing that the victim knows what is best for himself. We would rather accept the criticism for meddling than for abandoning the patient who needs help.

PSYCHIATRIC ASPECTS OF SEXUAL PROBLEMS

Sexual deviation and perversion: If abnormal sexual behavior could readily and accurately be defined, then perhaps society would be much better able to deal with it. The problems of sexual deviation and sexual perversion are so deeply imbedded in medieval morality, religious hysteria, and legal condemnation that even enlightened psychiatrists are often unable to deal appropriately with these problems. Theoretically, sexual deviation and perversion may be any sexual act which is obnoxious or repulsive to an observer. However, since most sexual activity is not performed in public or in the presence of an observer, whatever sexual activity is performed cannot be considered perverse as long as it is not considered so by the participants.

It seems reasonable to assume that virtually everyone has a covert interest in the unusual aspects of sexuality. Those men and women who derive their major sexual gratification in activity other than normal coitus, probably represent the group whom society can refer to as sexual deviants and their activity as perverse. Almost any type of activity imaginable can and probably does accompany normal coitus, but this cannot and should not be considered pathologic. What is deviant or perverse depends on what is "normal," a term which we are unable to define.

By this definition, there is more sexual perversity in men than women, but this may be due to the constraining effect society places on women and the passive role they are forced to assume in the sex act. Specific forms of sexual deviation include pedophilia (sexual activity with children), fetishism (sexual fixation on certain parts of the body such as hair, or on certain objects of clothing such as shoes), transvestism (sexual gratification from wearing clothing of the opposite sex), exhibitionism (gratification from displaying one's genitals in public or before others), voyeurism (sexual pleasure from watching others perform sexually—the classic "peeping

Tom"), and sado-masochism (achievement of sexual pleasure by inflicting or experiencing pain). The list can continue. It ultimately is limited only by what has been described often enough to have a name, but the human imagination has no bounds and it is certain that other forms of sexual perversion exist.

Society should distinguish between those acts of sexual deviation and perversion which are actual threats to others or to the public welfare, and those which are simply annoying or unpleasant or which only arouse the anxiety of the public. It seems reasonable that society should legally intervene if the activity involves coercion or violence, if it involves a minor, or perhaps if it occurs in public. These acts are entirely different from the annoyances of a peeping Tom or the unpleasant fright when confronted by an exhibitionist, although it is not unreasonable to assume that an impressionable child or a very fragile adult may be emotionally devastated by such a nonviolent experience.

Those criminal sexual acts which occur among two or more consenting adults in private are a classic example of a crime without a victim (except perhaps society). But if society is so offended by these acts, it might stop straining to hear the neighbors and put away its binoculars, and the crime will rapidly vanish.

The treatment of sexual deviation and perversion is difficult and sometimes futile. Much depends on how the individual views his unusual behavior. It is sometimes associated with a profound sense of shame and disgust despite the gratification and pleasure it provides. In these cases, if the individual voluntarily seeks help, there is a great deal that can be done. If the individual enjoys his habits, if they provide his sole source of gratification, if he is oblivious to the shame and if he is dragged into therapy by his family or the courts, it seems reasonable to assume that he will rarely benefit from psychiatric treatment.

Homosexuality: It is likely that there is some homosexuality in all of us. In some, the homosexuality is greater than the heterosexuality and the characteristic pattern is then apparent. In most people the heterosexuality predominates. Some unusual people are able to enjoy both aspects; they may marry, have children, and enjoy homosexual activity as well. Heterosexual people can sometimes revert (not regress) to homosexual behavior under periods of stress or prolonged isolation as in prisons, in the Army, and in boarding schools.

Society considers homosexuality "abnormal" if the homosexual behavior is persistent or repetitious beyond puberty. We use the word "abnormal" with caution. In view of the established social mores or existing laws, and in consideration of many psychiatric theories, the homosexual is suffering from a complex pathologic disease regardless of how it is derived; whether he has it forced on him, or he acquires it, or he is born that way. Most homosexuals would disagree, and more enlightened social, religious, and medical groups also deny that homosexuality is a pathologic entity at all. They feel that the only problem is that of society which is unable to accept anything but heterosexual behavior as normal.

Despite these reasonable assertions, the fact is that many homosexuals have considerable emotional and adjustment problems, far greater than suffered by the heterosexual population. A realistic view, however, is that society's attitude and condemnation of homosexual behavior and the emotional turmoil which it creates is, in fact, responsible for a large part of these emotional problems.

Many homosexuals don't want psychiatric treatment. Many have treatment thrust upon them by anxious parents, misguided guidance counselors, and vindictive courts. There has been some success with homosexuals who want to become heterosexual. Aversion therapy is a form of treatment where homosexual images are associated with painful "punishment" and heterosexual images are associated with pleasurable "reward." This method has enjoyed some success in deconditioning the homosexual, but very few therapists are convinced that this form of treatment does anything for the underlying homosexual attitudes and desires. The treatment may represent more the subconscious attitude of the therapist. It would appear more rational to assume that an individual should be able to voluntarily select his own sexual role—"normal or abnormal"—and that violent efforts to change it seem extreme. A motivated individual ought to be able to obtain successful therapy for sexual problems without having to fear violence or punishment.

Impotence and frigidity: Impotence and frigidity refer primarily to an inability to achieve orgasm during coitus, but the terms also describe an individual who cannot successfully function sexually or cannot obtain physical or emotional satisfaction from coitus. Transient impotence and frigidity are common and normal. They do not imply any underlying physical or psychologic disorder. Transient or intermittent sexual inability is sometimes a reflection of anxiety or depression, often a manifestation of preoccupation or fatigue or a sign of simple boredom with an unimaginative, unstimulating, or inept sexual partner.

If the impotence (in men) or the frigidity (in women) persists, there may be other problems. Occasionally, these are physical: a chronic illness, the result of some drug or medicine, sometimes chronic excessive alcohol, or rarely an unusual urologic or gynecologic disorder. Most of the time the impotence or frigidity is a manifestation of some psychologic problem. It sometimes is the result of guilt or anxiety about the whole sex act, or perhaps guilt associated with infidelity. Fear or hostility of one of the partners may result in sexual inability. A castrating woman will make a man impotent with a casual remark to belittle him. In some people impotence and frigidity may be a sign of homosexuality. The frigid woman is sometimes angry about being used only as a sex object. Some people reject sex as dirty or accept it reluctantly without pleasure only to perform a duty. Some people are responsive to one partner but not another.

The treatment for chronic impotence or frigidity is very difficult but can be successful. A whole lifetime of fears, superstitions, and misconceptions may have to be corrected. A whole course in sexual technique may have to be initiated. Social problems and living arrangements may have to be changed and contraceptive advice is often necessary. Hormones and aphrodisiacs are of absolutely no value.

ALCOHOLISM

For the many public officials and anxious parents in America who are worried about the "drug problem," a look into their own liquor cabinets (and their own medicine chests) may yield a better perspective on where the "drug problem" may have originated.

If a general pattern of an alcoholic can be formulated, it is that of an individual with low or flagging self-esteem, who is continually being put down by his boss or his wife or his friends or his children, often in a very subtle but pervasive fashion, who drinks too much because it may relieve some of the anxiety and pain and humiliation.

Not everyone who drinks, and not everyone who drinks to excess, is an alcoholic. The quantity of alcohol, the frequency of drinking, the propensity to get drunk, the nature of what is consumed, are all relatively unimportant factors in identifying an alcoholic. There is what is thought of as an alcoholic pattern which is strangely reproducible in different people in different parts of the country despite their different backgrounds. A list which characterizes the pattern of alcoholism, although it has some real limitations and is in many ways an oversimplification, may be useful in recognizing the pattern of alcoholism in your friends, your family, and possibly yourself. This section tries to avoid moralistic overtones, but so much of what is written and said about alcoholism reflects puritan morality that it is difficult to discuss the problem without appearing to paraphrase Alcoholics Anonymous or the Women's Christian Temperance Union.

- There is a gradual increase in the frequency of alcohol use along with subtle changes in the life style of the alcoholic.
- An alcoholic may begin a pattern of drinking alone and sneaking drinks, perhaps to fool others and perhaps to fool himself about how much he is drinking.
- The same goes for gulping drinks. It is harder to keep track of how many and how much.
- A gradual development of alcohol tolerance may develop; more is needed to achieve the same effect.
- Blackouts or periods of brief amnesia may appear during a period of excess use.
- A physiologic or psychologic change may develop. (Although the pattern never progresses this distinctly and in such a rigid chronologic order, the "problem drinker" above may become the "alcohol addict" below.)
- The alcohol addict often starts regular drinking in the morning (the eye-opener).
- Prolonged bouts of excess alcohol become more frequent and the pattern of binge drinking develops.
- A pattern of social disorganization develops. The alcoholic changes jobs, moves from place to place; marriages may deteriorate and financial problems increase.
- The addict begins to hide and hoard his supply.
- Paranoia develops. Perhaps this is an effect of alcohol on the brain; more likely it is the effect of society's attitude toward the alcoholic.
- Ultimately, as the alcohol consumption increases, a gradual decrease in the alcohol tolerance is noted. It takes less alcohol to produce the same effect.
- Finally, there is a gradual development of the physiologic changes in the body which result from the chronic ingestion of alcohol. Alcohol is a mild poison. It ultimately damages the liver, the brain, and the nervous system, and may damage the heart. Its effects can be fatal.

There are more than 5.5 million alcoholics in this country. These are the people who are drinking enough to interfere with or impair their lives, their jobs, their schoolwork, their state of health, their marriages, or whatever.

The treatment of a chronic alcoholic can be successful and gratifying, but, as with other problems, success may be more a measure of motivation than of any other factor. Treatment is difficult, frustrating, and often unsuccessful in many people simply for lack of motivation. The program of Alcoholics Anonymous is extremely effective, and either this form of counseling or some other type of psychologic support is essential in almost every treatment program. AA depends upon total abstinence and strong doses of moral judgment. Its program may be particularly useful in people with low self-esteem and a negative self-image, traits which are ordinarily difficult to overcome because they predispose to a sense of failure and a lack of confidence.

ADDICTION

The medical and pharmacologic problems of drug addiction are discussed in detail in the section on psychotropic drugs in Chapter 6. The psychiatric aspects are much more complex and controversial. Although some broad generalizations can be made about the psychologic aspects of addiction, the approach to the psychology of an addict must be highly individualized. The treatment has to be intensive and relentless. It is frustrating and difficult for the addict and the therapist as well. It can be successful despite the gloomy and depressing statistics, but the addict has to be strongly motivated and must be fortunate enough to have sympathetic, experienced, and compassionate help.

The best advice and most sensible treatment program we have seen comes from the autobiography of Malcolm X. "The addict first was brought to admit to himself that he was an addict. Secondly, he was taught why he used narcotics. Third, he was shown that there was a way to stop addiction. Fourth, the addict's shattered self-image, and ego, were built up until the addict realized that he had within, the self-power to end his addiction. Fifth, the addict voluntarily underwent a cold-turkey break with drugs. Sixth, finally cured, now an ex-addict completes the cycle by 'fishing' up other addicts whom he knows, and supervising their salvaging."*

This six-step program is impressive because it is the result of the experience of real people dealing with real addicts. It can be translated into any culture or any language; the message is clear, valid, and applicable to most addicts regardless of their backgrounds. There are fine points and subtleties which have to be incorporated into each individual's treatment, but the basics are there.

Amateur psychiatry is part of our daily conversation, and of our reaction to normal events, people, and situations. The psychiatrist in each of us is more apparent when we are dealing with someone who is "mixed up" or acting strangely or depressed. In this role, an amateur psychiatrist can be extremely effective and may offer the sympathy or the empathy or the advice or just the open ear to tide someone over a crisis. A well-meaning but inexperienced and misguided friend can sometimes do more harm than good, not only by delaying appropriate treatment, but by imposing his own hangups or problems on the anxious friend who is looking for help. We'd like to offer some advice for the amateur psychiatrist who might find himself giving treatment to a friend who is under stress.

Sometimes, the cause of someone's problem may be perfectly and embarrassingly obvious to you and to everyone else except the naïve sufferer. It is probably best to avoid brutally confronting him with this information; try to exercise discretion and tact.

Don't be too aggressive with your counseling or therapeutic maneuvers during a period of extreme stress or anxiety. First offer support to tide him over until the crisis has subsided; then he can more reasonably benefit from your efforts.

---

* *The Autobiography of Malcolm X,* with the assistance of Alex Haley. Grove Press, 1965.

Try to avoid premature interpretation of the problem. It may all seem so obvious to you, but the neurotic symptoms are sometimes due to very obscure and complex phenomena and may not be so obvious. An oversimplification can be more harmful than no advice at all.

Don't get angry or impatient if your patient can't or won't follow your advice or doesn't appear to get better once you have sorted it all out for him.

Some people function very well and are very happy and effective utilizing a set of defenses or rationalizations or excuses to explain or ignore certain phenomena. Don't be too quick to point out these defenses or to tear them down unless you are able to support your now-demolished patient or can offer him a new set of defenses to carry him through the next day or the next crisis.

Sometimes you may feel unable or uncomfortable about your amateur psychiatry. Or it may be clear that the patient needs professional advice. The following guidelines should be of some use. Professional advice is necessary when:

> there is even a remote possibility that a person may harm himself or others;

> his symptoms, whether they be anxiety or depression or whatever, don't seem to be getting any better with your informal therapy;

> paranoid, suspicious, or accusative behavior or thinking is more than just a small part of the problem;

> disturbances of mood, thinking, or behavior are prolonged, out of proportion to their apparent cause, or seem unusual or bizarre;

> irrational fears and phobias are so severe or profound as to seriously disable an individual or limit his effectiveness;

sexual activities cause anguish or shame or create a threat to others;

alcohol excess progresses from problem drinking to alcohol addiction; or

physical dysfunction or pain which have no basis in organic illness are interfering with normal activity.

When you decide to seek or advise professional help, you should know who is who in the psychiatric pecking order. A psychiatrist is a physician; he has gone to medical school and had specialty training in psychiatry. None of the other members of the psychiatric team has gone to medical school and, although a medical degree is of questionable value in many instances, it represents a generally accepted set of paper credentials and at least a minimum level of training. A clinical psychologist has graduate training in psychology but not in a medical school. He has usually a master's degree or a Ph.D. in psychology. Psychiatric social workers are trained in social work and then have special clinical experience in psychiatric problems. A large number of other professionals comprise the psychiatric team, each contributing his own skills to different problems or different facets of an individual complicated psychiatric problem. These professionals include psychiatric nurses, vocational counselors, school guidance counselors, religious advisers, and marriage counselors. On the sidelines are a whole spectrum of pseudo-professionals, quacks, charlatans, mediums, soothsayers, and astrologers, who should be ignored or avoided if you value sanity.

Now that you know who is who, the next question is where and how. Unfortunately, money is a big consideration, and where you turn depends on how much you can afford. If you can manage the financial burden and it seems appropriate, you can start with the private psychiatrist or psychologist, but this may not be appropriate for you regardless of how much you are willing to pay.

Perhaps a good place to start, if you can't deal with a private psychiatrist or psychologist in his office, is at one of the many community mental health centers. These are designed as an alternative to the state mental hospitals which conjure up the horrible image of the snake pit. The community mental health centers hope to avoid long-term institutionalization, to avoid long-term separation of the patient from his family and his familiar environment, and to provide psychiatric out-patient care where it is needed in the community. It is here that you may be able to get quickly whatever professional help is necessary at a cost you may be able to afford.

7 Food, Nutrition, and Obesity

There has been a deluge of nonsense written about food recently. Confusion, misinformation, and misunderstanding have always existed about the foods we eat and the relationship of food to health, but the turmoil of recent years appears to have compounded the problems with the recognition of new "solutions" to the world's food supply and new "problems" created thereby. We are reluctant to add to the confusion and will try to offer as dispassionate and factual an approach as possible, recognizing that the subject is laden with much passion and little fact and that ultimately we are indulging in our own prejudices.

Anyone who buys, prepares, or eats food is having a problem keeping well-informed about nutrition and is at a loss to sift the facts from the theories when even the experts disagree. How can anyone without an advanced degree in nutrition, toxicology, biochemistry, and medicine, who is besieged with the claims and threats of Madison Avenue or the food crusaders or the "nutrabiddies" and then warned and alarmed by the consumer advocates and ecologists, deal intelligently with the concepts of weight reduction, malnutrition, vitamin deficiencies, pellagra, vitamin C, macrobiotics, organic foods, pesticides, chemical additives, calories and proteins, brown rice and brown sugar, yoghurt and wheat germ, or DDT and fluoridation. Everyone is trying to tell everyone else what to eat and what not to eat, and there are as many theories and programs as the reader has patience to indulge in.

We have thousands of years of human experience with food and eating served up with a generous helping of myth, black magic, taboos, fantasy, and old wives' tales. An overwhelming supply of emotion, superstition, and folklore interferes with and cripples the food habits of the poorly nourished world. Eating and food are still problems and a source of serious concern for twentieth-century man. As with smoking and drinking, eating and food have recently become something else to add to our long list of things to worry about. The rational and irrational fears of heart disease and cancer, the deification of slimness, and the inconsistencies of food advertising and food safety reinforce the problem. Nowhere is the contradiction more profound than in food advertising. Television portrays bountiful tables and elegant slim housewives working in modern suburban kitchens for millions of people who have not. Husbands grow amorous over cardboard instant mashed potatoes, and children squeal with delight as they consume the latest plastic pudding.

If you are convinced with fanatical zeal that your way is the right way, the only way, the true way to eat and be healthy, happy, and sane, we ask you to read patiently and with an open mind, since any of a number of approaches may be quite consistent with good nutrition and good health.

BASICS OF NUTRITION

These two simple statements are likely to incur the anger and disbelief of every good "nutritionologist" who has written the volumes of suggestions which have successfully confused you up to now:

> Good nutrition is almost inescapable in America today without paying too much attention to any rules, tables, or charts.

> The elements of good nutrition are simple and uncomplicated.

Three conditions are needed for good nutrition:

> *Adequate funds.* If you are prudent and if you cook for yourself, you can do it for about $25 to $30 per person per month, and less per person as the size of the family

increases. Money makes it easier to eat well. When the wallets and the refrigerator are empty, good nutrition is more of a challenge.

Availability of food stores. We take no responsibility for those who will eat only what they themselves can grow or are living off berries and mountain water.

Avoidance of rigid patterns or fads. You will be malnourished if you insist on only egg whites or watermelon rinds.

Food is composed of six constituents: water, fats, carbohydrates, proteins, vitamins, and minerals.

The last three constituents, proteins, vitamins, and minerals, are the only things you could possibly get deficient in (this assumes, by the way, that you don't have some complicated and unusual intestinal or metabolic disease which impairs your digestive or absorptive capacity). Calories are not food, but a measure of the amount of energy that can be derived from food. Most of your calories come from carbohydrates and fats (sugars and starches and fatty food). People with inadequate funds often have to rely on high-calorie food (carbohydrate or fat) rather than on high-quality food (protein) since carbohydrates and fats are usually cheaper. It is a paradox to find poor people who are overweight but still seriously malnourished. They aren't getting enough of the necessary, but more expensive, food in their diet: the proteins, vitamins, and minerals.

The standard approach to nutrition taught in most American schools is absurd. Students memorize charts and tables and fear the development of a list of dreadful and obscure diseases as a penalty for failure to comply. The solution, however, is not in the individual's total recall of tabulations of vitamin content of various foods. It simply is unrealistic to expect people to memorize lists of foods and calories. The solution is also not the standard "basic four" or the "basic seven" food groups

(groups like green vegetables, milk products, etc.) which we were taught in high school biology or from the handouts of the school nurse. This is partly because an increasingly large number of foods are prepared in a factory and you can't see and don't know about the milk or flour or whatever that goes into them. And people will not, cannot, and need not, bother with maintenance of mental charts of food which they have eaten or neglected for each day.

We work on the assumption that most foods are good, some are obviously better and more nutritious (e.g., brown rice and vegetables), and that the easiest approach to good nutrition is variety. This is a bit of an oversimplification, so be careful. It obviously assumes that your variety is not merely switching from potato chips to corn chips. It assumes that, without conscious effort, you consume reasonably high-quality foods and that milk, vegetables, eggs, cheese, meat, and all the other "good" things are part of your standard diet.

Your capacity to provide a reasonable diet for yourself and your family is limited only by five conditions. You will have difficulty in eating properly

> if food and eating are a religion for you, or if they are a major part of your religion and are modified by your religious principles, or if you have the zeal and conviction about certain foods that a teetotaler has about alcohol or a vegetarian about meat; or,

> if you have some particular illness or problem such as diabetes or a stomach ulcer, in which case much of what we say may not be applicable or wise; or,

> if you have a weakness for, or tendency to adopt, new fads, or to follow trends or advertising; or

> if your finances are limited or non-existent and you are not eating regularly; or,

> if vanity is your direct or indirect motivation in food consumption, either by making food a status symbol or

by making your figure more important than your state of health.

If your diet is not being too strongly influenced or affected by these factors, and if you get a reasonable variety in your diet, you will get enough protein, vitamins, and minerals to avoid any deficiencies and you can cross malnutrition off your list of things to worry about.

GOOD FOOD ON A LOW BUDGET

There is a segment of the population in the U.S. which must daily face realistically the financial problems of good nutrition. This is particularly a problem if children must be fed. What kinds of good foods are cheap and how can limited resources yield the best nutritional value? A reasonable approach would be based on the following foods:

Milk and milk products. Skim milk is the same as whole milk but excludes the excess fat and vitamins A and D. It is cheaper than whole milk. In most parts of the country vitamins A and D are added back to the skim milk; their addition should not involve any additional cost. Don't buy skim milk which has not been fortified with vitamins A and D. Non-fat dry (powdered) milk is even cheaper, may be just as good, and needs only water to be reconstituted. (The value of powdered milk depends on the process by which it was prepared. Some preparative methods heat the milk and destroy a substantial amount of the biological value of the milk protein. It would be useful if the label told you how the milk is dried —spraying is good; heat rolling is bad—but labels don't identify the process. If you buy powdered milk you take some risk on the value of the milk protein.) Powdered milk is also low in vitamins A and D but strange regulations may prevent the addition of these vitamins to powdered milk in various places. (You might be able to get vitamin-fortified powdered milk in your area. Read the label.) Even without the vitamins, powdered milk is one of the best nutritional bargains once you get used to the flavor.

Breads and cereals. This refers not only to breads and cereals but to macaroni, flour, and other related foods made from rice, oats, wheat, barley, corn, etc. Your purchases of these foods should be influenced by some important considerations.

The more highly processed, convenient, and ready-to-eat foods are more costly.

Whole-grain cereals and flour are superior to processed grains and flour products (like white bread). Whole wheat or oats give you a lot of good nutrition for a relatively low price.

All "processed" breads and cereal products or anything made with grains which have been "treated" and do not contain the whole grain, should be enriched, fortified, or restored with the nutritional factors which have been removed if they are to retain their nutritional value. Be careful, though, because many commercial cakes, pastries, and convenience foods are not prepared with enriched flour. When you purchase these products, you lose the nutritional factors which have been removed and you pay more money for less nutritional, albeit more convenient food. You may assume that if the bakery is using enriched flour it will be on the label, and that if it is not labeled enriched, fortified, or restored, then processed or inferior flour has been used. The cost of enrichment is so small that if there is any extra cost for the enrichment, you are getting cheated.

The question of what vitamins, enrichment, or fortification to put back into milled or processed flour is an important one. As far as is known the enrichment or restoration maintains the characteristics of the milled flour which make it so desirable for baking and this enrichment returns all of the "significant" factors which have been lost in the milling process. The assertion is often made that, since not everything is replaced, some subtle or unknown nutritional constituent is being lost. This is a very reasonable argument, but it is clear that the absence of whatever it is that is being lost has no obvious effect on human health since enriched, fortified flour supports life as well as does whole flour. That the "lost factors" may have a subtle influence over many years cannot be established or denied, but we think it unlikely that a trace amount of any as yet to be discovered substances is going to have any miraculous curative or health maintaining properties.

Many of the cold breakfast cereals are heated during the process of making flakes and the like. This heating may impair the biological effectiveness of the protein. As with powdered milk, there is no way of telling about the preparative process from the label. You should assume that the cold breakfast cereals contain substantially less useful protein than is claimed on the label because much of the protein is put into a form which makes it biologically less valuable. With even the best cold cereal, you are getting not much more than the vitamins and minerals (often a good, but expensive vitamin pill) and the carbohydrate (which you don't need).

Beans probably do produce an increased amount of intestinal gas, but this is a small price to pay for a relatively inexpensive high-protein, highly nutritious food. Kidney beans, lima beans, lentils, split peas and soybeans are excellent cheap foods. It will take some imagination to put these into dishes that can regularly sustain your appetite. Consider, however, that the poor of most of the world have survived for all these generations primarily because they have had some kind of bean protein as a dietary staple.

This pattern of milk and milk products, breads and cereals, and beans might leave you low in vitamin C. Citrus fruits are not the only source of vitamin C. Beans or any of a number of vegetables, including potatoes (a potato contains about half as much vitamin C as the equivalent amount of grapefruit) will be more than adequate. If you are going on a real starvation or impoverished diet or if you eat only irregularly and poorly, you should consider some inexpensive multiple-vitamins, one each day. The cheapest will do as well as the advertised brands, but it's worth taking a minute to compare labels. Other than in extreme conditions, vitamin supplements are probably a waste of money and we do not recommend them for normal people.

DISASTER FOOD PLANNING

Special attention ought to be given to those circumstances in which an individual finds himself in a disaster, crisis, or emergency and cannot take advantage of normal channels of food distribution, or does so with very limited funds or at great personal risk. The approach to this problem depends on the duration and how much planning and storage can be done in anticipation. Adjustments can be made, depending on the specific conditions, but certain generalizations are useful in any case.

> Water supply should be assured. In whatever form of liquid, about two quarts per person per day are necessary.
>
> In the absence of any food after an extended period of time, there will soon be a need for salt—about 2 grams (a third of a teaspoon) per day. Most normal diets easily supply this, and supplements to a normal diet are not necessary except when sweating is excessive or starvation occurs. Excessive salt intake will increase thirst, so be cautious if water is in short supply.
>
> The basics of a minimal diet will be bread, beans, and milk products, with as much variety as possible within these groups. This will sustain life for prolonged periods if adequate quantities are consumed.

Vitamin supplementation probably is not necessary for periods of as much as a month on the bread-beans-milk diet. Beyond that time any multi-vitamin pill will do. The first vitamin to be depleted on a starvation diet will usually be vitamin B_1 (thiamin).

The best foods for stockpiling are dried milk, powdered eggs, dried beans and peas, canned meats and fish, and dried cheese. Add to this flour (enriched or whole), rice, dried potatoes, sugar, fats (canned butter or margarine), and oils. Canned water may be needed.

There is no perfect food. In general, different foods eaten together are better than a comparable caloric amount of a single food eaten alone. The body inefficiently utilizes incomplete foods and most foods alone are incomplete. The inadequacies of one good food can usually be complemented by the attributes of another to create a more complete mixture and the waste of poorly utilized food can be avoided. Bread and cheese for lunch and for dinner is far superior to twice as much bread for lunch and twice as much cheese for dinner.

VITAMIN AND VITAMIN SUPPLEMENTS

If you eat a fairly varied and regular diet, you don't need a vitamin supplement. Vitamins are probably the most over-utilized medicine on the drugstore shelves in America today. They have been pushed and promoted for the cure of a wide variety of ailments which are reminiscent of the itinerant quack peddler pushing his nerve tonic from the back of a covered wagon. In fact, vitamins can cure virtually nothing other than vitamin deficiencies, and their value in healing wounds, treating fatigue, insomnia, backaches, arthritis or preventing the common cold is probably fraudulent or questionable at the very least.

A total absence of some vitamins in experimental diets for prolonged periods of time produces no detectable disease in adults, and some vitamins may, in fact, be necessary only for growing children. The most fashionable vitamin today is vitamin E, and there are dozens of books available proclaiming its miraculous powers. It has been claimed that vitamin E will do most things, from curing impotence to preventing heart attack. As of this writing, there has been no human disease which can be prevented by vitamin E in whatever dose you take and only one rare human ailment (a strange type of anemia in premature infants) which can be cured by vitamin E. Its absence in the diet of certain laboratory animals has produced sterility, and it has been called the anti-sterility vitamin, but since it is virtually impossible for man to get a vitamin E deficient diet (the vitamin is ubiquitous), it is difficult to attribute human sterility to the absence of vitamin E. The claim that vitamin E prevents heart attacks is an absurd oversimplification of an extremely complex phenomenon; taking vitamin pills will not prevent or alter the progress of heart disease, which is the result of so many interrelated processes including at the very least your weight, your sex, your total diet, your cigarette smoking habits, your degree of physical activity, or the age of your parents when they died.

We suspect that the "experts" who are pushing vitamin E are more interested in selling books than in facts, and the purity of their motives is as questionable as the cigarette company's giving out free samples.

Thousands, perhaps millions, of Americans are convinced, however, that vitamins help them get better. This is adequate testimony to the gullibility of people and the fact that emotional and psychological factors play so large a role in an individual's feelings of well-being. Most diseases get better by themselves. Most therapeutic efforts can make the patient feel better (psychological) but offer little more curative assistance than sugar pills. It is fortunate that vitamins probably are relatively harmless and relatively inexpensive. It is difficult to condemn so benign a pill when it might be replaced on the druggist's shelves by something more toxic and probably more expensive. If people insist on taking pills, vitamins are as good as anything if taken in proper doses.

It does not necessarily follow that if a little is good, a lot is better. Larger than recommended doses can cause serious problems, and the huge doses of vitamin C suggested by some reputable scientists have been shown to produce abortions in experimental animals and diarrhea in susceptible individuals; they can produce heart failure in patients who need to restrict their salt intake, and can substantially modify the acid-alkali balance which will be a problem in individuals with lung or kidney disease. Moreover, people who consume very large amounts of vitamin C develop very efficient mechanisms for excreting the unusual amounts. When they discontinue their high intake, the excretory mechanisms continue to operate and the normal levels consumed now get excreted too rapidly, causing serious vitamin C depletion and even scurvy in people consuming ordinary amounts. How long it takes for the overexcretion to return to normal is not known.

Who does need vitamins besides those who are predisposed to malnutrition? Perhaps we are too critical of vitamins and their excessive use and we should hasten to point out that some people, albeit not many, do need vitamins.

- If you are a strict vegetarian, if you eat no meat or meat products, and no dairy products and no eggs, and you *never* cheat, you will probably become deficient in vitamin B12 after about five years and may need a small supplement to keep you healthy and prevent a rare form of anemia. Even then, you'll only need a millionth of a gram a day (or 30 billionths of an ounce) to prevent the anemia. If you accidentally eat anything containing meat or milk, you've spoiled it all, and now you probably won't need vitamin B12 for another few years.

- If you are on a weight-reducing diet and your food intake is limited or very selected and repetitious, you might benefit from a multiple vitamin capsule during the siege on the excess pounds.

- Many doctors give women vitamin supplements during

pregnancy. The main benefit appears to be to prevent the anemia often seen in young women. The constituents of the vitamin pill which are needed are iron and calcium; these are not vitamins but minerals.

- Many young women are anemic (sometimes called low, weak, or thin blood) because of blood loss during menstrual periods. If your periods are very heavy and you aren't feeling as spry as you used to, you might benefit from iron pills. But remember, iron is good only for an iron-deficiency anemia, not all types of anemia, and not for any of the dozens of other things which might cause fatigue in a young woman.
- Some people recovering from serious illness or surgery often have diminished appetite and can get slightly vitamin deficient at a time when they can ill afford to be deficient in anything. Sometimes a multiple vitamin capsule is of some help; but as we noted before, a lack of vitamins usually produces no evident disease in adults.
- If you drink your calories in the form of alcohol, your food intake is probably substandard and you might benefit from tossing down a vitamin or two with the morning eye-opener.
- If you are very poor, if you eat only every so often, or are just getting by, you may need a vitamin supplement.
- If you are obliged to eat prison or institutional food where the chef and management know as much about nutrition as they appear to know about penology, you are probably eating a nonvaried diet and you may be getting vitamin deficient. Some of the vitamin deficiency may be related to the fact that an institutional diet is just dull, unappetizing, and the deficiency may be a result of inadequate intake rather than poor quality food.
- If your diet is marginal or irregular or if you are worried about it, vitamin pills (in ordinary doses) won't hurt. They are a good source of nutrients and are a cheap form of added insurance.

ORGANIC FOODS

Organic foods are grown and prepared with minimum modification of their natural form and without chemicals or synthetic additives. Tons of complex chemicals, pesticides, hormones, preservatives, and artificial colorings, sweeteners, and flavors are added to the food consumed in America, and comparable amounts of other substances are removed in various stages of the processing and preparation of food. Organic foods try to avoid the problems possibly created by these manipulations. As a result, the organic foods are often thought, among other things, to taste better. Taste is, of course, very much an individual matter and is so much a culturally acquired characteristic that it does not appear reasonable to make blanket judgments about taste. In some cases the artificial flavors and chemicals have created foods which are, in general, much more acceptable to the American palate regardless of how plastic this taste is thought to be by some.

Organic foods, however, are substantially more expensive, a serious problem for many. They also store less successfully than their non-organic counterparts which have various preservation mechanisms incorporated into them. No less important is the recognition that the world's food supply depends, to a very large extent, on the chemicals used to process and preserve food. Were the chemicals not used, famine would be everywhere on the earth. Assuming the use of existing food production techniques, no amount of organic fertilizer could produce the quantities of food now needed in the world.

Most important about organic foods, though, is the issue of how much they add to one's health. There is serious concern over the safety of the countless additives placed in food, much of it there for commercial rather than quality considerations. There is serious concern also about what may be removed from food during the commercial preparative process. It is obvious that too little is known about these very complicated issues and the shabbiness of the studies of the safety of various additives, and the commercial rather than altruistic reasons for their addition (or deletion), raise many serious and sincere questions.

If there is any doubt at all about additives, they should not be included in food despite the fact that there is very little evidence that they do any harm. It is preferable to err on the side of caution. On the other hand, there is equally little evidence that natural or organic foods are significantly better for your health. Much of the reported value of organic foods derives from the obvious but often neglected fact that the great bulk of human disease is related to an emotional or psychological state of mind rather than to a specific organic cause. To the extent that natural foods can improve this spiritual state and thereby make people feel better, they are obviously magnificent health givers. Too often, however, the delicate line between spirit and body is lost and mystical powers are conferred upon organic foods or their manipulation which do not appear justified. Anecdotes can easily be made into generalizations and personal experiences are too often elaborated into principles and pronouncements which appear equally unjustified. The non sequitur and the miracle cure is the commonplace in books on organic food ("I once knew a man who had arthritis for twenty-two years and started eating five dozen walnuts a day. Within three weeks he was playing the piano. Therefore, walnuts cure arthritis"). We are concerned about this phenomenon of what we call the "therefore effect" and the fuzzy thinking that allows the oversimplification of complex things ("Fasting allows the body to cleanse itself of poisons"), and the too easy identification of cause and effect and their relationship to food consumed.

MACROBIOTIC DIETS

An extension of the use of organic food is the development of macrobiotic diets. This pattern of food consumption uses certain foods and ascribes certain qualities not only to the foods but to the combinations of the foods, to the way in which they are prepared and eaten, to the life style which is created by these patterns, and to the therapeutic value these manipulations are said to have.

These diets use foods which are basically similar to those used in organic diets balancing qualities of Yin and Yang in food consumption patterns. A series of diets are outlined which, as one progresses from the lower levels to higher levels, are associated with increased awareness, a spiritual awakening, and enrichment of the mind.

We have no objection to the use of the various foods, the quality of the foods, and certainly none with the life style implicit in the macrobiotic diets. We are convinced that much spiritual enrichment can be derived from a sincere devotion to this existence, and as with organic food, the therapeutic benefits which can be derived from a macrobiotic life can be remarkable in resolving many of the ills of mankind.

We urge, however, that great care be utilized in the application of the higher-level diets. They are seriously deficient in the bare minimum nutritional needs of humans. They can produce major nutritional problems and the frequency of scurvy, anemias, protein, iron, and calcium deficiencies, starvation, and even death solely as a result of prolonged adherence to high-level macrobiotic diets is now significant enough to cause some concern for the health, if not the life of those consuming these diets.

Finally, we are very cautious about the therapeutic qualities of these diets in the treatment of serious physical disease which occasionally occur. We do not believe that the use of high-level diets can cure or prevent heart disease or cancer, and we deplore the use of these diets and the use of compresses, plasters, stupes, and external massage for the treatment of all illness. The most serious consequence of the use of macrobiotic diets may be not only in the delay of seeking appropriate treatment for those diseases which can be effectively treated by standard procedures (e.g., diabetes, appendicitis), but may be in the untimely death of those who neglect therapy.

APHORISMS ON FOOD AND EATING

1. *De gustibus non est disputandum*—there is no dispute concerning taste. This is something which many of the food crusaders and self-appointed popular nutrition experts fail to take into consideration when they warn you about the dangers of eating this or skipping that. If you like the taste of salami, go ahead and eat salami, even though they tell you about all the junk and "bad things" that go into making it. Life is too short to worry about these things. Eating should be a pleasure and not a chore.

2. The basis of good nutrition is very simply a varied diet. Any repetitious or highly restricted diet may be nutritionally deficient after a variable period of time.

3. Canned or frozen foods are excellent, particularly when fresh foods are out of season.

4. Convenience foods are usually more convenient but they are substantially more expensive than unprocessed foods.

5. Some foods are nutritionally better when eaten raw, but many other foods are better for you when cooked. Most foods retain their nutritional value when cooked or prepared properly, but overcooking will destroy much nutritional value and often the taste as well.

6. Some people don't like to eat meat for a variety of reasons, including their abhorrence of killing other animals. We acknowledge this as a legitimate reason for being vegetarian (see Aphorism 7). Without meat, variety becomes even more important to assure that some of the vitamins and minerals normally found primarily in meat are consumed in adequate amounts. Some vegetarians do eat milk and eggs and for them the problem is less severe.

7. Man is an omnivore: he eats meat and vegetable naturally and with equal facility. There is nothing unnatural or dangerous about eating meat. Eating meat has never been shown to cause any illness, does not predispose to somnolence or sloth, cannot conceivably be the "cause of all man's ail-

ments," does not make man make war and does not make people violent (some of the most vicious, primitive tribes are vegetarians). Meat is, however, a very expensive and inefficient source of protein and will certainly become increasingly unavailable as the world's population increases.

8. Children and pregnant women need milk. No one else needs it but it is good food for anyone. If you drink milk, the non-fat or skim milk is as good as whole milk and it is lower in calories, lower in unnecessary animal fats, and less expensive.

9. Sugar and carbohydrates do not cause diabetes.

10. Most people would do well to eat less sugar in the form of candy, cake, and pastries, eat more green vegetables, eat fewer eggs, eat less "red meat" and more "white meat" (poultry, fish), eat less animal fat and more vegetable oils, eat less salt and eat fewer calories. Note that we stress the terms *less* and *more* and not *none* or *only*. Eat what you like but try to avoid excesses.

11. Although not established with certainty, saturated fats (animal fats) probably tend to predispose to early atherosclerosis and heart disease. It seems logical to try to minimize animal fats (hard or saturated fats) and replace them with vegetable or fish oils (see the discussion on diet and heart disease in Chapter 3).

12. Sugar makes things taste better and it probably can't harm you, but it has little to offer nutritionally except calories. If you must have sugar, brown or unprocessed sugar may at least contain some trace minerals, has a slightly different taste, and may have slightly better nutritional value than the refined white sugar. Its price, which is usually much higher than white sugar, would appear to vitiate this trivial benefit.

13. We do not believe that special rejuvenative or spiritual values ascribed to various food preparations or diets can be established.

14. Birdseed and honey diets rise and fall from time to time, and it is easy to find some crackpot touting the unique value of pomegranate seeds or an all brown-rice and water

diet. Ignore them or we shall all be eating alfalfa sprouts and little else.

15. While it offends us from a purely esthetic and emotional viewpoint to note that you can purchase cream without cream and beef stroganoff without meat, there probably is nothing intrinsically bad or harmful in such synthetic foods, and we may find that as the population grows, we will be increasingly obliged to turn to synthetic foods and seaweed to feed all the people.

16. A great deal is known about nutrition but much more is unknown, confused, and incorrect. As consumers of food, we should insist on the most careful supervision of food growing and processing to keep the poisons to an absolute minimum; we should be careful to separate the real problems that warrant attention and concern from the unsupported claims and mouthings of the food cranks.

OBESITY AND WEIGHT REDUCTION

Obesity is esthetically unappealing, and it is associated with a poorer state of health. It has been well demonstrated that obesity predisposes to heart disease, high blood pressure, diabetes, and orthopedic problems. The fat man will statistically die five to ten years before his thinner brothers. On a more practical and immediate note, obesity causes fatigue simply because a man who is fifty pounds overweight is burdened with the extra weight just as if he were carrying a fifty-pound knapsack all day.

Some people are overweight because there is something wrong with their glands. These people are medical rarities. Occasional endocrine disorders, and rarely a brain tumor or brain damage, may produce an abrupt increase in appetite and consequent weight gain.

Some people can't lose weight despite the fact that they "eat like a bird." These people sometimes delude themselves and usually they are eating bird-like portions of very high-calorie foods, or bird-like portions twenty-four hours a day, or bird-like portions for a very large bird. There are dozens of reasons why people can't lose weight or stick to their diet, varying from the charming ("Today is my birthday") to the absurd ("I'm so weak I can't work").

There are dozens of diets available for everyone to try—the high-protein diet, the Mayo diet, the drinking man's diet, etc. None of these helps to establish the necessary and desirable eating habits required to sustain the weight loss, and they are almost invariably followed by rebound overeating and weight gain. There are endless numbers of treatments for obesity, including hypnosis, hormones, drugs, psychotherapy, and a weird variety of mechanical and electrical devices. Their abundance attests to their ineffectiveness and man's inability to conquer the demands of his appetite. The best diet is simply a low-calorie diet. For the vast majority of fat people, it is basically a matter of balancing calorie intake against calorie output. If you eat 3,000 calories worth of food and you utilize 2,000 calories to go about your normal activities, there is a surplus of 1,000 calories available to be stored in the body, usually in the form of body fat. When stored in the body as fat, the 1,000 calories weigh about a quarter of a pound, and if you eat 1,000 calories more than you use every day for four days, you are one fat pound ahead. If you need 2,000 calories to get through the day and eat only 1,000 calories, the reverse is true: you take the necessary 1,000 calories from your fat stores either from your belly or from your hips or wherever you keep it hidden and you've lost a quarter of a pound. A 3,500 to 4,000 calorie deficit over whatever period it occurs produces about one pound weight loss. Dieting is simply a matter of eating less calories than you use. For purposes of weight reducing, the body cannot recognize whether the calories come from a drinking man's diet, a steak and banana diet, or whatever mystical diet you find to reduce the calorie intake. Many people fail at weight reduction despite their adherence to a diet because they increase the quantity of allowed or low-calorie foods and thereby increase the calorie count. A simple and absolutely reliable method of weight reduction which does not require any charts, calorie counting, or special diet is to continue on your regular diet and cut the quantity of each food in half; instead of two eggs have just one, or eat a half instead of a whole sandwich. This allows you to continue eating the foods you usually eat. You automatically cut the calories in half and if your appetite can stand the strain, and your activities or calorie demands are unchanged, the weight will invariably fall. A diet which contains less than 900 calories a day is impractically difficult to follow, is sometimes associated with metabolic and medical side effects, and does not prepare the dieter for the lifelong aspects of dietary management.

Two other major factors interfere with satisfactory weight reduction. One is motivation and the second is patience. You can usually expect to fail in a weight reducing program unless you are highly motivated by some very tangible factors. You are combating years of overindulgence, and modifying your eating habits will not come easily, unless you really want to or have to. Don't bother starting on a diet unless you seriously plan to continue on it and plan to succeed. And don't bother starting unless your plans include a reevaluation of your eating habits and your attitudes toward food. It's just too much hard work losing weight and then allowing the weight to creep up again as you fall back into your old indulgent ways.

The second ingredient in a weight-reducing plan is patience. Losing pounds takes time and a sensible and realistic weight-reduction program will result in not more than about a five-pound weight loss a month. You can expect a greater loss the first weeks or month perhaps because of increased enthusiasm and greater motivation, but also probably because of increased loss of some excess water which is often retained in obese people. But after the initial surge of success don't get discouraged if the rate of reduction slows down. You can't lose fifty pounds in three weeks. It is very important to set a realistic goal for yourself before you start. Decide on what weight you want to and can realistically achieve, and plan on losing no more than five pounds a month toward that goal. Nothing is quite so discouraging as failing to achieve unrealistic goals. Remember it has taken you years to accumulate the excess fat and it is unrealistic to expect to shed it in a few weeks.

We don't mean to give the impression that losing weight is easy and if you eat less food you will thereby simply lose weight. This approach is generally correct, but for individuals with specific eating habits, varying degrees of motivation, temptation, and distractions it is sadly naïve and inadequate. There are certain general factors which often increase the difficulty of weight reduction, but you should not let these deter you or rationalize these as excuses for your lack of success.

- Some people have an excess number of "fat cells" which were produced or created in their childhood. If you were a fat kid, your chances of losing weight and keeping thin are slim.
- Generally, people from fat families tend to remain fat. Whether it is because of thoroughly ingrained bad eating habits or a genetic predisposition to obesity is not clear, but if your parents and siblings are fat, you may find it more difficult to lose weight. This also should not be an excuse, however, because fat people from fat families can lose weight if they are determined to do so.
- The older you get, the more difficult it is to lose weight. Again, the intransigence of bad eating habits over many years may be an important factor, and this should be a stimulus to you to start early and make it easy for yourself.

If you start on a weight-reducing diet, don't ignore the value of competition, mutual support, and group therapy. About a third of those participating in group weight reducing plans lose twenty pounds or more. Another third continue with the group but don't lose any weight. The final third drops out. Almost all have regained the lost weight in a year or two. It helps if your spouse or other members of the family diet with you. It increases the motivation, it eliminates temptation, and it simplifies food preparation. The essence of group weight reduction programs is group therapy and the added stimulus of competition and the increased gratification with success.

A word also about weight-reducing pills and medication, particularly the amphetamines. Some doctors promise more successful weight reductions with the addition of regular medications or injections. The medications often include a combination of a type of thyroid extract, a digitalis preparation, a diuretic, and a form of amphetamine. This is a dangerous mixture and it takes very careful control and a strong, healthy individual to tolerate the side effects of these drugs. The thyroid extract has little effect in the doses given since it causes a feedback decrease in the output of your own thyroid and the net effect is zero. In excessive doses, the thyroid will increase your metabolism, make you very "hyper" and very uncomfortable. Digitalis stimulates and strengthens a sick heart, but it is dangerous in someone who has a normal heart and it has serious and potentially fatal side effects in improper doses. Too much digitalis will make you sick and you will lose your appetite, but the risk is substantial and unacceptable. The diuretics will promote excretion of water through the kidneys and bladder if there is any significant water retention, and it will produce an artificial and transient weight loss of excess body water which is usually quickly reversed when the pills are discontinued. The diuretics also have serious side effects and should not be taken without careful supervision. Finally, the amphetamines, which are hardly ever indicated, have dubious value and very serious side effects. They tend to decrease the appetite, but this effect lasts only temporarily for a few weeks, and a chronic fat man with a usual fat man's appetite can easily overcome this effect unless he is highly motivated. If this is the case, the amphetamines are not necessary. The amphetamines are stimulants, or pep pills, they can be addictive, and the dangers of amphetamines, particularly for weight reduction, cannot be overemphasized. There are many amphetamine-like drugs which are supposed to be more effective and have fewer side effects. Not true. There is no convincing evidence that they are any better or any safer.

Injections of chorionic gonadotropins or other pituitary hormones have no effect on weight reduction, excess fat, or appetite control. Weight reduction should be carried out without the benefit of any pills or shots which are of questionable value at best and have serious, potentially fatal side effects. We strongly recommend that you avoid any weight-reducing program or scheme that routinely employs any medication as an adjunct to dieting, even if it is administered by a doctor. Furthermore, the maintenance of weight loss requires at least some changes in your eating habits. Unless you are prepared to commit yourself to that change sometime early on in the weight-reducing program, you will never sustain your weight loss and pills won't help.

A sensibly graduated and regular exercise program should be part of every plan to lose weight. It uses up more calories, it helps tone up the flabby muscles, and generally makes you feel better. Vigorous exercise tends to decrease the appetite, but some people come back from the morning jog in the park ravenously hungry. Exercise alone without restricting calories generally won't work as a weight-reducing plan since the increase in calorie expenditure from the exercise is almost always associated with subtle increase in food intake.

You can see a psychiatrist if you are desperate and everything else fails. He may make you feel better about your being fat and help you adjust to it, but the psychiatrist's couch is rarely a satisfactory approach to weight reduction. You may hold your infantile oral urges responsible for your appetite and eating habits, but psychotherapy won't be able to make any substantial changes. Psychiatrists from the behaviorist school claim some success in aversion therapy when bad eating habits are unlearned and food and eating is associated with unpleasant stimuli. Its long-term benefits remain to be established.

We have come to some realistic and unhappy conclusions about obesity:

> Obesity is a very complex phenomenon, and sometimes blaming overweight on overeating is an unjustifiable oversimplification.
>
> You can lecture, threaten, and warn, and all the unsympathetic and authoritarian admonitions will only make a fat person feel uncomfortable, unloved, and guilty, but will not make him lose weight any faster.
>
> The most sensible approach to weight reduction is a gradual and balanced and lifelong reduction in calorie intake which is nutritionally adequate and which is based on one's own tastes and life style.
>
> Any plan which involves crash dieting, bizarre or extreme diets, or medications, will at best produce only a temporary weight reduction, and any plan which doesn't include a lifelong commitment to dietary control is doomed to fail.
>
> Exercise programs and group efforts at weight reducing are of small but definite value.
>
> Most people who lose weight tend to regain it in a variable amount of time.
>
> Repeated and unsuccessful efforts to lose weight or maintain weight reduction are sometimes more realistically managed by helping the obese patient accept and adapt to his obesity, rather than add guilt and a sense of lingering frustration and anxiety to his already troubled psyche.

8 Medical Supplies and Equipment

What to Get

There is no simple formula or standard first-aid pack of medical supplies, equipment, and drugs. What you take with you or arrange to have available depends entirely on what you will use it for and who will do the using. The needs of two college girls traveling through Europe for the summer are vastly different from the needs of a group of students planning a sit-in at the dean's office or a young couple who have just moved into a small apartment in downtown big city, or the group planning a two-week hiking trip into desolate back country.

Recognizing the limitations of our own inability to list what should be among your supplies, we nevertheless do just that, relying heavily on your intelligence, experience, perspective, and judgment to adapt the list of medicines and medical equipment to your needs and skills.

Without giving the impression of being too orthodox, too structured, or too medical, we would like to urge a little bit of anticipation and planning and the calm methodical gathering of one's resources well in advance of whatever you are planning. Unfortunately, this anticipatory gathering is often difficult and frustrating for people who are otherwise intelligent and flexible. It is sad but true that if you leave everything for the last minute, or worse yet, if you leave everything to chance, you will probably not have what you want when you need it.

The difficulty of gathering of resources stems, in part, from one of America's common myths, the fantasy of the magic potion—that some miracle can happen if a skilled magician (i.e., a physician) judiciously selects and administers a secret elixir. Put a doctor and a patient together, throw in some pills, shake, and presto!, out emerges good health. This is characteristic of the public's obsession with panaceas. The overreliance on pills, the unrealistic expectation that "a shot" will cure what ails you, and the impossibility of identifying such pills leads to the frustration and often abandonment of rational self-care efforts by rational people. Since they don't know which pills to take, they take a bit of everything or nothing at all. "If only I knew which pills (supplies, equipment, etc.) to take along, every contingency could be met and dispatched with full resolution and restitution."

We would like to adopt a more realistic view. We have found (1) that relatively few medical problems need specific or complex therapy, (2) that people who do stock medicine chests or take first-aid kits prepare too much and are burdened with the weight of a lot of unnecessary junk, and (3) that what is prepared or taken is poorly selected and too often based on the traditional and inappropriate Red Cross first-aid approach.

We would like to suggest that you organize your thinking with three simultaneous considerations in mind: How mobile or how stationary will you and your medical supplies have to be? What kind of situation and problems do you anticipate? What are your skills and experience?

Mobility: Are the medicines and equipment for use at home or at the ski cabin, or will they have to move with you around Europe or on your back on the hike up the mountain or at an encounter with the police?

The problems of a home medical kit are relatively simple; bulk and weight are no consideration. Home medical supplies tend to accumulate passively. This is regrettable, since the items which are crucially needed at the one right time are often depleted or not available or stale and decaying. Don't get too obsessive and morbid about it, but it may be worth your while to have a look around to see what you have and what you need and perhaps bring it up to date.

If you are going to carry it all on your back or in your suitcase or, more important still, if you need to have medical supplies for a demonstration, sit-in, picket, or whatever, and if you anticipate a possibility of violence or tear gas, the medical kit must be designed to be small in bulk and light in weight; the contents must be chosen with more discrimination and care. In general, the lists which follow are slightly oriented toward preparations for a demonstration, but home or traveling supplies can easily be adapted from the recommended lists with accommodations and adjustments made for conditions of need, family age, isolation, and the state of health.

What do you need it for? We can conceive of a number of variables which should influence your selection of drugs and equipment. The variations are almost infinite. We offer a partial checklist which you should keep in mind.

What are you planning to do?
How long do you anticipate the need?
What is the state of health of the participants?
Will you be stationary or moving?
Is it for day or nighttime activity?
How long will it last?
How much time do you have to get it together?
How accessible will additional supplies be at a later time?
How far will you be from competent professional assistance?
Do you anticipate violence?
Is there any possibility of confrontation with the authorities? (Who are the authorities? How experienced are they? How angry and how disciplined are they?)

You will obviously have to rely on your good sense, judgment, and experience as you adapt the kits which we suggest below to your individual circumstances.

What are your skills and experience? The spectrum extends from a frightened hysteric who faints at the sight of blood, or gets a headache when anyone is in pain, to the highly skilled and experienced physician with nerves of steel and inexhaustible stamina. Whatever your ability and experience, it is important that you assess them honestly and objectively. Too often, the arrival of the first-aid man is accompanied by a sense of relief among the helpless bystanders and by a quiet sense of horror as he, and everyone else, realizes that he is in over his head and doesn't know what he is doing.

Don't take what you can't use or aren't familiar with. Don't expect to figure it out when you get there. Either get familiar with it now or leave it home.

We have organized three types of supply kits.

Type A: This is a compact kit and can be carried by anyone who anticipates any problems at all. It should enable you to deal with the problems of your immediate companions and yourself.

Type B: This too is a portable kit but it assumes that you have some kind of useful medical experience and the medical responsibility for a group of people.

Type C: The size of this kit suggests that some professional skills are available. Its size and scope can obviously vary, but we generally think of this as a stationary unit or something to be carried in a truck. It is emergency oriented although it could be adapted for routine field medical station use. It may involve a moderate to substantial financial investment.

Each of the kits is described in detail below. A number of items are marked with an asterisk: this notes those items which would normally be used only by a person with some experience in their use. The experience may, in many instances, be easily acquired, and the details of the use can often be readily handled by a non-physician. For a number of items we have not included dosages and sizes since this varies so much with individual circumstances. We assume that a person preparing the kit is familiar enough with its contents to select those sizes which he knows how to use. Where dosages or sizes can be usefully specified, we have done so. We have listed the drugs by their most familiar name, whether it be a trade or generic name. This does not imply any endorsement of any item. We assume that any drug listed as a trade name which can be obtained as a generic equivalent should be so obtained. The money saved can be put to better purposes at no loss in effectiveness. Many of the medications specified are available with a prescription only. We haven't found this legal distinction particularly useful, but we rather depend on the asterisks as we describe above. It matters little to us how you get the medications but it might matter to the police or district attorney who will object if you are prescribing or dispensing medications without a license. If possible, medications should be kept in their prescription container on the assumption that they are to be used only for the person and purpose for which they were prescribed. Narcotics and those special drugs which require a special narcotics license demand a great deal of care. It is not against the law to be in possession of properly prescribed legal narcotics (some, like heroin, are not legal under any circumstances). It is against the law to possess those narcotics (even the legal ones) unless you have a license or they are prescribed for your use. If you want to keep a narcotic or a strong pain killer in your kit, you are taking a risk of being arrested for possession of a narcotic unless you have a proper prescription.

In each case, if you don't know what it is and how to use it, or if you feel uncomfortable in using it—don't take it.

TYPE A—PERSONAL SUPPLY KIT

The list includes those things which are small, simple conveniences and those which may be lifesaving or prevent serious disability. It is oriented toward younger people and their life style. (It does not, for example, include cardiac drugs. These are listed in the Type B kit.)

EQUIPMENT

Gauze pads. These are the sterile square pads of woven cotton. They are useful for covering and cleaning wounds, lacerations, burns, etc. They come in various sizes: 4-inch squares are probably best—smaller than that is too small to be generally useful.

Roller bandage. This is a rolled-up gauze pad. You can wind it around a limb or a head to cover a wound or hold a splint in place. Use the 2-inch or 4-inch variety. Both the roller bandage and the gauze pads are better if they come in a sterile package. There is no sense in adding a dirty dressing to a dirty wound.

Adhesive tape has many uses and is invaluable. The 2-inch width can be torn lengthwise if necessary.

Band-Aids. Take an assortment of sizes.

Cotton balls or absorbent cotton. These should be taken soaking wet in a small watertight plastic container or bag. They can be used to wash your eyes after tear gas.

Ace (elastic) bandage. The 3-inch type is very useful for supporting an injured ankle or wrist or for holding things together or in place. Be careful: don't wind it too tight.

Alcohol sponges or swabs. These come in small waterproof packages. They can be used to clean and partly sterilize a wound.

Flashlight. Take fresh or extra batteries. You will be in trouble very quickly at night with weak batteries.

Tourniquet. A belt, necktie, roller bandage, or similar object will do for tying around an arm or leg just tight enough to stop bleeding if it can't be stopped with simple pressure alone.

Airway. This is a simple question-mark-shaped device that fits into the mouth of an unconscious person, over his tongue, and helps to keep the breathing passages open. Get one that can be used for mouth-to-mouth resuscitation. If you don't know how to use it, take a few minutes to figure it out or get someone to show you.

Scissors or a knife. Useful, but be careful. As with any of a number of other bits of equipment, it leaves you open for a charge of carrying a concealed weapon.

*Stethoscope. If you go to the trouble of carrying this, you should know what you are listening to.

*Syringes, needles. A variety of sizes for administering some of the medications listed below. Again, it involves the

problem of the charges of carrying a concealed weapon or narcotics paraphernalia.

MEDICATIONS

Keep all medications labeled carefully. If you are carrying a prescription medication, keep it in the prescription container. If not, you stand an increased chance of getting some kind of drug charge added to an already complicated indictment.

Your own personal medications. Take along enough of the medications you must take routinely. Items such as insulin, anticonvulsants, birth control pills, blood pressure pills, asthma medications, etc., may be unavailable, difficult to obtain, or seriously delayed if you get busted. It's a good idea to carry medical certification of the medications that you need.

Aspirin. Anything stronger as a pain killer will need a prescription. Adults can take two or three aspirins every three to four hours.

**Stronger analgesics.* Codeine, morphine, or Demerol if you have a narcotics registration or prescription. Talwin (30 mg injected or 50 mg orally) is not very potent but may be adequate, and while it does need a prescription, it doesn't require narcotics registration.

Salt tablets. These are critically important in hot, sweaty weather. Figure about one or two half-grain tablets for every glass of water.

**Epinephrine.* 1 ml of 1:1000 solution. This may be useful for some cardiac emergencies, not for treating asthma.

**Parenteral and oral tranquilizers.* Valium and Thorazine are useful. Valium is useful also in controlling seizures. The dosages depend on the circumstances.

**Anti-asthma medications.* Tear gas can elicit asthma in even mild or unsuspected asthmatics. An oral drug combination like Tedral or Quadrinal is useful for mild cases only. A nebulizer, like an Isuprel mistometer may be more effective. For a bad attack you need injected epinephrine or intravenous or rectal aminophylline.

**Nalline.* This is effective in diagnosis and treatment of an overdose of opiates and related synthetic drugs. These drugs include heroin, morphine, codeine, methadone, and many others. Nalline is useless, and may even be dangerous, in any bad trip not caused by an opiate (see Chapter 6).

Anti-seizure medications. The Valium that you have among your tranquilizers is excellent.

Tetracaine, ophthalmic ointment or drops 0.5%. A little will do a lot for a tear-gassed eye. Be certain, though, that the eye is thoroughly washed and not otherwise injured. A few drops of ophthalmic fluorescein (1 per cent) is very useful to determine if there is any corneal damage. It is essential that any eye anesthetized with something like tetracaine be patched shut for at least four to six hours. Remember that an anesthetized eye does not have a normal blink response and cannot protect itself from the miscellaneous debris flying about.

Insect repellent. Some kind of insect powder or lotion is very comforting if you are going to be in among insects.

Water. You'll have to take some to wash out tear gas, and for a dozen other things. Take a canteen unless you are certain of a water supply. A large supply of water will be needed for most things, but water is very heavy.

TYPE B—PORTABLE SUPPLY KIT

This is going to be much heavier and bulkier and assumes that the person responsible has more than minimal skills. Again, it assumes that you don't take what you and your team don't know how to use. We've included some of the emergency drugs which might be applicable to a more diverse population. We have included some aches-and-pains medicines and some of the drugs which might be used in the treatment of a cardiac emergency. Our experience has shown that these problems become substantial in any large crowd where tensions are high, walking is long, exhaustion is common, or where very hot or very cold weather provide additional challenges.

In addition to each of the items in the Type A Kit (and in some cases a more generous supply) we suggest the following:

EQUIPMENT

Large pad dressings. The big 8-inch squares or 10-inch by 36-inch variety can cover almost any wound and can pad a splinted limb.

Paper towels. Very convenient.

Cotton-tipped applicators. The prepackaged sterile type.

Eye patches. An eye should be patched after you anesthetize it. These are convenient but a gauze pad (4-inch square) will do almost as well.

Splints. Optional. You can almost always use something makeshift, but a wide splint (more than 3 inches) is really best and can be obtained in portable varieties. The inflatable splints are very useful and compact.

*Syringes and needles. A small assortment of sterile disposable types should do.

*Intravenous (IV) equipment. You should give some consideration to a small bottle of 5 per cent dextrose and some IV tubing.

*Suture kit. This should not be used unless more definitive treatment is not available at all. The suture kit should contain gauze pads, scissors, forceps, and needle holder. You should have an assortment of suture material (3-0 to 5-0 silk). It also implies that you have a local anesthetic (1 per cent or 2 per cent lidocaine), needles and syringes and a method of cleaning or sterilizing the skin.

Forceps. Take them if they aren't part of your suture kit.

Gloves. Sterile rubber gloves in suitable sizes.

Safety pins. Small and surprisingly useful.

*Surgical knife and blade. There are very few reasons to take this along. There should be one in your tracheostomy kit, if you have one. If not, a clean sharp pocket knife will sometimes do very well.

Tongue depressors. These are useful for many things besides depressing tongues. A finger or a teaspoon will do fine for depressing a tongue.

Clinical thermometer. This is most important, particularly in dealing with heat stroke.

* *Blood pressure equipment.* Like a stethoscope, it's useful only if it tells you something that you can do something about.

**Endotracheal tube.* One step beyond the airway (above) and one step before the tracheostomy kit (below).

**Laryngoscope.* This is probably the only way you'll be able to use an endotracheal tube. Don't take it if you don't take an endotracheal tube.

**Portable tracheostomy kit.* Listed only with great reluctance, it may be lifesaving in skillful hands. It is assumed you will do a tracheostomy between the thyroid and cricoid cartilage (cricothyrotomy) with insertion of an adequate airway. Insertion of large gauge needles alone does not provide for adequate air exchange for very long.

Hand-operated bag and mask for ventilation. Be certain that this fits or has an adapter for your endotracheal tubes and airways.

70% isopropyl alcohol. A small container of this, or some other antiseptic, will be useful if things have to be kept clean or if equipment must be prepared for reuse.

A *safety razor* and a few *razor blades* will be helpful if you are going to suture a hairy scalp wound.

Paper and pencil. Simple records can be a hassle but can save much agony in litigation. We suggest that you do not ask for, and do not use, a patient's name but assign him a number and give him a copy of his number for future reference. (See Chapter 2 on legal considerations.)

MEDICATIONS

Smelling salts. The small breakable vials of ammonia are very useful for rousing the unrousable and for various faints, swoons, and the vapors.

Neosporin or Bacitracin ointment. This can be used in the treatment of superficial infections on the skin. It should be applied only after the infected area has been washed thoroughly and allowed to dry.

Benadryl (50 mg) or *Pyribenzamine* (50 mg) can be taken every four hours to treat an allergy. Either may cause some drowsiness and should not be used while driving or if you have to stay alert.

Hydrocortisone.

Ipecac syrup (not the tincture). It is sometimes necessary to get the patient to vomit if he has just taken an overdose of something. One or two tablespoons of ipecac will induce vomiting; so will a finger placed in the back of the throat. Vomiting should not be induced in a person who is not fully conscious, nor should you induce vomiting in someone who has ingested lye or a solvent such as gasoline or benzine. A stomach tube may be necessary to empty the stomach in these cases. This is included in Kit C.

Tetanus toxoid should be liberally available and liberally used, 0.5 ml intramuscularly in anyone who has a contaminated wound. If the wound is seriously contaminated tetanus antitoxin may be necessary (see Chapter 5).

*Cardiac drugs. Assuming you have someone with a heart attack, a myocardial infarct, or pulmonary edema, the following might prove useful: Digoxin, Isuprel, lidocaine, atropine, nitroglycerin, ethacrynic acid, morphine, sodium bicarbonate, propranolol, and Levophed. In this case you'd better know what you are doing.

Snakebite kit. Convenient kits are available if you are going into the woods. Directions are included in the kit.

TYPE C—STATIONARY SUPPLY KIT

This is not really a kit but almost a portable emergency room. It may involve a moderate to substantial expense. The expense of this elaborate equipment implies that it will be used or available more than just once; it should be responsibly stored and available the next time it is needed—even on very short notice.

The equipment in this kit involves all of what is included in the Type A and Type B kits. The optional things listed there should now be included. More generous supplies of various items should be available and greater variety of some (e.g., various needles and syringes and oral and injectable medications) should be added.

This kit need not be stationary but can be assembled in the back of a station wagon or panel truck. The station wagon is fine if you'll be treating patients on the ground outside. The panel truck has the advantage of more security and privacy, but you take a big loss in poor lighting and ventilation.

A stationary (or semi-stationary) outfit has some very big advantages if you don't need mobility. It is much less of a haphazard affair and often much more comfortable for the patient. It has an air of authority which makes it a little less likely to be harassed by police, particularly if it is properly identified. (We have found that even prior clearance and "proper" identification for first-aid stations and medical personnel is no guarantee againt police harassment.) Most important, though, given enough time, a stationary set-up can be plugged into a water line, power line, telephone line, and even conceivably, a sewer line. Never underestimate the water supply problem. Water is needed for much more than just the treatment of tear gas injuries and hand washing. Failure to assure an adequate supply of water will leave you high and dry almost as soon as you start. Arrangements for water should be a critical part of your planning.

If you establish a stationary medical unit you should have some kind of vehicle for transporting the seriously sick or injured or the dead and dying to a hospital which presumably has facilities greater than yours.

Don't, by the way, be put off by the cost and difficulty in securing a generous stationary facility. With a lot of hustling and tact and the right approach, much can be accomplished. Comments on how to go about obtaining the necessary equipment are included in the next section.

EQUIPMENT

(Unless you have a supply of electricity, it is going to be very difficult operating your portable electrical equipment.

"Portable" may mean only that it is movable. It may still have to be plugged in.)

Stretchers, cots, blankets. You'll need blankets even if it is summertime. Washable blankets are best.

*A portable electrocardiogram machine is an enormous convenience. You will need someone qualified to interpret the results.

*A cardiac defibrillator is an expensive piece of equipment, but if it is available it is a useful thing to have.

Portable suction apparatus and tubing.

A stomach tube and tubing for gastric lavage.

An oxygen tank and the appropriate control valves.

*An obstetrical kit. People have babies at strange times.

Urinalysis testing equipment. For sugar and acetone.

*Ophthalmoscope—otoscope. With fresh batteries.

Intravenous solutions—dextrose, saline, and plasma.

Soap—The strong antibacterial kind to generously use with your generous supply of water.

MEDICATIONS

Now you can start including some optional drugs. People are always running out of the medicines they take regularly and need as maintenance treatment. You should be prepared to treat non-emergency routine problems. The listing below is not complete but does include a few of the medications that our experience suggests will be necessary.

Birth-control pills. It is amazing how many women forget them. You ought to have a few varieties and dispense only enough to tide a woman over.

*Anti-seizure pills. Dilantin, Valium, and phenobarbital should do it.

*Anti-hypertensive pills. Reserpine and any of the thiazides.

*Anticoagulants and related drugs. Coumadin and vitamin K.

*Anti-asthma pills. Tedral and/or Quadrinal.

*Diabetic medications. Insulin (regular and NPH) and some of the oral drugs.

Antibiotics. Among other things you may see someone with syphilis or gonorrhea. You'll need some penicillin (oral and parenteral) and tetracycline. The urinary infections will generally need a sulfa drug such as Gantrisin.

Donnatal and any kind of antacid.

Neo-synephrine nasal spray (¼ per cent), This may help clear a stuffed nose and may help in slowing a nosebleed.

Lomotil. This is an excellent drug for diarrhea; one or two tablets after each episode of diarrhea to a maximum of eight per day. If you can't get any (you'll need a prescription), you can use tincture of opium (also needs a prescription) or kaopectate.

Oil of cloves. This is good temporary relief for a toothache. It is an effective local anesthetic.

Where to Get It

To get small quantities of medical supplies or equipment for personal or family use, you will need only a good pharmacy or surgical supply house with necessary prescriptions in hand from a cooperative doctor.

Getting large quantities of some of the material and equipment, particularly those listed in Kit B or Kit C, can require some imagination and resourcefulness; more so if you are on a tight budget. But the resourcefulness of determined people is infinite. We offer some suggestions on how and where to get large quantities of the medical supplies you may need, but we don't presume to have exhausted all the potential donors.

It should first be understood that sponsors of profit-making events should be required to provide adequate medical facilities, adequate supportive staff, and transportation (including helicopter evacuation, if necessary). If you represent a nonprofit group effort (for example, providing emergency medical care during a demonstration), there are some agencies who might be able to help, either willingly or with some gentle coercion. The discussions with these official or semi-official agencies can realistically only be handled by a physician; without the authenticity he can lend to a group effort, you are unfortunately negotiating from a very weak position.

The big supplies, the large quantities, and the major equipment are the major problem, and we'll consider these first.

MAJOR PROVIDERS OF FREE SUPPLIES

Your local, friendly health department. These people will not be inclined to help because of their commitment, their dedication, their sympathy or their tradition of high-quality public service. They might help because individuals among them may be basically good and in a position to help, or they can be gently manipulated into offering assistance.

The manipulation requires care and depends on circumstances. Our experience, for example, in Washington, D.C., may be unusual but is worth a try. When 250,000 people march on the Capitol or 5,000 camp at Resurrection City for two months, the city simply can't ignore it. Someone high enough at the Health Department knows that an outbreak of hepatitis or a few "preventable" deaths among the demonstrators, worse still among the police, will be very difficult to explain to a suddenly self-righteous mayor, city council, or grand jury. This official also knows that realistically he is powerless to do anything about it; he doesn't have the personnel, the imagination, the enthusiasm, and the flexibility to take care of the problem. Here's where the bargain is made. In Washington, the local chapter of the Medical Committee for Human Rights provides the personnel and organizational framework; the city provides supplies, medications, and equipment.

Not every city has a chapter of MCHR (many do, see Appendix 1), but most cities can gather a few dedicated professionals to manage some of the medical problems. And not every city has a health department that can be made to understand its responsibility or the potential difficulty it might be in. The approach, however, is worth considering. It's a mutually beneficial arrangement.

(The entire question of just whose responsibility it is to take care of those people who are sick or injured remains unanswered. The purists will argue that medical activities such as those outlined above are merely bailing out the health department and it makes it even easier for them to do nothing, to avoid or delay reform, and to continue to side-step the problem of providing medical care for the people. We do not dispute the validity of this argument. The purists may sit back, do nothing, and be right, but we are not for a moment convinced that the rectitude of their convictions will move the health department one bit, nor, unfortunately, will it provide medical services to the sick and injured.)

The Hospital Emergency Room. This is a variant of the local health department. Generally, one hospital is going to bear the brunt of a large number of casualties from a demonstration—and they know it. Their proximity, prominence, or public financing makes them the likely place to which the sick and injured will repair.

The hospital must be convinced that you will help them, in effect, provide them with additional personnel and take the load off their overworked emergency room if they will provide you with supplies and equipment for you to establish mobile or field aid stations.

You are not simply ripping off the hospital. You are offering them an honest and real service. If you approach it right you might be able to convince them of this.

The Red Cross. Our experience with the Red Cross suggests a slightly different approach. They have a worse track record than even most primitive city health departments, but they generally have an enormous respository of money, supplies, and equipment which they are saving for the next tornado or earthquake. Their vulnerability is shame, publicity, and exposure; they can be blackmailed. An anecdote from Resurrection City will illustrate this point. When we first approached the Red Cross for supplies, they expressed feigned concern but allowed that this was not their responsibility. They wished us well. We did get them to attend a meeting of various health and hospital agencies to discuss our plans for the forthcoming arrival of the Poor People's March. When it came the turn of the Red Cross to discuss its plans, its representative proudly announced that the Red Cross would provide all the Band-Aids and tongue depressors that were needed. The room was silent. Even the commissioner of health recognized the absurdity of their offer. The Red Cross had given us our ammunition. Ultimately, they too saw their vulnerability (we didn't even have to threaten them with exposure), and they eventually realized that their storehouse had a few extra cots, stretchers, and blankets. Reason prevailed.

It's such a hassle with the Red Cross, though, that in our experience it isn't worth it unless you're desperate or you have someone with enough time and curiosity to see what they'll say.

Free Clinics. There are probably 500 free clinics of every sort and description all over the country. A partial list is included in Appendix 2.

The free clinics usually have supplies and personnel and might well be able to help. They invariably are short of funds, however, and if you use theirs it means that they have to scrounge a bit more or someone else goes without.

MARGINAL PROVIDERS—BUT FREE

Your doctor friends can sometimes help. They might be able to lend you some equipment or donate some supplies or medications. (Don't forget that they are going to be the people who will negotiate with the health department. They might also help locate sources of supplies in remote places which would be otherwise unnoticed.)

The local MCHR chapters (see Appendix 1) are organizations of health workers; doctors, nurses, lab technicians, hospital workers, etc., who can often provide a great deal of assistance in organizing medical supplies for a forthcoming event. The sooner they are brought in, the better for all.

Some church groups and an occasional labor union can be extremely helpful in selected instances. Usually local churches or unions are aware of activities that their national groups might sponsor. Some churches have special clinics (e.g., in migrant farm labor areas) in this country in addition to missionary activities abroad. The Seventh Day Adventists have at least one thoroughly equipped and staffed medical van which travels to various parts of the country in response to special needs. (They provided excellent services at Resurrection City.)

Donations, if solicted on behalf of medical needs, are often easily obtained and generously given. Your yield depends on how systematic you want to be and the circumstances of your solicitation. In the riot in Washington, D.C., in 1968, a fair number of cash contributions were received by MCHR simply because it was announced on the radio that the group was establishing medical facilities for people who were arrested, burned out, or otherwise in need. Scores of people will contribute bits and pieces of supplies to a medical unit when the word goes out that things are running a little short. These contributions, however, tend to be general pieces of equipment: blankets, lanterns, candles, etc. Generous, but not to be relied upon if you are stocking your medical kit.

Don't overlook *drugstores,* or particularly drugstore chains. For the right kind of event they have been very generous in Washington with contributions of supplies.

Drug samples. This is included more for the sake of completeness than because we think much of it. Most drug companies do send samples to physicians, but the samples are not those of the staples or well-established standard drugs. They're generous with what they are pushing this month and it usually is their newest product and not aspirin, morphine, or penicillin. Gathering samples from individual physicians is also a big job. We've tried contacting the drug companies for corporate drug contributions; some will supply whichever of their products you request, but most will send along a generous sample of the current featured item.

PURCHASING SUPPLIES

If you have to purchase supplies, don't buy anything retail if you can avoid it. Most physicians receive catalogues from wholesale drug companies and you certainly should start here if you have the time and a minimum (usually $10) order.

If you're stuck, the local drugstore will have most of what you need. They should have most of the non-asterisked supplies and medications. If a medication has an asterisk you'll probably need a prescription or have to get it at a medical supply house. If you have to rely on the drugstore, we assume that you're stocking a Type A or a small Type B kit.

One final word. If you're borrowing any equipment, return it cleaned and reasonably close to its original state. You'll never get it again, if you're planning on a next time, unless you get it back to its owner. Donors get very touchy if the stretcher was used for firewood or if someone ripped off the $2,000 electrocardiograph machine.

Appendices

I. Chapters of the Medical Committee for Human Rights

ARIZONA

TUCSON
4122 East 6th Street
Tucson 85711

ARKANSAS

LITTLE ROCK
West Side Clinic
4311 Barrow Road
Little Rock 72204

CALIFORNIA

DAVIS
927 Gregory Place
Davis 95616
Tom Schragg

FRESNO
1407 N. Van Ness Avenue
Fresno 93728
Larry Sheehy

ISLA VISTA
811 Camino Pesadero #40
Isla Vista 93017
David Bearman

LOS ANGELES
129 Fraser
Santa Monica 90405
213-399-4811
Heleena Van Raan

PALO ALTO
c/o P.O. Box 7677
San Francisco 94119
415-548-7572
Michael Schneider

SACRAMENTO
4915 South Land Park Drive
Sacramento 94522
916-442-2306
Mark Murray

SAN DIEGO
P.O. Box 99011
San Diego 92109
714-488-2216
Jeoffrey Gordon

SAN FRANCISCO—BAY AREA
P.O. Box 7677
San Francisco 94119
415-548-7572
Linda Morse

COLORADO

CENTER
P.O. Box 458
Center 81125
Martha Higdon

DENVER
291 South Pearl #6
Denver
303-744-7656
Cheryl Parker & Bob Ratner

CONNECTICUT

HARTFORD
1823 Asylum Avenue
Hartford 06116
Liz Gunderson

NEW HAVEN
333 Cedar Street
New Haven 06520
203-387-8772
Art Mazer

DISTRICT OF COLUMBIA

WASHINGTON
2506 Cliffbourne
Washington
202-667-6277
Jackie Kelly

FLORIDA

GAINESVILLE
16½ NW 20th Drive
Gainesville 32601
904-378-4297
Margaret Megill

JACKSONVILLE
124 East Adams Street
Jacksonville 32202
904-356-8357
Duvall County Legal Aid Assn.

MIAMI
3190 Florida Avenue
Coconut Grove 33133
305-446-4691
Bill Shore

GEORGIA

ATLANTA
371 Amal Drive, SW #5
Atlanta 30315
404-627-0947
Beatrice Gray

AUGUSTA
1549 Craig Street
Augusta 30904
404-736-0432
Robert Wyatt

HAWAII

HONOLULU
2006 Oswald Street
Honolulu 96816
808-732-5197
Marjorie Benning

ILLINOIS

CARBONDALE
c/o Carbondale Free Clinic
104 E. Jackson
Carbondale 62901
618-549-5633
Joel Lee

CHAMPAIGN-URBANA
104 West Mumford
Urbana 60801
217-344-5543
Anita Pisciotte

CHICAGO
710 South Marshfield
Chicago 60612
312-243-4137
DiDi Halkin

DANVILLE
1106 North Logan
Danville 61832
217-443-0585
Gene VanderPort

FREEPORT
215 East Stephenson
Freeport 61032
815-232-9316
LaMorn Morris

IOWA

DES MOINES
841 6th Avenue #B-1
Des Moines 50309
Michael Griffen

KENTUCKY

LEXINGTON
458 West 3rd Street
Lexington 40508
606-254-9855
Bob Young

LOUISIANA

NEW ORLEANS
P.O. Box 30362
New Orleans 70130
504-522-9978
Dan Blumenthal

MARYLAND

BALTIMORE
3022 North Calvert
Baltimore 21218
301-467-2327
Ellen Siegel

MASSACHUSETTS

BOSTON
c/o Old Cambridge Baptist Church
1151 Massachusetts Avenue
Cambridge 02138
617-492-6247
Rena Lieb

WORCESTER
820 Main Street
Worcester 01601
Dr. & Ms. A. Saxton

MICHIGAN

ANN ARBOR
1323 West Huron
Ann Arbor 48103
313-761-9556
Connie Sprauer

DETROIT
8824 Fenkell
Detroit 48238
313-342-8355
Edna Watson

MINNESOTA

MINNEAPOLIS
825 North Lilac Drive
Minneapolis 55422
612-545-4250
Cathy and Jack Carson

MISSOURI

COLUMBIA
1032 South Park #2
Columbia 65201
Daniel Taylor

KANSAS CITY
Department of Pediatrics
24th at Gilham Road
Kansas City 64108
816-471-0626
Jerome Grunt

ST. LOUIS
6106 McPherson
St. Louis 63112
314-863-6790
Peter Muckerman

NEW JERSEY

NEWARK
49 Monticello Avenue
Newark 07100
201-373-6931
Jane Katz

NEW YORK

BUFFALO
115 Lafayette
Buffalo 14213
716-885-8158
Richard Duffy

ITHACA
14 German Cross Road
Ithaca 14856
607-277-3268
Jack Salmon

QUEENS-NASSAU
270-05 76th Avenue
LIJ Social Services
New Hyde Park 11040
212-343-6700
Lenny Guardino

ROCHESTER
Crittenden Blvd., Strong Memorial
Rochester 14620
716-442-0049
Barry Lachman

NEW YORK
137A West 14th Street
New York 10014
212-924-0894
Naomi Appel

STONY BROOK, L.I.
Building G, Health Science Center
SUNY
Stony Brook 11790
516-751-4508
Judy Kahn

SYRACUSE
509 South Beech
Syracuse 13210
315-478-5681
Diane Cass

NORTH CAROLINA

DURHAM
4505 Ryan
Durham 27704
919-477-0938
Paul Bermanzohn

FAYETTEVILLE
P.O. Box 5101, Eutow Station
Fayetteville 28301
919-868-2202
Jay Lockard

OHIO

ATHENS
Coburn Road
Shade 45776
614-696-1229
Andrea Schmidt

CINCINNATI
3344 Vine Street
Cincinnati 45220
513-751-1439
Ken Casey

CLEVELAND
2753 Hampshire Road
Cleveland Hts 44106
216-231-8456
Marilyn Silverman

COLUMBUS
4679 Dundee Avenue
Columbus 43227
Dorothy Kavanaugh

SPRINGFIELD
320 Baltimore Place
Springfield 44226
513-325-9637
Bob Lange

Medical Committee for Human Rights

OKLAHOMA

OKLAHOMA CITY
1619 NW 27th
Oklahoma City   73106
405-525-6249
Dana Brian

OREGON

PORTLAND
2536 NE 20th Avenue
Portland   97212
503-288-2497
Sol and Gerri Peck

PENNSYLVANIA

HARRISBURG
P.O. Box 1272
Harrisburg   17108
Denny Rock

PHILADELPHIA
1307 Samson
Philadelphia   19147
215-EV6-6114
Donna Calame

PITTSBURGH
617 Empire Building
Pittsburgh   15222
412-731-6813
Kay Fitts

RHODE ISLAND

PROVIDENCE
Providence Health Center
228 Thurber Avenue
Providence
401-781-5153
Mike Gerhardt

SOUTH CAROLINA

COLUMBIA
P.O. Box 11399
Columbia   29211
803-254-9903
Janet Jenkins

TENNESSEE

KNOXVILLE
1914 Andy Holt Avenue
Knoxville   37961
U. of Tenn. Health School
615-522-8260
Ruth Eng

MEMPHIS
1300 Medical Towers
969 Madison Avenue
Reg Med Program
Memphis   38104
James Couch

NASHVILLE
4023 Hydes Ferry Pike
Nashville   37218
615-255-3896
Ed Risby

TEXAS

DALLAS
3974 Cortez Drive
Dallas   75220
214-351-1858
Patti Larson

HOUSTON
2551 North MacGregor Way
Houston   77004
713-523-1445
Kim Shinkoskey

SAN ANTONIO
P.O. Box 13341
San Antonio   78213
512-732-5197
Emily Homonoff

UTAH

SALT LAKE CITY, UTAH
6453 South 3rd East
Midvale 84047
801-266-1408
Wes Tator

WASHINGTON

SEATTLE
4727 46th NE
Seattle 98294
206-LA3-1190
John Holcenberg

TACOMA
P.O. Box 94055
Tacoma 98494
206-SK2-1617
Stephen Geary

WEST VIRGINIA

BLUEFIELD
Route #2, Box 382
Bluefield 24701
Reg. Occup. Resp. Proj.
Wesley Mason

MORGANTOWN
321 Ridgewood
Morgantown 26505
304-292-7663
Robb Burlage

WISCONSIN

MADISON
1335 North Wingra Drive
Madison 53715
608-255-3647
Lewis Leavitt

MILWAUKEE
2473 West Highland
Milwaukee 53233
414-933-2617
Jeanne Weisman

II. Free Clinic Directory*

ALASKA

ANCHORAGE
The Anchorage Open Door Clinic
112 W. 5th Ave.
Anchorage, Alaska 99501

ARIZONA

PHOENIX
Terros, Inc.
1229 N. 1st Street
Phoenix, Arizona 85004
William K. Ponder, Executive Director

CALIFORNIA

ALHAMBRA
Chinese Community Free Clinic
3000 West Ramona Rd.
Alhambra, California 91803
attn: Mr. James Yong

Open Door Clinic
1209 South Sixth St.
Alhambra, California 91801
attn: Don La Perna

ANAHEIM
Free Clinic of Orange County
504 N. Anaheim Blvd.
Anaheim, California 92805
attn: Dean Reinemann

ARCATA
Humboldt Open Door Clinic
P.O. Box 367
Arcata, California 95521
attn: Don Sampson

BALDWIN PARK
Baldwin Park Free Clinic
4488 North Stewart Ave.
Baldwin Park, California 91706
attn: David G. Martinez

BELLFLOWER
Hawaiian Gardens Youth Clinic
22101 Norwalk Blvd.
Bellflower, California 90706

BERKELEY
Berkeley Free Clinic
2339 Durant Ave.
Berkeley, California

George Jackson People's Free Health Clinic
3236 Adeline Street
Berkeley, California

---

* This list of clinics was compiled by Jerome L. Schwartz of Berkeley, California, from the files of the National Free Clinic Council. For a summary of clinic characteristics see Dr. Schwartz's report, "Preliminary Observations of Free Clinics," in *The Free Clinic: A Community Approach to Health Care and Drug Abuse* (Eds., David E. Smith, David J. Bentel and Jerome L. Schwartz), STASH Press, Beloit, Wisconsin, 1971, pp. 143-206.
We are very grateful to Dr. Schwartz for his permission to publish this list.

COMPTON
American Indian Free Clinic
526 East Oaks Street
Compton, California   90221
attn: Rev. E. Sarracino

CORONA
Corona Free Clinic
821 S. Main Street
Corona, California   91720
attn: Rev. Richard C. Hall

COSTA MESA
Youth Problem Center
132 E. 18th Street
Costa Mesa, California   92627
attn: Bob Aldrich

DALY CITY
Our Lady of Guadalupe Health Center
6705 Mission Street
Daly City, California   94014

ESCONDIDO
Escondido Community Clinic
401 North Spruce Street
Escondido, California   92025
attn: Dr. Oliver Thomas

HUNTINGTON BEACH
Huntington Beach Free Clinic
222 Fifth Street
Huntington Beach, California   92647

IMPERIAL BEACH
Imperial Beach Free Clinic
150 Palm Ave.
Imperial Beach, California   92032
attn: John Farnum

ISLA VISTA
Isla Vista Community Service Center

Medical Clinic—Suite C
970 Embarcadero Del Mar
Isla Vista, California   93017
attn: David Bearman, M.D.

LAGUNA BEACH
Laguna Beach Free Clinic
424 Gelneyre Street
Laguna Beach, California   92651
attn: Mary Stack

LA PUENTE
East Valley Free Clinic
15256 Fair Grove Ave.
La Puente, California   91745
attn: Howard Jackson

LONG BEACH
Long Beach Free Clinic
1228 Pine Ave.
Long Beach, California   90813
attn: Ron Lofstrom

LOS ANGELES
Bridge Back Free Clinic
4771 South Main Street
Los Angeles, California   90037
attn: Roy Evans

El Barrio Free Clinic
5016 E. Whittier Blvd.
Los Angeles, California   90022
attn: Gloria Arellanes

Hollywood-Sunset Free Clinic
3324 Sunset Blvd.
Los Angeles, California   90026
attn: Mark Clein

Imperial Heights Youth Clinic
10616 South Western Ave.
Los Angeles, California

Koinonia Free Clinic
c/o Bethel Lutheran Church
5750 W. Olympic Blvd.
Los Angeles, California   90017
attn: Gordon Larson

Los Angeles Free Clinic
115 North Fairfax Ave.
Los Angeles, California 90036
attn: Lenny Somberg

Midtown Free Clinic
940¾ Menlo Ave.
Los Angeles, California 90006
attn: M. Yoshio Tsukiyama

Northeast Youth Clinic
2032 Marengo Street
Los Angeles, California

People's Free Clinic
3223 S. Central
Los Angeles, California 90011

San Vincente Youth Clinic
621 North San Vicente
Los Angeles, California 90036

Southside Community Free Clinic
1101 West Jefferson
Los Angeles, California 90007
attn: Paul Polk

Younger Generation
10616 South Western Ave.
Los Angeles, California
attn: Dr. Kani

MANHATTAN BEACH
South Bay Free Clinic
1807 Manhattan Beach Blvd.
Manhattan Beach, California
  90266
attn: Bruce Lagatree

MENDOCINO
Health Center of the Mendocino
  Coast
P.O. Box 944
Mendocino, California 95460
attn: Pamela Hudson

NORTH HOLLYWOOD
North Hollywood Free Clinic
5224 Lankershim Blvd.
North Hollywood, California
  91601
attn: Barbara Feiner

OAKLAND
Black Panther Community Clinic
1048 Peralta
Oakland, California 94600

Clinica De La Raza
1415 Fruitvale
Oakland, California

East Oakland Health Alliance
8501 E. 14th
Oakland, California

OXNARD
Oxnard Free Clinic
200 Enterprise
Oxnard, California 93030
attn: Diana J. May

PALO ALTO
Community for the People's
  Medical Center
P.O. Box 3205
Palo Alto, California
attn: Marty Kalishman, M.D.

PASADENA
Foothill Free Clinic
35 S. Raymond
Pasadena, California 91105
attn: John Binkley

POMONA
Pomona Open Door Clinic
861 North Park Ave.
Pomona, California 91766
attn: Jim Oliver

PORTERVILLE
Salud
Coyle Colony
1243 East Date Ave.
Porterville, California   93257

RIVERSIDE
Youth Service Center of Riverside, Inc.
3847 Terracina
Riverside, California   92506

SACRAMENTO
Aquarian Effort Free Clinic
4500 47th Avenue
Sacramento, California   95824
attn: Dr. Gordon Runnels

SAN DIEGO
Beach Area Free Clinic
3705 Mission Blvd.
San Diego, California

Chicano Free Clinic
1809 National Ave.
San Diego, California

Oceanside Community Action Corp. Free Clinic
605 San Diego Street
Oceanside, California   92054

San Diego Community Crisis Center
3004 Imperial Ave.
San Diego, California   92102
attn: John Robbins

SAN FRANCISCO
Asian Community Health Clinic
799 Pacific Street
San Francisco, California   94109
c/o Mr. Johnson Kam

Blackman's Free Clinic
689 McAllister Street
San Francisco, California

Centra de la Saluda para Gente
2990 22nd Street
San Francisco, California   94114
attn: Corey Weinstein

Everyman's Free Clinic
120 Church Street
San Francisco, California   94114
attn: Bert Meyer, M.D.

Haight-Ashbury Free Medical Clinic
558 Clayton Street
San Francisco, California   94117
attn: Dr. David Smith

SAN PEDRO
Harbor Free Clinic
524 W. 6th Street
San Pedro, California   90731
attn: Ted Peterson

SANTA ANA
Community Health Clinic
c/o PAN C-R-O All Color Resource Organization
1431 West Fourth St.
Santa Ana, California   92703

SANTA BARBARA
Freedom Community Clinic
c/o 1363 Tunnel Road
Santa Barbara, California   93105

SANTA FE SPRINGS
Santa Fe Springs Youth Clinic
9255 Pioneer Blvd.
Santa Fe Springs, California

SANTA MONICA
Ex-Helps Center
1533 Euclid
Santa Monica, California   90404
attn: Katie Campbell

SIMI VALLEY
Free Clinic of Simi Valley

1725 Deadora Street
Simi Valley, California 93065
attn: Fred Bauermeister

TUSTIN
Rap Center
285 E. Main St., Suite #12
Tustin, California
attn: Karen Morton

VAN NUYS
Van Nuys Youth Clinic
14340 Sylvan Street
Van Nuys, California 91401

VENICE
Salud/Venice Health Clinic
1625 Washington
Venice, California

Venice Community Family Health Center
316 South Lincoln Blvd.
Venice, California 90291

Venice Youth Clinic
905 Venice Blvd.
Venice, California 90291

VENTURA
Ventura Free Clinic
32 North Ash
Ventura, California 93001

VISTA
Vista Free Clinic
645 Mercantile
Vista, California 92083
attn: Bill Raff

WOODVILLE
Salud Free Clinic
Road 16815 & Ave. 168
Woodville, California 93257

COLORADO

BOULDER
People's Clinic
999 Alpone
Boulder, Colorado

FORT COLLINS
Fort Collins Free Clinic
c/o Cecil Oakes, Jr., M.D.
P.O. Box 511
Fort Collins, Colorado 80521

CONNECTICUT

NEW HAVEN
Black Panther People's Clinic
35 Sylvan
New Haven, Connecticut
attn: Fran Carter

DISTRICT OF COLUMBIA

WASHINGTON
Anacostia Center for Medical Services
Good Hope Road
Washington, D.C.
attn: Dave Jackson

Washington Free Clinic
1556 Wisconsin Ave. N.W.
Washington, D.C. 20007
attn: Judy Seckler

FLORIDA

GAINESVILLE
Corner Drug Store
1128 S.W. 1st Avenue
Gainesville, Florida 32601
attn: Barbara Lemcke

GEORGIA

AUGUSTA
Hyde Park Health Clinic
c/o Clara Jenkins Elementary School

Dan Bowles Road
Augusta, Georgia

HAWAII

HONOLULU
Honolulu Free Clinic
319 Paoakalani Avenue
Honolulu, Hawaii   96815
attn: Dr. Paul Koons

Waikiki Drug Clinic
319 Paoakalani Avenue
Honolulu, Hawaii   96815
attn: Gregory Molica

IDAHO

POCATELLO
Pocatello Free Clinic
145 South Third
Pocatello, Idaho   83201
attn: Steven Robinson

ILLINOIS

CARBONDALE
Carbondale Free Clinic
104 E. Jackson
Carbondale, Illinois
attn: Joel M. Lee, Medical Coordinator

CHICAGO
Benito Jaurez People's Health Center
1831 S. Racine
Chicago, Illinois
attn: Maury Mendoze

Fritzi Englestein Free People's Health Center
2747 N. Wilton
Chicago, Illinois
attn: Kathy Sheehan

LADO
2353 W. North Avenue
Chicago, Illinois
attn: Mitchell L. Klein

Spurgeon Jake Winters Free People's Medical Care Center
3850 W. 16th
Chicago, Illinois
attn: Ronald "Doc" Satchel

Young Patriots Community Health Center
4408 N. Sheridan
Chicago, Illinois
attn: Doug Youngblood

FREEPORT
People's Health Center
215 E. Stephenson Street
Freeport, Illinois   61032
attn: John White, Coordinator

IOWA

DES MOINES
Mid-Iowa Drug Abuse Council
512 9th Street
Des Moines, Iowa   50309
attn: Bonnie Christensen, R.N.

IOWA CITY
Iowa City Free Medical Clinic
P.O. Box 1170
Iowa City, Iowa   52240
attn: Susan Krohmer

KANSAS

LAWRENCE
Headquarters
1546 Massachusetts
Lawrence, Kansas   66044

Reality, Inc.
380 Essex Street
Lawrence, Kansas

KENTUCKY

LEXINGTON
Grosvenor Street Zoo
305 Grosvenor Street
Lexington, Kentucky

LOUISIANA

NEW ORLEANS
Central City Neighborhood
 Health Clinic
3307 Freret Street
New Orleans, Louisiana

HEAD
1117 Decatur
New Orleans, Louisiana   70116

Health Committee of the Lower
 Ninth Ward
5426 North Galvez Street
New Orleans, Louisiana

MARYLAND

BALTIMORE
People's Free Medical Clinic
3028 Greenmount Ave.
Baltimore, Maryland   21218
attn: Howard Evans, Coordinator

PRINCE GEORGES COUNTY
Prince Georges County Free
 Clinic
c/o Jeff Chlebrikow
Dept. of Psychology
Catholic University of America
Washington, D.C.

MASSACHUSETTS

AMHERST
Amherst Free Clinic
c/o Philip A. Terrence
353 Northampton Road
Amherst, Massachusetts   01002

BOSTON
The Medical Service
1 Walnut Street
Boston, Massachusetts

CAMBRIDGE
Cambridge Free Clinic
10 Mt. Auburn Street
Cambridge, Massachusetts
 02139
attn: Dr. Joseph Brenner

PROVINCETOWN
Provincetown Drop-In Center
6 Gosnold Street
Provincetown, Massachusetts
 02657
attn: Eric Chivian, M.D., Director

MICHIGAN

ANN ARBOR
Free People's Clinic
302 E. Liberty
Ann Arbor, Michigan
attn: Nancy Lessin, Coordinator

DETROIT
Jeffries Clinic
Jeffries Housing Project
1451 Selden
Detroit, Michigan

Open City Free Clinic
Third Ave. and Canfield
Detroit, Michigan

EAST LANSING
Free Clinic
1416 "H" Street
Spartan Village
East Lansing, Michigan   48823
attn: Paul Koons, M.D.

MINNESOTA

COON RAPIDS
NUCLEUS
c/o Workshop, Inc.
2701 Northdale Blvd.
Coon Rapids, Minnesota 55303

MINNEAPOLIS
Beltrami Health Center
759 Pierces St. N.E.
Minneapolis, Minnesota 55413
attn: Pauline LaClaire

Cedar Riverside People's Center
2000 S. 5th Street
Minneapolis, Minnesota 55404
attn: Mary E. Lange

Fremont Community Clinic
2507 Fremont North
Minneapolis, Minnesota 55411
attn: David Schuman or Judy
  Dwyer

Southside Medical Clinic
116 E. 32nd Street
Minneapolis, Minnesota 55408

Teen-Age Medical Center
2425 Chicago Avenue South
Minneapolis, Minnesota

ST. PAUL
Westside Clinic
712 S. Robert Street
St. Paul, Minnesota

WYOMING
Lakes Community Medical Clinic
Wyoming 1, Minnesota
or c/o Susan Miller
Box 121
St. Francis, Minnesota 55070

MISSOURI

KANSAS CITY
Westport Free Health Clinic
3939 Wyandotte
Kansas City, Missouri 64111

NEBRASKA

OMAHA
Equilibria
4924 Poppleton and Saddle Creek
Omaha, Nebraska
attn: Donald Parkinson, M.D.

NEW MEXICO

ALBUQUERQUE
Albuquerque Free Clinic
1409 Hazeldine, S.E.
Albuquerque, New Mexico
  87106
attn: Cassell Carpenter

Taos Free Clinic
P.O. Box 190
Arroyo Seco
Taos, New Mexico 87514

NEW YORK

ALBANY
Washington Park Free Medical
  Clinic
332 Hudson
P.O. Box 19268
Albany, New York 12208

NEW YORK
Judson Mobile Health Unit
East Village
New York, New York
attn: June Finer, M.D.

St. Marks Free Clinic
44 St. Marks Place
New York, New York 10003
attn: Leon Fay

WOODSTOCK
Woodstock Free Clinic
General Delivery
Woodstock, New York
attn: Peter Walker

NORTH CAROLINA

DURHAM
Edgemont Community Clinic
1012 E. Main St.
Durham, North Carolina
attn: Dan McConnell

OHIO

CANTON
Canton Free Clinic
c/o Kathleen Essik
3724 Woodland Ave., N.W.
Canton, Ohio   44709

CINCINNATI
Cincinnati Free Clinic
P.O. Box 19268
Cincinnati, Ohio   45219
attn: Arnie Leff, M.D.

CLEVELAND
Near West Side People's Free Clinic
Parish House
W. 44th and Bridge
Cleveland, Ohio

The Free Medical Clinic of Greater Cleveland
2039 Cornell
Cleveland, Ohio   44106
attn: Gordon Freidman

COLUMBUS
Open Door Clinic
1985 Waldeck Ave.
Columbus, Ohio   43201
attn: Alex Katz

MENTOR
Free Clinic of Lake County
8683 Mentor Avenue
Mentor, Ohio   44060
attn: David R. Lima, Exec. Director

OREGON

COTTAGE GROVE
Cottage Grove Free Clinic
c/o Jay Crithley
1406 E. Washington Street
Cottage Grove, Oregon   97424

EUGENE
White Bird Sociomedical Aid Station
837 Lincoln Street
Eugene, Oregon   97401
attn: Frank Lemmons

PORTLAND
Fred Hampton's People's Health Clinic
109 N. Russell
Portland, Oregon

Outside In
1240 Southwest Salmon Street
Portland, Oregon   97205
attn: Eliot Grossman

Southeast Portland Medical Clinic
Laurelwood Methodist Church
S.E. 62nd and Holgate
Portland, Oregon

PHILADELPHIA
HELP Free Clinic
2310 Locust Street
Philadelphia, Pennsylvania
attn: Dr. Sid Schnoll

PITTSBURGH
Pittsburgh Free Medical Clinic
East End Christian Church

South Highland Avenue and
  Adler Street
Pittsburgh, Pennsylvania 15206
attn: John Pfahler, Jr., Medical
  Coordinator

TENNESSEE

MEMPHIS
North Memphis Community
  Health Organization
278 Greenlaw
Memphis, Tennessee
attn: Sharon McConnell

TEXAS

AUSTIN
The People's Free Clinic
2330 Guadalupe
Austin, Texas 78705

CORPUS CHRISTI
CCDAC Free Clinic
425 South Broadway
Corpus Christi, Texas 78401

EL PASO
El Paso Free Clinic
103 Montana
El Paso, Texas 79901
attn: Chuck Williams

HOUSTON
Carl B. Hampton Free Health
  Clinic
2828 Dowling
Houston, Texas

Fifth Ward Free Clinic Inlet
P.O. Box 133
Texas Southern University
3201 Wheeler
Houston, Texas 77004

SAN ANTONIO
San Antonio Free Clinic

107 North Cibolo
San Antonio, Texas
attn: Tom Payte, M.D.

VERMONT

BURLINGTON
People's Free Clinic
260 North Street
Burlington, Vermont 05401

VIRGINIA

VIRGINIA BEACH
Norfolk Free Clinic
811 Goldsboro Avenue
Virginia Beach, Virginia 23451
attn: M. K. Thompson

Virginia Beach Free Clinic
c/o Rev. Timothy Sniffen
Galilee Episcopal Church
P.O. Box 847
Virginia Beach, Virginia 23451

WASHINGTON

EVERETT
Karma Clinic
2807½ Hewitt Avenue
Everett, Washington 98201

SEATTLE
Country Doctor Clinic
402-15 15th Avenue E.
Seattle, Washington 98102
attn: Ann Sebeste

First Avenue Service Center
  Clinic
1203 1st Avenue
Seattle, Washington 98102
attn: Joany Bush

Fremont Women's Clinic
3413 Fremont Avenue N.
Seattle, Washington 98103
attn: Coe Axt

Georgetown Clinic
659 S. Lucille
Seattle, Washington 98108
attn: Kathy Karpela

High Point Clinic
6536 32nd Avenue, S.W.
Seattle, Washington 98126
attn: Marian Curry

Holly Park Clinic
13120 Van Asselt Ct.
Seattle, Washington
attn: Gloria Pugh

Kinatechitapi Indian Clinic
US Public Health Service Hospital
1131 S. 14th
Seattle, Washington 98114
attn: Bernie White Bear

Open Door Free Clinic
5012 Roosevelt N.E.
Seattle, Washington 98105
attn: John Green, M.D.

Park Lake Clinic
413 S. W. 113th Place
Seattle, Washington 98146
attn: Barbara Blakeley

Rainier Vista Clinic
4215 Sears Drive South
Seattle, Washington 98108
attn: Leisa Pearson, Director

Sidney Miller Clinic
1129 18th
Seattle, Washington 98122
attn: Vanetta Molson

Yesler Terrace Clinic
102 Broadway, #607
Seattle, Washington 98122
attn: David Loud

TACOMA
Tacoma Free Clinic
3812½ South Yakima
Tacoma, Washington 98408
attn: Scott Jackson, Director

WISCONSIN

CHAMPAIGN
Francis Nelson Health Center
1306 Carver
Champaign, Wisconsin 61820
attn: Elsie Easley

MADISON
Blue Bus Free Clinic
Johnson Street at Bassett
Madison, Wisconsin

MILWAUKEE
Guadalupe Children's Clinic
1112 South 3rd Street
Milwaukee, Wisconsin 53204

People's Free Health Center
946 N. 27th Street
Milwaukee, Wisconsin

Underground Switchboard
  Medical Clinic
St. Mary's Hospital Administration Bldg.
2390 N. Lake Drive
Milwaukee, Wisconsin 53211

III. Medical Fitness Standards for Appointment, Enlistment, and Induction

Section I. General

2–1. SCOPE

This chapter sets forth the medical conditions and physical defects which are causes for rejection for military service in peacetime.

2–2. APPLICABILITY

These standards apply to—

a. Male and female applicants for appointment as commissioned or warrant officers, or for enlistment in the U.S. Army, regardless of component.

b. Applicants for the Advanced Course Army ROTC, and other personnel procurement programs other than induction, where these standards are prescribed.

c. Registrants who undergo preinduction or induction medical examination pursuant to the Universal Military Training and Service Act (50 USC, Supplement IV, Appendix 454 as amended) except medical and dental registrants who are to be evaluated under chapter 8.

d. Male and female applicants for enlistment in the U.S. Air Force or Air Force Reserve.

e. Male applicants for enlistment or reenlistment in the U.S. Navy or Naval Reserve.

f. "Chargeable accessions" for enlistment in the U.S. Marine Corps or Marine Corps Reserve. See paragraph 12*d,* AR 601–270.

Section II. Abdomen and Gastrointestinal System

2-3. ABDOMINAL ORGANS AND GASTROINTESTINAL SYSTEM

The causes for rejection for appointment, enlistment, and induction are—

a. Cholecystectomy, sequelae of, such as postoperative stricture of the common bile duct, re-forming of stones in hepatic or common bile ducts, or incisional hernia, or post-cholecystectomy syndrome when symptoms are so severe as to interfere with normal performance of duty.

b. Cholecystitis, acute or chronic, with or without cholelithiasis, if diagnosis is confirmed by usual laboratory procedures or authentic medical records.

c. Cirrhosis regardless of the absence of manifestations such as jaundice, ascites or known esophageal varices, abnormal liver function tests with or without history of chronic alcoholism.

d. Fistula in ano.

e. Gastritis, chronic hypertrophic, severe.

f. Hemorrhoids.
  (1) External hemorrhoids producing marked symptoms.
  (2) Internal hemorrhoids, if large or accompanied with hemorrhage or protruding intermittently or constantly.

g. Hepatitis within the preceding 6 months, or persistence of symptoms after a reasonable period of time with objective evidence of impairment of liver function.

h. Hernia:
  (1) Hernia other than small asymptomatic umbilical or hiatal.
  (2) History of operation for hernia within the preceding 60 days.

i. Intestinal obstruction or authenticated history of more than one episode, if either occurred during the preceding 5 years, or if resulting condition remains which produces significant symptoms or requires treatment.

j. Megacolon of more than minimal degree, *diverticulitis, re-*

gional enteritis, and *ulcerative colitis. Irritable colon* of more than moderate degree.

    k. Pancreas, acute or chronic disease of, if proven by laboratory tests, or authenticated medical records.

    l. Rectum, stricture or prolapse of.

    m. Resection, gastric or of bowel; or gastroenterostomy; however minimal intestinal resection in infancy or childhood (*for example:* for intussusception or pyloric stenosis) is acceptable if the individual has been asymptomatic since the resection and if surgical consultation (to include upper and lower gastrointestinal series) gives complete clearance.

    n. Scars.
  (1) Scars, abdominal, regardless of cause, which show hernial bulging or which interfere with movements.
  (2) Scar pain associated with disturbance of function of abdominal wall or contained viscera.

    o. Sinuses of the abdominal wall.

    p. Splenectomy, except when accomplished for the following:
  (1) Trauma.
  (2) Causes unrelated to diseases of the spleen.
  (3) Hereditary spherocytosis.
  (4) Disease involving the spleen when followed by correction of the condition for a period of at least 2 years.

    q. Tumors. See paragraphs 2–40 and 2–41.

    r. Ulcer:
  (1) Ulcer of the stomach or duodenum, if diagnosis is confirmed by X-ray examination, or authenticated history thereof.
  (2) Authentic history of surgical operation(s) for gastric or duodenal ulcer.

    s. Other congenital or acquired abnormalities and defects which preclude satisfactory performance of military duty or which require frequent and prolonged treatment.

Section III. Blood and Blood-Forming Tissue Diseases

2-4. BLOOD AND BLOOD-FORMING TISSUE DISEASES

The causes for rejection for appointment, enlistment and induction are—

  a. Anemia:
    (1) Blood loss anemia—until both condition and basic cause are corrected.
    (2) Deficiency anemia, not controlled by medication.
    (3) Abnormal destruction of RBC's: Hemolytic anemia.
    (4) Faulty RBC construction: Hereditary hemolytic anemia, thallassemia and sickle cell anemia.
    (5) Myelophthisic anemia: Myelomatosis, leukemia, Hodgkin's disease.
    (6) Primary refractory anemia: Aplastic anemia, DiGuglielmo's syndrome.

  b. Hemorrhagic states:
    (1) Due to changes in coagulation system (hemophilia, etc.).
    (2) Due to platelet deficiency.
    (3) Due to vascular instability.

  c. Leukopenia, chronic or recurrent, associated with increased susceptibility to infection.

  d. Myeloproliferative disease (other than leukemia):
    (1) Myelofibrosis.
    (2) Megakaryocytic myelosis.
    (3) Polycythemia vera.

  e. Splenomegaly until the cause is remedied.

  f. Thromboembolic disease except for acute, nonrecurrent conditions.

Section IV. Dental

2-5. DENTAL

The causes for rejection for appointment, enlistment, and induction are—

a. Diseases of the jaws or associated tissues which are not easily remediable and which will incapacitate the individual or prevent the satisfactory performance of military duty.

b. Malocclusion, severe, which interferes with the mastication of a normal diet.

c. Oral tissues, extensive loss of, in an amount that would prevent replacement of missing teeth with a satisfactory prosthetic appliance.

d. Orthodontic appliances. See special administrative criteria in paragraph 7–12.

e. Relationship between the mandible and maxilla of such a nature as to preclude future satisfactory prosthodontic replacement.

Section V. Ears and Hearing

2–6. EARS

The causes for rejection for appointment, enlistment, and induction are—

a. Auditory canal:
   (1) Atresia or severe stenosis of the external auditory canal.
   (2) Tumors of the external auditory canal except mild exostoses.
   (3) Severe external otitis, acute or chronic.

b. Auricle: Agenesis, severe; or severe traumatic deformity, unilateral or bilateral.

c. Mastoids:
   (1) Mastoiditis, acute or chronic.
   (2) Residual or mastoid operation with marked external deformity which precludes or interferes with the wearing of a gas mask or helmet.
   (3) Mastoid fistula.

d. Meniere's syndrome.

e. Middle ear:
   (1) Acute or chronic suppurative otitis media. Individuals with a recent history of acute suppurative otitis media will not be accepted unless the condition is healed and a

sufficient interval of time subsequent to treatment has elapsed to insure that the disease is in fact not chronic.

(2) Adhesive otitis media associated with hearing level by audiometric test of 20 db or more average for the speech frequencies (500, 1000, and 2000 cycles per second) in either ear regardless of the hearing level in the other ear.

(3) Acute or chronic serous otitis media.

(4) Presence of otic perforation in which presence of cholesteatoma is suspected.

(5) Repeated attacks of catarrhal otitis media; intact greyish, thickened drum(s).

f. Tympanic membrane:

(1) Any perforation of the tympanic membrane.

(2) Severe scarring of the tympanic membrane associated with hearing level by audiometric test of 20 db or more average for the speech frequencies (500, 1000, and 2000 cycles per second) in either ear regardless of the hearing level in the other ear.

g. Other diseases and defects of the ear which obviously preclude satisfactory performance of duty or which require frequent and prolonged treatment.

2–7. HEARING

(See also para. 2–6.)

The cause for rejection for appointment, enlistment, and induction is—

Hearing acuity level by audiometric testing (regardless of conversational or whispered voice hearing acuity) greater than that described in table I, appendix II. There is no objection to conducting the whispered voice test or the spoken voice test as a preliminary to conducting the audiometric hearing test.

Section VI. Endocrine and Metabolic Disorders

2–8. ENDOCRINE AND METABOLIC DISORDERS

The causes for rejection for appointment, enlistment, and induction are—

a. Adrenal gland, malfunction of, of any degree.
   b. Cretinism.
   c. Diabetes insipidus.
   d. Diabetes mellitus.
   e. Gigantism or acromegaly.
   f. Glycosuria, persistent, regardless of cause.
   g. Goiter:
      (1) Simple goiter with definite pressure symptoms or so large in size as to interfere with the wearing of a military uniform or military equipment.
      (2) *Thyrotoxicosis.*
   h. Gout.
   i. Hyperinsulinism, confirmed, symptomatic.
   j. Hyperparathyroidism and *hypoparathyroidism.*
   k. Hypopituitarism, severe.
   l. Myxedema, spontaneous or postoperative (with clinical manifestations and not based solely on low basal metabolic rate).
   m. Nutritional deficiency diseases (including sprue, beriberi, pellagra, and scurvy) which are more than mild and not readily remediable or in which permanent pathological changes have been established.
   n. Other endocrine or metabolic disorders which obviously preclude satisfactory performance of duty or which require frequent and prolonged treatment.

Section VII. Extremities

2-9. UPPER EXTREMITIES

(See para. 2-11.)

The causes for rejection for appointment, enlistment, and induction are—

   a. Limitation of motion. An individual will be considered unacceptable if the joint ranges of motion are less than the measurements below (app. IV).
      (1) *Shoulder:*
         (*a*) Forward elevation to 90°.
         (*b*) Abduction to 90°.

417 † Standards for Appointment, Enlistment, and Induction

  (2) *Elbow:*
    (*a*) Flexion to 100°.
    (*b*) Extension to 15°.
  (3) *Wrist:* A total range of 15° (extension plus flexion).
  (4) *Hand*: Pronation to the first quarter of the normal arc. Supination to the first quarter of the normal arc.
  (5) *Fingers:* Inability to clench fist, pick up a pin or needle, and grasp an object.
 b. *Hand and fingers:*
  (1) Absence (or loss) of more than ⅓ of the distal phalanx of either thumb.
  (2) Absence (or loss) of distal and middle phalanx of an index, middle or ring finger of either hand irrespective of the absence (or loss) of little finger.
  (2.1) Absence of more than the distal phalanx of any two of the following fingers, index, middle finger or ring finger, of either hand.
  (3) Absence of hand or any portion thereof except for fingers as noted above.
  (4) Hyperdactylia.
  (5) Scars and deformities of the fingers and/or hand which impair circulation, are symptomatic, are so disfiguring as to make the individual objectionable in ordinary social relationships, or which impair normal function to such a degree as to interfere with the satisfactory performance of military duty.

 c. *Wrist, forearm, elbow, arm, and shoulder:* Healed disease or injury of wrist, elbow, or shoulder with residual weakness or symptoms of such a degree as to preclude satisfactory performance of duty.

2–10. LOWER EXTREMITIES

(See para. 2–11.)

The causes for rejection for appointment, enlistment, and induction are—

 a. *Limitation of motion.* An individual will be considered unac-

ceptable if the joint ranges of motion are less than the measurements listed below (app. IV).
  (1) *Hip.*
    (*a*) Flexion to 90°.
    (*b*) Extension to 10° (beyond 0).
  (2) *Knee.*
    (*a*) Full extension.
    (*b*) Flexion to 90°.
  (3) *Ankle.*
    (*a*) Dorsiflexion to 10°.
    (*b*) Plantar flexion to 10°.
  (4) *Toes.* Stiffness which interferes with walking, marching, running, or jumping.
 b. *Foot and ankle.*
  (1) Absence of one or more small toes of one or both feet, if function of the foot is poor or running or jumping is precluded, or absence of foot or any portion thereof except for toes as noted herein.
  (2) Absence (or loss) of great toe(s) or loss of dorsal flexion thereof if function of the foot is impaired.
  (3) Claw toes precluding the wearing of combat service boots.
  (4) Clubfoot.
  (5) Flatfoot, pronounced cases, with decided eversion of the foot and marked bulging of the inner border, due to inward rotation of the astragalus, regardless of the presence or absence of symptoms.
  (6) Flatfoot, spastic.
  (7) Hallux valgus, if severe and associated with marked exostosis or bunion.
  (8) Hammer toe which interferes with the wearing of combat service boots.
  (9) Healed disease, injury, or deformity including hyperdactylia which precludes running, is accompanied by disabling pain, or which prohibits wearing of combat service boots.

- (10) Ingrowing toe nails, if severe, and not remediable.
- (11) Obliteration of the transverse arch associated with permanent flexion of the small toes.
- (12) Pes cavus, with contracted plantar fascia, dorsiflexed toes, tenderness under the metatarsal heads, and callosity under the weight-bearing areas.

c. *Leg, knee, thigh, and hip.*
- (1) Dislocated semilunar cartilage, loose or foreign bodies within the knee joint, or history of surgical correction of same if—
  - (a) Within the preceding 6 months.
  - (b) Six months or more have elapsed since operation without recurrence, and there is instability of the knee ligaments in lateral or anteroposterior directions in comparison with the normal knee or abnormalities noted on X-ray, there is significant atrophy or weakness of the thigh musculature in comparison with the normal side, there is not acceptable active motion in flexion and extension, or there are other symptoms of internal derangement.
- (2) Authentic history or physical findings of an unstable or internally deranged joint causing disabling pain or seriously limiting function. Individuals with verified episodes of buckling or locking of the knee who have not undergone satisfactory surgical correction or if, subsequent to surgery, there is evidence of more than mild instability of the knee ligaments in lateral and anteroposterior directions in comparison with the normal knee, weakness or atrophy of the thigh musculature in comparison with the normal side, or if the individual requires medical treatment of sufficient frequency to interfere with the performance of military duty.

d. *General.*
- (1) Deformities of one or both lower extremities which have interfered with function to such a degree as to prevent the individual from following a *physically active* vocation

in civilian life or which would interfere with the satisfactory completion of prescribed training and performance of military duty.
  (2) Diseases or deformities of the hip, knee, or ankle joint which interfere with walking, running, or weight bearing.
  (3) Pain in the lower back or leg which is intractable and disabling to the degree of interfering with walking, running, and weight bearing.
  (4) Shortening of a lower extremity resulting in any limp of noticeable degree.

2–11. MISCELLANEOUS

(See also para. 2–9 and 2–10.)

The causes for rejection for appointment, enlistment, and induction are—

  a. *Arthritis.*
  (1) Active or subacute arthritis, including Marie-Strumpell type.
  (2) Chronic osteoarthritis or traumatic arthritis of isolated joints of more than minimal degree, which has interfered with the following of a physically active vocation in civilian life or which precludes the satisfactory performance of military duty.
  (3) Documented clinical history of rheumatoid arthritis.
  (4) Traumatic arthritis of a major joint of more than minimal degree.

  b. *Disease of any bone or joint,* healed, with such resulting deformity or rigidity that function is impaired to such a degree that it will interfere with military service.

  c. *Dislocation,* old unreduced; substantiated history of recurrent dislocations of major joints; instability of a major joint, symptomatic and more than mild; or if, subsequent to surgery, there is evidence of more than mild instability in comparison with the normal joint, weakness or atrophy in comparison with the normal side, or if the individual requires medical treatment of sufficient frequency to interfere with the performance of military duty.

d. *Fractures.*
  (1) Malunited fractures that interfere significantly with function.
  (2) Ununited fractures.
  (3) Any old or recent fracture in which a plate, pin, or screws were used for fixation and left in place and which may be subject to easy trauma, i.e., as a plate tibia, etc.

e. *Injury of a bone or joint* within the preceding 6 weeks, without fracture or dislocation, of more than a minor nature.

f. *Muscular paralysis,* contracture, or atrophy, if progressive or of sufficient degree to interfere with military service.

f.1 *Myotonia congenita.* Confirmed.

g. *Osteomyelitis,* active or recurrent, of any bone or substantiated history of osteomyelitis of any of the long bones unless successfully treated 2 or more years previously without subsequent recurrence or disqualifying sequelae as demonstrated by both clinical and X-ray evidence.

h. *Osteoporosis.*

i. *Scars,* extensive, deep, or adherent, of the skin and soft tissues or neuromas of an extremity which are painful, which interfere with muscular movements, which preclude the wearing of military equipment, or that show a tendency to break down.

j. *Chondromalacia,* manifested by verified history of joint effusion, interference with function, or residuals from surgery.

Section VIII. Eyes and Vision

2–12. EYES

The causes for rejection for appointment, enlistment, and induction are—

a. *Lids.*
  (1) Blepharitis, chronic more than mild. Cases of acute blepharitis will be rejected until cured.
  (2) Blepharospasm.
  (3) Dacryocystitis, acute or chronic.

(4) Destruction of the lids, complete or extensive, sufficient to impair protection of the eye from exposure.
(5) Disfiguring cicatrices and adhesions of the eyelids to each other or to the eyeball.
(6) Growth or tumor of the eyelid other than small early basal cell tumors of the eyelid, which can be cured by treatment, and small nonprogressive asymptomatic benign lesions. See also paragraphs 2–40 and 2–41.
(7) Marked inversion or eversion of the eyelids sufficient to cause unsightly appearance or watering of eyes (entropion or ectropion).
(8) Lagophthalmos.
(9) Ptosis interfering with vision.
(10) Trichiasis, severe.

b. *Conjunctiva.*
(1) Conjunctivitis, chronic, including vernal catarrh and trachoma. Individuals with acute conjunctivitis are unacceptable until the condition is cured.
(2) Pterygium:
  (a) Pterygium recurring after three operative procedures.
  (b) Pterygium encroaching on the cornea in excess of 3 millimeters or interfering with vision.

c. *Cornea.*
(1) Dystrophy, corneal, of any type including keratoconus of any degree.
(2) Keratitis, acute or chronic.
(3) Ulcer, corneal; history of recurrent ulcers or corneal abrasions (including herpetic ulcers).
(4) Vascularization or opacification of the cornea from any cause which interferes with visual function or is progressive.

d. *Uveal tract.* Inflammation of the uveal tract except healed traumatic choroiditis.

e. *Retina.*
(1) Angiomatoses, phakomatoses, retinal cysts, and other congenito-hereditary conditions that impair visual function.

(2) Degenerations of the retina to include macular cysts, holes, and other degenerations (heredity or acquired degenerative changes) and other conditions affecting the macula. All types of pigmentary degenerations (primary and secondary).
(3) Detachment of the retina or history of surgery for same.
(4) Inflammation of the retina (retinitis or other inflammatory conditions of the retina to include Coat's disease, diabetic retinopathy, Eales' disease, and retinitis proliferans).

f. Optic nerve.
(1) Congenito-hereditary conditions of the optic nerve or any other central nervous system pathology affecting the efficient function of the optic nerve.
(2) Optis neuritis, neuroretinitis, or secondary optic atrophy resulting therefrom or documented history of attacks of retrobulbar neuritis.
(3) Optic atrophy (primary or secondary).
(4) Papilledema.

g. Lens.
(1) Aphakia (unilateral or bilateral).
(2) Dislocation, partial or complete, of a lens.
(3) Opacities of the lens which interfere with vision or which are considered to be progressive.

h. Ocular mobility and motility.
(1) Diplopia, documented, constant or intermittent from any cause or of any degree interfering with visual function (i.e., may suppress).
(2) Diplopia, monocular, documented, interfering with visual function.
(3) Nystagmus, with both eyes fixing, congenital or acquired.
(4) Strabismus of 40 prism diopters or more, uncorrectable by lenses to less than 40 diopters.
(5) Strabismus of any degree accompanied by documented diplopia.
(6) Strabismus, surgery for the correction of, within the preceding 6 months.

i. Miscellaneous defects and diseases.
   (1) Abnormal conditions of the eye or visual fields due to diseases of the central nervous system.
   (2) Absence of an eye.
   (3) Asthenopia, severe.
   (4) Exophthalmos, unilateral or bilateral.
   (5) Glaucoma, primary or secondary.
   (6) Hemianopsia of any type.
   (7) Loss of normal pupillary reflex reactions to light or accommodation to distance of Adies syndrome.
   (8) Loss of visual fields due to organic disease.
   (9) Night blindness associated with objective disease of the eye. Verified congenital night blindness.
   (10) Residuals of old contusions, lacerations, penetrations, etc., which impair visual function required for satisfactory performance of military duty.
   (11) Retained intra-ocular foreign body.
   (12) Tumors. See $a(6)$ above and paragraphs 2–40 and 2–41.
   (13) Any organic disease of the eye or adnexa not specified above which threatens continuity of vision or impairment of visual function.

2–13. VISION

The causes for medical rejection for appointment, enlistment, and induction are listed below. The special administrative criteria for officer assignment to Armor, Artillery, Infantry, Corps of Engineers, Signal Corps, and Military Police Corps are listed in paragraph 7–15.

a. Distant visual acuity. Distant visual acuity of any degree which does not correct to at least one of the following:
   (1) 20/40 in one eye and 20/70 in the other eye.
   (2) 20/30 in one eye and 20/100 in the other eye.
   (3) 20/20 in one eye and 20/400 in the other eye.

b. Near visual acuity. Near visual acuity of any degree which does not correct to at least J–6 in the better eye.

c. Refractive error. Any degree of refractive error in spherical equivalent of over −8.00 or +8.00; or if ordinary spectacles cause discomfort by reason of ghost images, prismatic displacement, etc.; or if an ophthalmological consultation reveals a condition which is disqualifying.

d. Contact lens. Complicated cases requiring contact lens for adequate correction of vision as keratoconus, corneal scars, and irregular astigmatism.

Section IX. Genitourinary System

2–14. GENITALIA

(See also para. 2–40 and 2–41.)

The causes for rejection for appointment, enlistment, and induction are—

a. Bartholinitis, Bartholin's cyst.

b. Cervicitis, acute or chronic manifested by leukorrhea.

c. Dysmenorrhea, incapacitating to a degree which necessitates recurrent absences of more than a few hours from routine activities.

d. Endometriosis, or confirmed history thereof.

e. Hermaphroditism.

f. Menopausal syndrome, either physiologic or artificial if manifested by more than mild constitutional or mental symptoms, or artificial menopause if less than 13 months have elapsed since cessation of menses. In all cases of artificial menopause, the clinical diagnosis will be reported; if accomplished by surgery, the pathologic report will be obtained and recorded.

g. Menstrual cycle, irregularities of, including menorrhagia, if excessive; metrorrhagia; polymenorrhea; amenorrhea, except as noted in *f* above.

h. New growths of the internal or external genitalia except single uterine fibroid, subserous, asymptomatic, less than 3 centimeters in diameter, with no general enlargement of the uterus. See also paragraphs 2–40 and 2–41.

i. Oophoritis, acute or chronic.

j. Ovarian cysts, persistent and considered to be of clinical significance.

 k. Pregnancy.
 l. Salpingitis, acute or chronic.
 m. Testicle(s). (See also para. 2–40 and 2–41.)
  (1) Absence or nondescent of both testicles.
  (2) Undiagnosed enlargement or mass of testicle or epididymis.
  (3) Undescended testicle.
 n. Urethritis, acute or chronic, other than gonorrheal urethritis without complications.
 o. Uterus.
  (1) Cervical polyps, cervical ulcer, or marked erosion.
  (2) Endocervicitis, more than mild.
  (3) Generalized enlargement of the uterus due to any cause.
  (4) Malposition of the uterus if more than mildly symptomatic.
 p. Vagina.
  (1) Congenital abnormalities or severe lacerations of the vagina.
  (2) Vaginitis, acute or chronic, manifested by leukorrhea.
 q. Varicocele or hydrocele, if large or painful.
 r. Vulva.
  (1) Leukoplakia.
  (2) Vulvitis, acute or chronic.
 s. Major abnormalities and defects of the genitalia such as a change of sex, a history thereof, or complications (adhesions, disfiguring scars, etc.) residual to surgical correction of these conditions.

2–15. URINARY SYSTEM

(See para. 2–8, 2–40, and 2–41.)

The causes for rejection for appointment, enlistment, and induction are—

 a. Albuminuria if persistent or recurrent including so-called orthostatic or functional albuminuria.

 b. Cystitis, chronic. Individuals with acute cystitis are unacceptable until the condition is cured.

c. *Enuresis* determined to be a sympton of an organic defect not amenable to treatment. (See also para. 2–34c.)

d. *Epispadias or hypospadias* when accompanied by evidence of infection of the urinary tract or if clothing is soiled when voiding.

e. *Hematuria, cylindruria,* or other findings indicative of renal tract disease.

f. *Incontinence* of urine.

g. *Kidney.*
   (1) Absence of one kidney, regardless of cause.
   (2) Acute or chronic infections of the kidney.
   (3) Cystic or polycystic kidney, confirmed history of.
   (4) Hydronephrosis or pyonephrosis.
   (5) Nephritis, acute or chronic.
   (6) Pyelitis, pyelonephritis.

h. *Penis,* amputation of, if the resulting stump is insufficient to permit micturition in a normal manner.

i. *Peyronie's disease.*

j. *Prostate gland,* hypertrophy of, with urinary retention.

k. *Renal calculus.*
   (1) Substantiated history of bilateral renal calculus at any time.
   (2) Verified history of renal calculus at any time with evidence of stone formation within the preceding 12 months, current symptoms or positive X-ray for calculus.

l. *Skeneitis.*

m. *Urethra.*
   (1) Stricture of the urethra.
   (2) Urethritis, acute or chronic, other than gonorrheal urethritis without complications.

n. *Urinary fistula.*

o. *Other diseases and defects of the urinary system* which obviously preclude satisfactory performance of duty or which require frequent and prolonged treatment.

Section X. Head and Neck

2-16. HEAD

The causes for rejection for appointment, enlistment, and induction are—

  a. Abnormalities which are apparently temporary in character resulting from recent injuries until a period of 3 months has elapsed. These include severe contusions and other wounds of the scalp and cerebral concussion. See paragraph 2–31.

  b. Deformities of the skull in the nature of depressions, exostoses, etc., of a degree which would prevent the individual from wearing a gas mask or military headgear.

  c. Deformities of the skull of any degree associated with evidence of disease of the brain, spinal cord, or peripheral nerves.

  d. Depressed fractures near central sulcus with or without convulsive seizures.

  e. Loss or congenital absence of the bony substance of the skull except that The Surgeon General may find individuals acceptable when—

  (1) The area does not exceed 2.5 centimeters square, and does not overlie the motor cortex or a dural sinus.
  (2) There is no evidence of alteration of brain function in any of its several spheres (intelligence, judgment, perception, behavior, motor control, sensory function, etc.).
  (3) There is no evidence of bone degeneration, disease, or other complications of such a defect.

  f. Unsightly deformities, such as large birthmarks, large hairy moles, extensive scars, and mutilations due to injuries or surgical operations; ulcerations; fistulae, atrophy, or paralysis of part of the face or head.

2-17. NECK

The causes for rejection for appointment, enlistment, and induction are—

  a. Cervical ribs if symptomatic, or so obvious that they are found on routine physical examination. (Detection based primarily on X-ray is not considered to meet this criterion.)

   b. Congenital cysts of branchial cleft origin or those developing from the remnants of the thyroglossal duct, with or without fistulous tracts.

   c. Fistula, chronic draining, of any type.

   d. Healed tuberculosis lymph nodes when extensive in number or densely calcified.

   e. Nonspastic contraction of the muscles of the neck or cicatricial contracture of the neck to the extent that it interferes with the wearing of a uniform or military equipment or so disfiguring as to make the individual objectionable in common social relationships.

   f. Spastic contraction of the muscles of the neck, persistent, and chronic.

   g. Tumor of thyroid or other structures of the neck. See paragraphs 2-40 and 2-41.

Section XI. Heart and Vascular System

2-18. HEART

The causes for rejection for appointment, enlistment, and induction are—

   a. All organic valvular diseases of the heart, including those improved by surgical procedures.

   b. Coronary artery disease or myocardial infarction, old or recent or true angina pectoris, at any time.

   c. Electrocardiographic evidence of major arrhythmias such as—

   (1) Atrial tachycardia, flutter, or fibrillation, ventricular tachycardia or fibrillation.

   (2) Conduction defects such as first degree atrio-ventricular block and right bundle branch block. (These conditions occurring as isolated findings are not unfitting when cardiac evaluation reveals no cardiac disease.)

   (3) Left bundle branch block, 2d and 3d degree AV block.

   (4) Unequivocal electrocardiographic evidence of old or re-

cent myocardial infarction; coronary insufficiency at rest or after stress; or evidence of heart muscle disease.

 d. *Hypertrophy or dilatation of the heart* as evidenced by clinical examination or roentgenographic examination and supported by electrocardiographic examination. Care should be taken to distinguish abnormal enlargement from increased diastolic filling as seen in the well-conditioned subject with a sinus bradycardia. Cases of enlarged heart by X-ray not supported by electrocardiographic examination will be forwarded to The Surgeon General for evaluation.

 e. *Myocardial insufficiency* (congestive circulatory failure, cardiac decompensation) obvious or covert, regardless of cause.

 f. *Paroxysmal tachycardia* within the preceding 5 years, or at any time if recurrent or disabling or if associated with electrocardiographic evidence of accelerated AV conduction (Wolff-Parkinson-White).

 g. *Pericarditis; endocarditis; or myocarditis,* history or finding of, except for a history of a single acute idiopathic or Coxsackie pericarditis with no residuals.

 h. *Tachycardia* persistent with a resting pulse rate of 100 or more, regardless of cause.

2-19. VASCULAR SYSTEM

The causes for rejection for appointment, enlistment, and induction are—

 a. *Congenital or acquired lesions of the aorta and major vessels,* such as syphilitic aortitis, demonstrable atherosclerosis which interferes with circulation, congenital or acquired dilatation of the aorta (especially if associated with other features of Marfan's syndrome), and pronounced dilatation of the main pulmonary artery.

 b. *Hypertension* evidenced by preponderant blood pressure readings of 150-mm or more systolic in an individual over 35 years of age or preponderant readings of 140-mm or more systolic in an individual 35 years of age or less. Preponderant diastolic pressure over 90-mm diastolic is cause for rejection at any age.

 c. *Marked circulatory instability* as indicated by orthostatic hypotension, persistent tachycardia, severe peripheral vasomotor disturbances and sympatheticotonia.

d. Peripheral vascular disease including Raynaud's phenomena, Buerger's disease (thromboangiitis obliterans), erythromelalgia, arteriosclerotic and diabetic vascular diseases. Special tests will be employed in doubtful cases.

e. Thrombophlebitis.
(1) History of thrombophlebitis with persistent thrombus or evidence of circulatory obstruction, or deep venuos incompetence in the involved veins.
(2) Recurrent thrombophlebitis.

f. Varicose veins, if more than mild, or if associated with edema, skin ulceration, or residual scars from ulceration.

2-20. MISCELLANEOUS

The causes for rejection for appointment, enlistment, and induction are—

a. Aneurysm of the heart or major vessel, congenital or acquired.

b. History and evidence of a congenital abnormality which has been treated by surgery but with residual abnormalities or complications, *for example:* Patent ductus arteriosus with residual cardiac enlargement or pulmonary hypertension; resection of a coarctation of the aorta without a graft when there are other cardiac abnormalities or complications; closure of a secundum type atrial septal defect when there are residual abnormalities or complications.

c. Major congenital abnormalities and defects of the heart and vessels unless satisfactorily corrected without residuals or complications. Uncomplicated dextrocardia and other minor asymptomatic anomalies are acceptable.

d. Substantiated history of rheumatic fever or chorea within the previous 2 years, recurrent attacks of rheumatic fever or chorea at any time, or with evidence of residual cardiac damage.

Section XII. Height, Weight, and Body Build

2-21. HEIGHT

The causes for rejection for appointment, enlistment, and induction are—

  a. For appointment.
    (1) *Men.* Regular Army—Height below 66 inches or over 78 inches. However, see special administrative criteria in paragraph 7-13.
    Other—Height below 60 inches or over 78 inches.
    (2) *Women.* Height below 58 inches or over 72 inches.
  b. For enlistment and induction.
    (1) *Men.* Height below 60 inches or over 78 inches.
    (2) *Women.* Height below 58 inches or over 72 inches.

2-22. WEIGHT

The causes for rejection for appointment, enlistment, and induction are—

a. Weight related to height which is below the minimum shown in table I, appendix III for men and table II, appendix III for women.

b. Weight related to age and height which is in excess of the maximum shown in table I, appendix III for men and table II, appendix III for women. See chapter 7 for special requirements pertaining to maximum weight standards applicable to women enlisting for and commissioned from Army Student Nurse and Army Student Dietician Programs.

2-23. BODY BUILD

The causes for rejection for appointment, enlistment, and induction are—

a. Congenital malformation of bones and joints. (See para. 2-9, 2-10, and 2-11.)

b. Deficient muscular development which would interfere with the completion of required training.

c. *Evidences of congenital asthenia* (slender bones; weak thorax; visceroptosis; severe, chronic constipation; or "drop heart" if marked in degree).

d. *Obesity.* Even though the individual's weight is within the maximum shown in table I or II, as appropriate, appendix III, he will be reported as medically unacceptable when the medical examiner considers that the individual's weight in relation to the bony structure and musculature, constitutes obesity of such a degree as to interfere with the satisfactory completion of prescribed training.

Section XIII. Lungs and Chest Wall

2-24. GENERAL

The following conditions are causes for rejection for appointment, enlistment, and induction until further study indicates recovery without disqualifying sequelae:

a. *Abnormal elevation of the diaphragm* on either side.

b. *Acute abscess* of the lung.

c. *Acute bronchitis* until the condition is cured.

d. *Acute fibrinous pleurisy,* associated with acute nontuberculous pulmonary infection.

e. *Acute mycotic disease* of the lung such as coccidioidomycosis and histoplasmosis.

f. *Acute nontuberculous pneumonia.*

g. *Foreign body in trachea or bronchus.*

h. *Foreign body of the chest wall* causing symptoms.

i. *Lobectomy,* history of, for a nontuberculous nonmalignant lesion with residual pulmonary disease. Removal of more than one lobe is cause for rejection regardless of the absence of residuals.

j. *Other traumatic lesions* of the chest or its contents.

k. *Pneumothorax,* regardless of etiology or history thereof.

l. *Recent fracture* of ribs, sternum, clavicle, or scapula.

m. *Significant abnormal findings* on physical examination of the chest.

2-25. TUBERCULOUS LESIONS

(See also para. 2-38.)

The causes for rejection for appointment, enlistment, and induction are—

 a. *Active tuberculosis* in any form or location.

 b. *Pulmonary tuberculosis,* active within the past 5 years.

 c. *Substantiated history or X-ray findings* of pulmonary tuberculosis of more than minimal extent at any time; or minimal tuberculosis not treated with a full year of approved chemotherapy or combined chemotherapy and surgery; or a history of pulmonary tuberculosis with reactivation, relapse, or other evidence of poor host resistance.

2-26. NONTUBERCULOUS LESIONS

The causes for rejection for appointment, enlistment, and induction are—

 a. *Acute mastitis,* chronic cystic mastitis, if more than mild.

 b. *Bronchial asthma,* except for childhood asthma with a trustworthy history of freedom from symptoms since the 12th birthday.

 c. *Bronchitis,* chronic with evidence of pulmonary function disturbance.

 d. *Bronchiectasis.*

 e. *Bronchopleural fistula.*

 f. *Bullous or generalized pulmonary emphysema.*

 g. *Chronic abscess of lung.*

 h. *Chronic fibrous pleuritis* of sufficient extent to interfere with pulmonary function or obscure the lung field in the roentgenogram.

 i. *Chronic mycotic diseases* of the lung including coccidioidomycosis; residual cavitation or more than a few small-sized inactive and stable residual nodules demonstrated to be due to mycotic disease.

 j. *Empyema,* residual sacculation or unhealed sinuses of chest wall following operation for empyema.

 k. *Extensive pulmonary fibrosis* from any cause, producing dyspnea on exertion.

l. Foreign body of the lung or mediastinum causing symptoms or active inflammatory reaction.

m. Multiple cystic disease of the lung or solitary cyst which is large and incapacitating.

n. New growth of breast; history of mastectomy.

o. Osteomyelitis of rib, sternum, clavicle, scapula, or vertebra.

p. Pleurisy with effusion of unknown origin within the preceding 5 years.

q. Sarcoidosis. See paragraph 2–38.

r. Suppurative periostitis of rib, sternum, clavicle, scapula, or vertebra.

Section XIV. Mouth, Nose, Pharynx, Trachea, Esophagus, and Larynx

2–27. MOUTH

The causes for rejection for appointment, enlistment, and induction are—

a. Hard palate, perforation of.

b. Harelip, unless satisfactorily repaired by surgery.

c. Leukoplakia, if severe.

d. Lips, unsightly mutilations of, from wounds, burns, or disease.

e. Ranula, if extensive. For other tumors see paragraphs 2–40 and 2–41.

2–28. NOSE

The causes for rejection for appointment, enlistment, and induction are—

a. Allergic manifestations.
  (1) Chronic atrophic rhinitis.
  (2) Hay fever if severe; or if not controllable by antihistamines or by desensitization, or both.

b. Choana, atresia, or stenosis of, if symptomatic.

c. Nasal septum, perforation of:
  (1) Associated with interference of function, ulceration of crusting, and when the result of organic disease.

(2) If progressive.
(3) If respiration is accompanied by a whistling sound.
   d. Sinusitis, acute.
   e. Sinusitis, chronic, when more than mild:
      (1) Evidenced by any of the following: Chronic purulent nasal discharge, large nasal polyps, hyperplastic changes of the nasal tissues, or symptoms requiring frequent medical attention.
      (2) Confirmed by transillumination or X-ray examination or both.

2–29. PHARYNX, TRACHEA, ESOPHAGUS, AND LARYNX

The causes for rejection for appointment, enlistment, and induction are—

a. Esophagus, organic disease of, such as ulceration, varices, achalasia; peptic esophagitis; if confirmed by appropriate X-ray or esophagoscopic examinations.

b. Laryngeal paralysis, sensory or motor, due to any cause.

c. Larynx, organic disease of, such as neoplasm, polyps, granuloma, ulceration, and chronic laryngitis.

d. Plica dysphonia ventricularis.

e. Tracheostomy or tracheal fistula.

2–30. OTHER DEFECTS AND DISEASES

The causes for rejection for appointment, enlistment, and induction are—

a. Aphonia.

b. Deformities or conditions of the mouth, throat, pharynx, larynx, esophagus, and nose which interfere with mastication and swallowing of ordinary food, with speech, or with breathing.

c. Destructive syphilitic disease of the mouth, nose, throat, larynx, or esophagus. (See para. 2–42.)

d. Pharyngitis and nasopharyngitis, chronic, with positive history and objective evidence, if of such a degree as to result in excessive time lost in the military environment.

Section XV. Neurological Disorders

2-31. NEUROLOGICAL DISORDERS

The causes for rejection for appointment, enlistment, and induction are—

a. *Degenerative disorders.*
  (1) Cerebellar and Friedreich's ataxia.
  (2) Cerebral arteriosclerosis.
  (3) Encephalomyelitis, residuals of, which preclude the satisfactory performance of military duty.
  (4) Huntington's chorea.
  (5) Multiple sclerosis.
  (6) Muscular atrophies and dystrophies of any type.

b. *Miscellaneous.*
  (1) Congenital malformations if associated with neurological manifestations and meningocele even if uncomplicated.
  (2) Migraine when frequent and incapacitating.
  (3) Paralysis or weakness, deformity, discoordination, pain, sensory disturbance, intellectual deficit, disturbances of consciousness, or personality abnormalities regardless of cause which is of such a nature or degree as to preclude the satisfactory performance of military duty.
  (4) Tremors, spasmodic torticollis, athetosis or other abnormal movements more than mild.

c. *Neurosyphilis* of any form (general paresis, tabes dorsalis, meningovascular syphilis).

d. *Paroxysmal convulsive disorders,* disturbances of consciousness, all forms of psychomotor or temporal lobe epilepsy or history thereof except for seizures associated with toxic states or fever during childhood up to the age of 12.

e. *Peripheral nerve disorder.*
  (1) Polyneuritis.
  (2) Mononeuritis or neuralgia which is chronic or recurrent and of an intensity that is periodically incapacitating.
  (3) Neurofibromatosis.

f. Spontaneous subarachnoid hemorrhage, verified history of, unless cause has been surgically corrected.

Section XVI. Psychoses, Psychoneuroses, and Personality Disorders

2-32. PSYCHOSES

The causes for rejection for appointment, enlistment, and induction are—

Psychosis or authenticated history of a psychotic illness other than those of a brief duration associated with a toxic or infectious process.

2-33. PSYCHONEUROSES

The causes for rejection for appointment, enlistment, and induction are—
 a. *History of a psychoneurotic reaction* which caused—
  (1) Hospitalization.
  (2) Prolonged care by a physician.
  (3) Loss of time from normal pursuits for repeated periods even if of brief duration, or
  (4) Symptoms or behavior of a repeated nature which impaired school or work efficiency.

 b. *History of a brief psychoneurotic reaction* or nervous disturbance within the preceding 12 months which was sufficiently severe to require medical attention or absence from work or school for a brief period (maximum of 7 days).

2-34. PERSONALITY DISORDERS

The causes for rejection for appointment, enlistment, and induction are—
 a. *Character and behavior disorders,* as evidenced by—
  (1) Frequent encounters with law enforcement agencies, or antisocial attitudes or behavior which, while not a cause for administrative rejection, are tangible evidence of an

impaired characterological capacity to adapt to the military service.

(2) Overt homosexuality or other forms of sexual deviant practices such as exhibitionism, transvestism, voyeurism, etc.

(3) Chronic alcoholism or alcohol addiction.

(4) Drug addiction.

b. Character and behavior disorders where it is evident by history and objective examination that the degree of immaturity, instability, personality inadequacy, and dependency will seriously interfere with adjustment in the military service as demonstrated by repeated inability to maintain reasonable adjustment in school, with employers and fellow-workers, and other society groups.

c. Other symptomatic immaturity reactions such as authenticated evidence of enuresis which is habitual or persistent, not due to an organic condition (para. 2–15c) occurring beyond early adolescence (age 12 to 14) and stammering or stuttering of such a degree that the individual is normally unable to express himself clearly or to repeat commands.

d. Specific learning defects secondary to organic or functional mental disorders.

Section XVII. Skin and Cellular Tissues

2–35. SKIN AND CELLULAR TISSUES

The causes for rejection for appointment, enlistment, and induction are—

a. Acne. Severe, when the face is markedly disfigured, or when extensive involvement of the neck, shoulders, chest, or back would be aggravated by or interfere with the wearing of military equipment.

b. Atopic dermatitis. With active or residual lesions in characteristic areas (face and neck, antecubital and popliteal fossae, occasionally wrists and hands), or documented history thereof.

c. Cysts.

(1) *Cysts, other than pilonidal.* Of such a size or location as to interfere with the normal wearing of military equipment.

(2) *Cysts, pilonidal.* Pilonidal cysts, if evidenced by the presence of a tumor mass or a discharging sinus.

d. *Dermatitis factitia.*

e. *Dermatitis herpetiformis.*

f. *Eczema.* Any type which is chronic and resistant to treatment.

f. *Elephantiasis or chronic lymphedema.*

g. *Epidermolysis bullosa; pemphigus.*

h. *Fungus infections,* systemic or superficial types: If extensive and not amenable to treatment.

i. *Furunculosis.* Extensive, recurrent, or chronic.

j. *Hyperhidrosis* of hands or feet: Chronic or severe.

k. *Ichthyosis.* Severe.

l. *Leprosy.* Any type.

m. *Leukemia cutis; mycosis fungoides; Hodgkins' disease.*

n. *Lichen planus.*

o. *Lupus erythematosus* (acute, subacute, or chronic) or any other dermatosis aggravated by sunlight.

p. *Neurofibromatosis* (Von Recklinghausen's disease).

q. *Nevi or vascular tumors:* If extensive, unsightly, or exposed to constant irritation.

r. *Psoriasis* or a verified history thereof.

s. *Radiodermatitis.*

t. *Scars* which are so extensive, deep, or adherent that they may interfere with the wearing of military equipment, or that show a tendency to ulcerate.

u. *Scleroderma.* Diffuse type.

v. *Tuberculosis.* See paragraph 2–38.

w. *Urticaria.* Chronic.

x. *Warts, plantar,* which have materially interfered with the following of a useful vocation in civilian life.

y. *Xanthoma.* If disabling or accompanied by hypercholesterolemia or hyperlipemia.

z. Any other chronic skin disorder of a degree or nature which requires frequent outpatient treatment or hospitalization, interferes with the satisfactory performance of duty, or is so disfiguring as to make the individual objectionable in ordinary social relationships.

aa. Tattoos on any part of the body which in the opinion of the examining physician are obscene or so extensive on exposed areas as to be considered unsightly, are administratively disqualified.

Section XVIII. Spine, Scapulae, Ribs, and Sacroiliac Joints

2–36. SPINE AND SACROILIAC JOINTS

(See also para. 2–11.)

The causes for rejection for appointment, enlistment, and induction are—

a. Arthritis. See paragraph 2–11*a*.

b. Complaint of disease or injury of the spine or sacroiliac joints either with or without objective signs and symptoms which have prevented the individual from successfully following a physically active vocation in civilian life. Substantiation or documentation of the complaint without symptoms and objective signs is required.

c. Deviation or curvature of spine from normal alignment, structure, or function (scoliosis, kyphosis, or lordosis, spina bifida acculta, spondylolysis, etc.), if—

(1) Mobility and weight-bearing power is poor.

(2) More than moderate restriction of normal physical activities is required.

(3) Of such a nature as to prevent the individual from following a *physically active vocation* in civilian life.

(4) Of a degree which will interfere with the wearing of a uniform or military equipment.

(5) Symptomatic, associated with positive physical finding(s) demonstrable by X-ray.

d. Diseases of the lumbosacral or sacroiliac joints of a chronic type and obviously associated with pain referred to the lower extremities, muscular spasm, postural deformities and limitation of motion in the lumbar region of the spine.

 e. Granulomatous diseases either active or healed.

 f. Healed fracture of the spine or pelvic bones with associated symptoms which have prevented the individual from following a *physically* active vocation in civilian life or which preclude the satisfactory performance of military duty.

 g. Ruptured nucleus pulposus (herniation of intervertebral disk) or history of operation for this condition.

 h. Spondylolysis or spondylolisthesis that is symptomatic or is likely to interfere with performance of duty or is likely to require assignment limitations.

2–37. SCAPULAE, CLAVICLES, AND RIBS

(See also para. 2–11.)

The causes for rejection for appointment, enlistment, and induction are—

 a. Fractures, until well healed, and until determined that the residuals thereof will not preclude the satisfactory performance of military duty.

 b. Injury within the preceding 6 weeks, without fracture, or dislocation, of more than a minor nature.

 c. Osteomyelitis of rib, sternum, clavicle, scapula, or vertebra.

 d. Prominent scapulae interfering with function or with the wearing of uniform or military equipment.

Section XIX. Systemic Diseases and Miscellaneous Conditions and Defects

2–38. SYSTEMIC DISEASES

The causes for rejection for appointment, enlistment, and induction are—

 a. Dermatomyositis.
 b. Lupus erythematosus; acute, subacute, or chronic.
 c. Progressive systemic sclerosis.
 d. Reiter's Disease.
 e. Sarcoidosis.

f. Scleroderma, diffuse type.

g. Tuberculosis:
  (1) Active tuberculosis in any form or location.
  (2) Pulmonary tuberculosis. See paragraph 2–25.
  (3) Confirmed history of tuberculosis of a bone or joint, genitourinary organs, intestines, peritoneum or mesenteric glands at any time.
  (4) Meningeal tuberculosis; disseminated tuberculosis.

2–39. GENERAL AND MISCELLANEOUS CONDITIONS AND DEFECTS

The causes for rejection for appointment, enlistment, and induction are—

a. Allergic manifestations.
  (1) Allergic rhinitis (hay fever). See paragraph 2–28.
  (2) Asthma. See paragraph 2–26*b*.
  (3) Allergic dermatoses. See paragraph 2–35.
  (4) Visceral, abdominal, and cerebral allergy, if severe or not responsive to treatment.

b. Any acute pathological condition, including acute communicable diseases, until recovery has occurred without sequelae.

c. Any deformity which is markedly unsightly or which impairs general functional ability to such an extent as to prevent satisfactory performance of military duty.

d. Chronic metallic poisoning especially beryllium, manganese, and mercury. Undesirable residuals from lead, arsenic, or silver poisoning make the examinee medically unacceptable.

e. Cold injury, residuals of, (*example:* frostbite, chilblain, immersion foot, or trench foot) such as deep seated ache, paresthesia, hyperhidrosis, easily traumatized skin, cyanosis, amputation of any digit, or ankylosis.

f. Positive tests for syphilis with negative TPI test unless there is a documented history of adequately-treated lues or any of the several conditions which are known to give a false-positive S.T.S. (vaccinia, infectious hepatitis, immunizations, atypical pneumonia, etc.) or unless there has been a reversal to a negative S.T.S. during an appropriate followup period (3 to 6 months).

g. Filariasis; trypanosomiasis; amebiasis; schistosomiasis; un-

Physical Profile Functional Capacity Guide

Profile serial	P Physical capacity	U Upper extremities	L Lower extremities	H Hearing—Ears	E Vision—Eyes	S Psychiatric
1	Good muscular development with ability to perform maximum effort for indefinite periods.	No loss of digits, or limitation of motion; no demonstrable abnormality; able to do hand-to-hand fighting.	No loss of digits, or limitation of motion; no demonstrable abnormality; be capable of performing long marches, standing over long periods.	Audiometer average level each ear not more than 15 db @ 500, 1000, 2000 cps.. Not over 40 db at 4000 cps.	Uncorrected visual acuity 20/200 correctible to 20/20, in each eye.	No psychiatric pathology. May have history of a transient personality disorder.
2	Able to perform maximum effort over long periods.	Slightly limited mobility of joints, muscular weakness, or other musculo-skeletal defects which do not prevent hand-to-hand fighting and do not disqualify for prolonged effort.	Slightly limited mobility of joints, muscular weakness or other musculo-skeletal defects which do not prevent moderate marching, climbing, running, digging, or prolonged effort.	Audiometer average level not more than 20 db @ 500, 1000, 2000 cps and 50 db at 4000 cps in both ears, or 15 db at 500, 1000, 2000 cps and 30 db at 4000 in better ear.	Distant visual acuity correctible to 20/40–20/70, 20/30–20/100, 20/20–20/400.	Mild character and behavior disorders which may somewhat limit but do not impair duty performance. May have history of recovery from an acute psychotic reaction due to external or toxic causes unrelated to alcoholic or drug addiction.

3	Unable to perform full effort except for brief or moderate periods.	Defects or impairments which interfere with full function requiring restriction of use.	May have hearing level at 20 db with hearing aid by speech reception score, or acute or chronic ear disease not falling below retention standards.	Uncorrected distant visual acuity of any degree which is correctible not less than 20/40 in the better eye or an acute or chronic eye disease not falling below retention standards.	Satisfactory remission from an acute psychotic or neurotic disorder which permits utilization under specific conditions (assignment when out-patient psychiatric treatment is available or certain duties can be avoided).
4	Below Retention Standards.	Below Retention Standards.	Below Retention Standards.	Below Retention Standards.	Below Retention Standards.
Factors to be considered	Organic defects, age, build, strength, stamina, weight, height, agility, energy, muscular coordination, function, and similar factors.	Strength, range of motion, and general efficiency of upper arm, shoulder girdle and back, including cervical, thoracic, and lumbar vertebrae.	Strength, range of movement, and efficiency of feet, legs, pelvic girdle, lower back.	Auditory acuity, and organic disease of the ears.	Visual acuity, and organic disease of the eyes and lids.	Type, severity, and duration of the psychiatric symptoms or disorder existing at the time the profile is determined. Amount of external precipitating stress. Predisposition as determined by the basic personality makeup, intelligence, performance, and history of past psychiatric disorder impairment of functional capacity.

cinariasis (hookworm) associated with anemia, malnutrition, etc., if more than mild, and other similar worm or animal parasitic infestations, including the carrier states thereof.

h. Heat pyrexia (heatstroke, sunstroke, etc.): Documented evidence of predisposition (includes disorders of sweat mechanism and previous serious episode), recurrent episodes requiring medical attention, or residual injury resulting therefrom (especially cardiac, cerebral, hepatic, and renal).

i. Industrial solvent and other chemical intoxication, chronic including carbon bisulfide, tricholorethylene, carbon tetrachloride, and methyl cellosolve.

j. Mycotic infection of internal organs.

k. Mycositis or fibrositis; severe, chronic.

l. Residuals of tropical fevers and various parasitic or protozoal infestations which in the opinion of the medical examiner preclude the satisfactory performance of military duty.

Section XX. Tumors and Malignant Diseases

2–40. BENIGN TUMORS

The causes for rejection for appointment, enlistment, and induction are—

a. Any tumor of the—
  (1) Auditory canal, if obstructive.
  (2) Eye or orbit (see also para. 2–12a(6)).
  (3) Kidney, bladder, testicle, or penis.
  (4) Central nervous system and its membranous coverings unless 5 years after surgery and no otherwise disqualifying residuals of surgery or original lesion.

b. Benign tumors of the abdominal wall if sufficiently large to interfere with military duty.

c. Benign tumors of bone likely to continue to enlarge, be subjected to trauma during military service, or show malignant potential.

d. Benign tumors of the thyroid or other structures of the neck, including enlarged lymph nodes, if the enlargement is of such degree as to interfere with the wearing of a uniform or military equipment.

e. Tongue, benign tumor of, if it interferes with function.

f. Breast, thoracic contents, or chest wall, tumors, of, other than fibromata lipomata, and inclusion or sebaceous cysts which do not interfere with military duty.

f. For tumors of the internal or external female genitalia see paragraph 2–14*h*.

2–41. MALIGNANT DISEASES AND TUMORS

The causes for rejection for appointment, enlistment, and induction are—

a. Leukemia, acute or chronic.

b. Malignant lymphomata.

c. Malignant tumor of any kind, at any time, substantiated diagnosis of, even though surgically removed, confirmed by accepted laboratory procedures, except as noted in paragraph 2–12*a*(6).

Section XXI. Venereal Diseases

2–42. VENEREAL DISEASES

In general the finding of acute, uncomplicated venereal disease which can be expected to respond to treatment is not a cause for medical rejection for military service. The causes for rejection for appointment, enlistment, and induction are—

a. Chronic venereal disease which has not satisfactorily responded to treatment. The finding of a positive serologic test for syphilis following the adequate treatment of syphilis is not in itself considered evidence of chronic venereal disease which has not responded to treatment (para. 2–39*f*).

b. Complications and permanent residuals of venereal disease if progressive, of such nature as to interfere with the satisfactory performance of duty, or if subject to aggravation by military service.

c. Neurosyphilis. See paragraph 2–31*c*.

Section XXII. Vocational Waivers

2–43. VOCATIONAL WAIVERS

When an individual who fails to meet the medical standards listed in this chapter has demonstrated in the pursuit of his civilian occupation, profession, or avocation that he is likely to be able satisfactorily to perform the duties of a member of the Armed Forces, the medical examiner may recommend to the Surgeon General of the appropriate service that such an individual be accepted on waivers of medical fitness standards. Such cases shall be considered by the Surgeon General before a final decision is made.

IV. 4-F Memo

The Central Committee for Conscientious Objectors' (CCCO) "4F Memo," reproduced in part on the following pages, was revised and updated in April, 1972. Copies of the complete memo are available for thirty cents each (discounts for greater quantities) and additional draft-counseling information may be obtained from CCCO.

National Office: 2016 Walnut Street
Philadelphia, Pennsylvania 19103
(215) 568–7971

Midwest Office: 711 South Dearborn Street
Chicago, Illinois 60605
(312) 427–3350

Western Office: 140 Leavenworth Street
San Francisco, California 94102
(415) 441–3700

Information on Abolition of 1-Y Deferments

Under Selective Service Regulations effective December 10, 1971, the 1-Y classification has been eliminated. Class 4-F now includes those who would formerly have been 1-Y, unless scheduled for re-examination. All of the implications of this policy are not yet clear. Many men awaiting re-examination have been reclassified from 1-Y to 1-A or 1-H already. But any man now classified 1-Y or 1-A should expect to be called for re-examination if the local board's file copy (which he can inspect) of DD Form 62, Statement of Acceptability, from the physical where he was rejected, states "Re-examination believed justified (or **RBJ**) _____ months." If there is no such notation on his DD Form 62, he should be classified 4-F without re-examination. Any man who expects to be called for re-examination and believes he should be rejected again should submit to his local board or collect for the examination the strongest and most recent medical evidence he can.

A man is classified 4-F if he "is found under applicable physical, mental, and moral standards to be not qualified for service in the Armed Forces either currently, or in time of war or national emergency declared by the Congress. . . ." This memo discusses the procedures for men seeking 4-F classification.

Informing the Draft Board

At the time he registers for the draft, a man is required to fill out SSS Form 100, Registration Questionnaire. In addition to checking "Yes" in Series V, despite the form's suggestion that evidence should only be sent "when requested," he should describe any medical condition he has, on a *separate* piece of paper (so it can be forwarded to the AFEES later), and supporting documents from a doctor should be submitted to the local board as soon as possible. Even though one is classified 1-H and not yet required to send in evidence, he should do so as early as possible, in order to build up any medical history he may have.

If he is reclassified out of his initial 1-H, a man is required to inform his local board within 10 days of any change or new information which could change his classification. If he has a condition which could lead to a 4-F, not described when he filled out SSS Form 100, he should notify the local board in writing and submit complete documentation as soon as possible, even though he might not be examined soon. The local board must keep medical information in the man's file, and should send it to the AFEES when he is examined.

Confidentiality of records—Some men fear that if they send medical information to their draft boards it might become public. Legally a man's draft file is confidential. It is open only to officials and individuals authorized by a state or national director, and to the FBI for investigation of draft violations. Civilian health agencies can be notified of contagious diseases. The classification of every registrant is public, but the reasons and evidence are confidential. Because any person authorized by the registrant can examine his file, a few employers ask job applicants to sign forms authorizing file checks. A man should consider carefully before putting potentially damaging information in his file, though illegal release is probably rarer than many men fear. Some draft boards will return medical documentation to the physician who wrote it, on his request, after it has been evaluated by the proper medical authorities. A man who is concerned about his file being seen should ask his doctor to request the return of medical information.

Selective Service Appeals

If a man submits new information to his draft board which, if assumed to be true, would require the board to reclassify him, the board should reopen his classification. The board will then send the registrant a new classification card to inform him of its decision on the new information. The man then has personal appearance and appeal rights to contest the decision of the local board. When new medical information is sent in, however, local boards usually have not given 4-F classification or even reopened the man's classification to allow appeal rights. Some courts have ruled that boards must reopen in these circumstances, and a man in doubt about the law in his area should check with a reliable draft counselor. In general, though, whenever a man submits new medical information he should specifically request reopening of his classification. Although the local board will usually deny reopening, the request may serve to protect his rights if he ever goes to court.

Often a man is already classified 1-A when he is examined at the AFEES. If he is then found acceptable, or found unacceptable with "re-examination believed justified," he will not be reclassified, and will have no rights of appeal within the Selective Service System. If found acceptable while eligible for induction under the lottery, he might even receive an induction order in the same envelope as the Statement of Acceptability.

A man who believes he should receive a 4-F deferment should use all Selective Service appeal rights whenever he receives a classification as eligible for service (1-A, 1-A-O, or 1-O). To begin the appeal process, he should request a personal appearance before his local draft board within 15 days after an unsatisfactory classification card is mailed. At his personal appearance before his local board, the board members may be reluctant to evaluate medical evidence. But, under new regulations, a man is entitled to bring as many as three witnesses to his personal appearance; one or more of these could be physicians or other medical experts. The local board cannot refuse to hear a man's witnesses, though it is not yet clear how they will deal with medical evidence presented in this way. Though local and appeal boards are unlikely to classify a man 4-F if he has not been found unacceptable at an AFEES examination, he still has a right to use all appeals. Most importantly, *an order to report for induction or alternate service cannot be issued while appeals are pending.* A man may need this time to protest to Army officials after an AFEES examination, to explore other alternatives before an induction order is issued, or to contact an attorney.

Rejection Without Examination—Medical Interviews

A local board can reject a man directly, without sending him for examination, if it believes it has enough evidence. A man with a serious medical condition can ask the board in writing to schedule a medical interview and to classify him 4-F. Examples of such conditions are amputation of a limb, blindness, or diabetes. Some boards reject men for their police and court records without sending them to the AFEES for screening under the Army "moral standards."

Medical interviews. A local board may have an unpaid civilian doctor appointed as its medical advisor. The board may order a registrant to be interviewed by the medical advisor if it believes he has a medical condition listed in a special set of medical standards. A man may be able to get a medical interview if he sends a doctor's letter showing he has a serious medical condition, whether or not listed, since LBM 78 (section 3) states that "There are other conditions which would not be obvious but which upon receipt of valid documentary evidence, can be evaluated by the Medical Advisor . . ." and cites the list that follows as being merely "examples."

New Selective Service regulations seem to encourage local boards to make more use of medical advisors. However, since they are not legally bound to schedule medical interviews, most boards rarely grant them. Many men refused interviews later get 4-Fs after AFEES exams under the complete Army medical standards. Medical interviews are intended to save draft boards the delay and expense of sending men to the AFEES, rather than as a convenience for registrants.

When an interview is arranged, the man will receive SSS Form 219, Notice to Registrant to Appear for Medical Interview. A man ordered to a medical interview when he is living outside the area where his local board is can take the SSS Form 219 to a nearby draft board and ask for transfer. If there is difficulty in arranging an interview there or at his local board, the state director can be asked to schedule an interview with any medical advisor in the state. "If no Medical Advisor is available, the registrant must be sent to the Armed Forces Examining and Entrance Station." Whenever it is difficult for a board to hold a medical interview, it usually waits for the results of an AFEES exam instead.

The medical advisor should consider all reports provided, and may give the man "such examination as he deems necessary," but will not himself make X-rays or lab tests. The local board considers the medical advisor's report, and can then reclassify the man 4-F.

Even if he had a medical interview and was found acceptable there, a man cannot be ordered for induction until he has been ordered to the AFEES for a pre-induction physical.

State medical advisor. In some states there is a medical advisor to the state director who considers petitions from men who believe the local board has improperly failed to classify them 4-F. Sometimes the state medical advisor schedules re-examinations at the AFEES. For information, contact a local draft counselor.

Reporting for a Pre-Induction Examination

Before he can be drafted, a man must be sent SSS Form 223, Order to Report for Armed Forces Physical Examination. A pending personal appearance or appeal does not delay this order. The board will usually first send for examinations those men most likely to be drafted. A man must be given 15 days' advance notice of the date of his physical. He may be ordered to a physical while deferred or exempt if the board believes he will soon be reclassified available for service. Regardless of his classification, a registrant who receives an examination order is legally bound to report, with one exception. A man classified 1-O is not required to report for a pre-induction physical, but if he does not take one he is considered to be acceptable for civilian work.

Voluntary examinations. A man under age 26, regardless of his classification, can request a pre-induction physical by visiting or writing his local board, provided he has not yet had an Armed Forces physical. The regulations apparently allow even a man classified 1-H to try for a 4-F by requesting an exam. If he wants it transferred out of the local board area, his request should say where he wants to report and why. The local board will arrange for transfer to another board if necessary. The board ordering him for examination must set a date which is within 60 days of the time it receives the request, and must give him at least 15 days' notice to report. Voluntary examinations may be suspended by the Director of Selective Service during heavy draft board or AFEES workloads. Requesting an examination may allow a man to know where he stands long before he faces an induction order. It also gives him more time to try to get a re-examination if he is found acceptable. Before requesting an examination, one should send complete medical documentation to his draft board.

Transfer of an examination is available when a man lives far from his local board. He takes SSS Form 223 to a nearby draft board and requests transfer on a special form (SSS Form 230). Local boards have been instructed to make sure that transfers are to prevent "hardship," not just for delay. The man may be asked reasons for his presence in the transfer board's area and the date he will return to his local board area, and he should have evidence of a local address near the transfer board. He will be sent a new examination date by the transfer board, often after some delay. There are special procedures for physicals outside the U.S.—a man may have to travel hundreds of miles across foreign continents at his own expense.

Postponement of a pre-induction physical is available "in case of death of a member of the registrant's immediate family, extreme emergency involving a member of the registrant's immediate family, serious illness of the registrant, or other emergency beyond the registrant's control," for no more than 60 days, and "in case of imperative necessity" for another 60 days. Request should be made in writing to the board that issued the examination order. The state or national director can postpone a physical whenever persuaded this is necessary.

Records processing before examination. The local board

should send all medical records in the file to the AFEES before examination, usually in time to arrive at least three days early. Because boards often fail to send all the medical records to the AFEES, the registrant should plan ahead to take one copy of each medical report with him to the examination.

Special instructions. Local boards should send a "Special Notice" with the examination order, warning that contact lenses should not be worn 72 hours before the examination, to avoid holdover at the AFEES for up to three days. The note also tells men to bring any medical reports not already sent to the board. In some states, local boards also send men medical history or criminal record forms with the examination order, to be filled out before reporting to the AFEES.

Pre-Induction Physical at the AFEES

IMPORTANT: AFEES have very small staffs—often only two or three doctors at a given induction station on a given day. Armed Forces Examining and Entrance Stations conduct over one million physical examinations each year. Thus, examinations are not performed as carefully and completely as one might expect. A man tends to be "shuffled through" his physical as quickly as possible, unless he refuses to accept such treatment. A registrant must be prepared to speak up when he feels he has been examined poorly, his documentation has been overlooked, the results of a given examination have not been recorded accurately, or he has been treated unfairly in any way. At any point during his physical when he feels an AFEES examiner has made a mistake, the registrant should complain immediately. He should ask to be re-examined, or to have his documentation considered further. If a particular AFEES doctor is uncooperative, the man should request to see the chief of the medical examining section or the Commanding Officer of the AFEES. In addition, any man who has doubts about the validity of any physical examination should write down in complete detail exactly what happened at the examination, including the name of any AFEES physician or technician who he feels has examined him unfairly. If a man allows himself to be mistreated at his physical, he is the only one who will lose, for he will probably pass his physical.

Mental testing. Written tests are given to measure mental ability. The first is the Armed Forces Qualification Test (AFQT), a fifty-minute multiple-choice test. A man who gets an AFQT score of 30 or less is given a number of shorter tests in the Army Qualification Battery (AQB). In a borderline case, he is interviewed by an AFEES personnel psychologist. The AFEES can write for information on his education. A high school graduate should expect to be declared mentally acceptable regardless of his test scores.

The contents of the mental tests are classified, and proctors usually give men sitting next to each other different versions to prevent cheating. Anyone giving random or inconsistent answers is scored in the "Deliberate Failure Category," and is usually accepted.

Medical History Form. The first step in the medical examination is filling out Standard Form 93, Report of Medical History. SF 93 is a questionnaire asking about the man's present state of health in his own words, whether he has ever had any of more than 70 different medical problems, and whether he has been hospitalized or seen a doctor. It is important to answer this form very carefully, to get a complete examination.

In order to safeguard a man's rights against self-incrimination, the form no longer asks about homosexuality and drug use, nor about excessive use of alcohol. A man who believes he should be disqualified on these grounds must now volunteer the information. If possible, he might do so in terms of *tendencies,* rather than of presently continuing overt acts which might be illegal. A man with any questions should ask for an explanation.

Medical Examination Form. As a man undergoes his physical examination, various AFEES physicians will note their findings on Standard Form 88, Report of Medical Examination. It is important that a man check the comments on SF 88 as soon as they are written down, and if any of them are incorrect he should immediately bring them to the attention of the AFEES examiner who originally recorded them, and if necessary the chief of the medical examining section or the AFEES commander.

Medical examination. Each man is required to remove and check his clothes, except for shoes and shorts. He is processed along an assembly line of numbered stations. Though the order of the stations varies, each man should receive the standard tests. (Note that men classified 1-O are supposed to be given the same physical examination as all others.) All parts of the body are examined by sight or touch. Height is measured to the nearest quarter inch and weight to the nearest pound (a man with borderline measurements should bring a doctor's letter). Exercises are done to observe free movement of arms, legs, hips, and spine. The man gives a urine sample, sometimes under supervision of an examiner, which is tested only for glucose and albumin. A chest X-ray is taken. A blood sample is taken by a technician and checked for syphilis only (a hemophiliac should have a doctor's letter). Blood pressure and pulse are recorded in sitting position only. Heart and lungs are listened to with a stethoscope. Hearing is measured on an audiometer in a soundproof room or booth (results are sometimes checked with a lie detector). Eyesight is checked on a stereoscope, and any eyeglass prescription is recorded (if the prescription is unknown, the lenses are measured). Eye movements and color vision are checked. IMPORTANT: One should not expect any of these simple tests to reveal his disqualifying condition, but should rely instead on evidence brought along from civilian doctors.

No further examination is done unless indicated by evidence in the draft file, letters the man brings, his answers on the SF 93, or clear signs that he has something wrong with him.

Psychological problems. A report from a civilian doctor or therapist is essential for a man with psychological problems. Although draftees are examined physically at the AFEES, there is no routine psychological testing, only a questionnaire. There is often no psychiatrist at the AFEES, so the medical officers must do the best they can without specialized training.

Standard Form 93, Report of Medical History, asks whether the registrant ever had depression or excessive worry, nervous trouble of any sort, attempted suicide, etc. Only if a man checks "yes" to any of these, or gives further information about such problems as drug involvement, heavy drinking, or homosexuality, in the blank section reserved for "explanations," is he likely to be interviewed about psychiatric problems, either by the chief of the medical examining section, or by a psychiatric specialist. The examiner will try to guess whether the condition is serious, or whether the man is bluffing. Without letters from civilian specialists, checking a box on SF 93 does not usually lead to disqualification.

Special consultations with psychiatrists can be arranged by the AFEES. The man may be held over several days until the interview, but more likely will be called back for a special appointment.

The military considers some psychological conditions to be "moral" problems as well as medical conditions. Homosexuality, alcoholism, drug use, and frequent conflicts with authority are the most common examples.

Profiling. As a man is being examined, he carries along both SF 93 and SF 88. At the end of the examination, the physical profiling officer summarizes the results at the bottom of SF 88. At this point the registrant should be told if he has been found unacceptable for service. If he is not told, he can look at the codes on SF 88, item 76; if a *3* or *4* shows in the "PULHES" chart, he has been found unacceptable for physical or psychiatric reasons. If no *3* or *4* has been entered in the "PULHES" chart, then the man is being found medically acceptable for induction.

Holdovers and hospitalizations. Men are sometimes held over at the AFEES for special examinations, usually for not more than three days. The Army is required to furnish meals and lodging if necessary; a man asked to stay over may have to insist that the AFEES do so. If he lives near the AFEES he is sent home and asked to return. Hospitalization is authorized when necessary as part of the exam.

Additional documentation. If a man tells AFEES examiners that he could produce medical reports which would show he is not acceptable for service, he should be told to send them to his local board. The man is declared acceptable, and the AFEES considers the new papers at the time of induction unless the man requests special procedures earlier. The AFEES can write the local board, and through it ask for information from the man's school, a doctor or a hospital, but it rarely does, so the registrant should plan ahead to provide all records and use all procedures available.

Doubtful cases. When the AFEES needs more time or information to make a decision, it can declare "acceptability undetermined," send the man home, and notify him of the decision weeks or months later. In a "doubtful" case, AFEES officials can refer the medical records to the USAREC Surgeon, who in turn can refer them to the office of the Surgeon General.

Waivers. The medical fitness standards should be binding on the AFEES, and a man with a condition listed should be found unacceptable if he presents convincing evidence. AFEES examiners could formerly recommend acceptance of a man who was able to function well as a civilian, even if his condition was listed. This "vocation waiver" provision in the medical regulations was revoked on October 15, 1971.

Under the Medical Remedial Program (MREP), a man with certain minor medical problems leading to disqualification may be asked whether he would like to enlist or to volunteer for induction if he were found acceptable. If a man agrees to MREP, special tests can be carried out by recruiters, leading to a medical waiver, and the man can then enter the Armed Forces. Or he can decide to keep his 4-F instead; no one is required to seek an MREP.

Uncooperativeness. A man who refuses to cooperate with

one of the required steps of examination is warned that he is violating the law. If he persists, he is asked to make and sign a statement (but cannot be required to do so), and is sent home without transportation. He is then processed as if he had refused to report for examination. A man is not a noncooperator because he refuses to fill out or sign the Security Questionnaire, or to do janitorial or other work at the AFEES.

Examination Records

DD Form 62. After a man has taken his physical, the AFEES completes two copies of DD Form 62, Statement of Acceptability, and both copies are sent to the man's local board. One copy is then forwarded to the registrant. The DD Form 62 is normally the only official notification given to a man of whether he was found acceptable or unacceptable at his AFEES examination.

On the local board's copy of DD Form 62 there is a space labeled "Remarks" which is blacked out on the copy sent to the registrant. AFEES officials use this space to notify local boards if the AFEES thinks that the registrant should be reexamined. Thus on the local board copy of DD Form 62 a man will sometimes find such comments as "re-examination believed justified in 3 months" (or some other time period—often abbreviated "RBJ 3 mos"). A man can examine the local board copy of DD Form 62 in his draft file if he wishes. It is sometimes possible to make out a recommendation for re-examination on the registrant's own copy of the DD Form 62.

Other forms. The local board sends a copy of SSS Form 223, Order to Report for Armed Forces Physical Examination and all medical records in the draft file to the AFEES before examination. The AFEES returns this packet to the board with SF 93, SF 88, and DD Form 62, supposedly within 5 working days after the exam is completed, but delays are common.

Enlistment exams. Enlistees for all the military branches are also examined at the AFEES. The ordinary enlistment standards are the same as for induction. Medical records of enlistment exams should be sent by the AFEES to the state director of Selective Service, and if he chooses, to the local board. If a man fails an enlistment exam and has not yet had a preinduction physical under orders of his local board, he should write to his board, and if necessary to the state director, to ask that the results of the enlistment exam be obtained and any pre-induction examination order be canceled. If one passes an enlistment exam he should still be ordered to a pre-induction physical before he can be drafted, though this is sometimes violated.

Classification After Examination

Men found acceptable for induction. A man who is determined to be acceptable for induction, and who does not qualify for any deferment or exemption, will be classified 1-A, 1-A-O, or 1-O. If he is already in one of these classifications when he takes the physical, however, he will not be reclassified when he passes. The local board may not mail an induction order to a man who takes the physical, however, until it has sent him DD Form 62, Statement of Acceptability. After DD Form 62 has been mailed, the man may be ordered for induction if his lottery number has been reached.

Men found temporarily unacceptable for induction. A man who is rejected at an examination but "whose further examination or re-examination may be justified" is not classified 4-F. If he no longer qualifies for any other deferment or exemption he will be classified 1-A, and if he is already 1-A the local board will not reopen his classification. This 1-A classification is sometimes referred to as "1-A Unacceptable," "1-A Hold," or "1-A-H." Although classified 1-A, a man found temporarily unacceptable for induction cannot be drafted until he has been re-examined and found acceptable. When a man is later re-examined, if he is found acceptable, he is not entitled to a reopening of his classification or to the appeal rights that go with reopening, since his 1-A classification will not have changed. If a man is 1-A Unacceptable, with a lottery number below the cutoff announced by the Director of Selective Service, and he is still 1-A on December 31, he will enter the Extended Priority Selection Group on January 1 of the following year.

Selective Service officials have stated that a man who is found disqualified (even temporarily) at induction should receive a cancellation of his induction order rather than a postponement. A man found temporarily disqualified at a physical or induction, who is subsequently re-examined and found disqualified again, should then be reclassified 4-F by his local board, even if the doctors at the AFEES where he was re-examined believe he should be examined a third time.

It is not clear what medical problems are to be considered temporary. Presumably an acute illness or injury, such as a broken leg or mononucleosis, would fall into this category. Underweight, overweight, failure to meet minimum height standards, high blood pressure, and dental braces are considered temporary by some AFEES. A man who hopes to be found medically disqualified should try to submit medical evidence indicating as strongly as possible that he has a long-term or permanent problem.

Men found permanently unacceptable for induction. A registrant who is found permanently unacceptable for induction, with no "re-examination believed justified" on the local board copy of DD Form 62, should be classified 4-F.

A man classified 4-F should have his deferment as long as his disqualifying condition continues and medical standards do not change. A man with a 4-F who is ordered for re-examination should prepare new medical documentation and contact a draft counselor who may be aware of current re-examination policies. A man who is ordered for re-examination will receive a complete medical exam if he has not been examined at the AFEES in the previous year. Otherwise the exam will concentrate only on the conditions which led to the finding of unacceptability in the first place and any new evidence he submits.

Appealing a Finding of Acceptability

IMPORTANT: Selective Service does not postpone issuance of an induction order so that one may submit new medical information or request medical review, so any available Selective Service personal appearance and appeal procedures which delay issuance of an induction order should be used at the same time as the procedures described below. If a man has no Selective Service appeal rights, he should request medical review of his acceptability as soon as possible.

Presenting new medical information. Although local boards should reopen a man's classification if presented with medical evidence which, if true, would warrant a change in classification, in practice this is rarely done. What a man usually gets when he presents new medical evidence is either a "papers only" review of the medical evidence, or the Registrant Medical Reevaluation and Review System (RMRRS). Both of these procedures are described below.

"Papers only" review. When a local board decides to grant a registrant a "papers only" review, all of the medical records contained in the man's draft file are forwarded to the AFEES servicing the area of his local board. The AFEES considers the information presented to it and then reports any change in the registrant's status to the local board.

A man may request a "papers only" review of his medical acceptability if (1) since having taken a pre-induction physical, he has obtained further documentation of a claimed disqualifying condition, or (2) there has been a change in his physical condition since he took his pre-induction physical. A man who complains to his local board about the result of his AFEES examination but who does not submit new evidence may erroneously be given a "papers only" review. However, RMRRS is better than the "papers only" review for a man who wishes to challenge the findings of his AFEES examination, and it is important that a man request RMRRS before he is issued an induction order. Thus, a man should ask for a "papers only" review before requesting RMRRS only if he is sure that he cannot be ordered for induction in the near future.

The following procedures are suggested for a registrant trying to get a "papers only" review of his AFEES examination:

If he has time, he should examine SF 93 and SF 88 in his draft file at his local board and note any incorrect or incomplete findings on these forms. He should then write a letter to his local board which contains:

1) a request for a "papers only" review of his case and a reopening of his classification;

2) a statement that he passed an examination at the AFEES, giving date and location;

3) a description of how the examination was conducted at the point where his disqualifying condition should have been found and an explanation of why he feels that he was treated unfairly—a statement that the AFEES failed to give him an appropriate special consultation (for example, with an orthopedist or psychiatrist) if such a consultation should have been given and was not, the name of the AFEES examiner involved in the unfair treatment, etc.;

4) complete medical documentation, including if possible a doctor's letter about the condition in question written *after* the physical examination, any new X-rays or laboratory reports, and any other new information;

5) a brief summary of the medical evidence which is already in the file;

6) an indication of which sections of the medical standards apply.

Registrant Medical Reevaluation and Review System. A "papers only" review is unlikely to result in disqualification in most cases. A man who has tried it unsuccessfully, or who has reason to believe he will soon be issued an induction order, should immediately request Registrant Medical Reevaluation and Review System (RMRRS). Normally, a man is only allowed to use RMRRS once, unless there has been some significant change in his condition, so it is important to prepare carefully. The registrant's letter to his local board should include all the material suggested in the "papers only" review section, except that instead of asking for a "papers only" review, he should specifically request Registrant Medical Reevaluation and Review System. In addition, he should stress that he wishes to be given another AFEES examination.

A request sent to the local board for RMRRS, and all medical records, must be forwarded to the state director, who will determine if such a request is appropriate (in other words, if the man has used the RMRRS before, if he should be given a "papers only" review instead, etc.). If the state director decides that the RMRRS should be granted, he will then forward all records to the AFEES normally used by the registrant's local board. The AFEES will review the information presented, and a re-examination or special consultation will be scheduled if the AFEES deems it necessary. NOTE: If a man does not emphasize in his request for RMRRS that he wants to be re-examined, the AFEES may decide that another physical is not necessary.

A man will usually be ordered for re-examination at the AFEES servicing his local board. If he has taken a physical there before, he may want to transfer the examination to another AFEES, so that he is not examined by the same physicians who originally found him acceptable. Transfer procedures under RMRRS are the same as for pre-induction physicals.

After the AFEES has completed its examination, it will forward all medical information and records, and its own tentative determination of the man's acceptability, to the headquarters of the U.S. Army Recruiting Command (USAREC) in Hampton, Virginia. USAREC Headquarters, after reviewing the papers, makes a final determination of acceptability and sends the decision and its findings back through the AFEES, the state director, and the local board. The board notifies the registrant of the results (but he will have to examine his file at the local board to learn the reasons), and if his status has changed, issues a new Statement of Acceptability. If he is permanently disqualified, the board should reopen his classification and classify him 4-F at its next meeting. If he is disqualified only temporarily, he will not be reclassified, but will be re-examined as required by the AFEES, and cannot be inducted in the meantime.

Requests for RMRRS after issuance of an induction order. When a man under an induction order asks for review of his medical acceptability, he should be told by his local board to bring all his medical documentation with him to induction. At induction, he should get a physical inspection including tests or interviews necessary to review the condition. If these procedures cannot be finished that day, he may be kept at the AFEES as long as three days. After its examination, the AFEES should then obtain by telephone the final decision of USAREC Headquarters on his acceptability, but does not usually postpone induction so that USAREC can review the actual papers, except in some cases where a member of Congress has expressed interest. For this reason, it may be especially important for a man in this situation to report for induction early at an AFEES other than the one where he was first examined in order to have his condition inspected by a different specialist, and perhaps to have two chances of being disqualified.

A man facing induction should know beforehand what he will do if found acceptable. Some men, particularly those thinking of refusing induction or starting habeas corpus proceedings, will want to contact a lawyer.

Complaints about AFEES administration. If a man goes through the RMRRS procedure and does not get the desired change in classification, he may still be able to protest the way his original physical or his reevaluation was administered. He should not expect, however, that such a protest will always be useful. The man may write a letter explaining how his physical was improper in any of the following ways:

1) Administration—items of medical history, examination, or medical documentation not properly considered, required items of the examination not correctly entered on the proper forms, or improper treatment by AFEES personnel during examination.

2) Examination procedures—hasty or incomplete handling of portions of the examination or omissions of parts of the examination, testing procedures, laboratory studies, or X-rays.

3) Facilities—faulty examination equipment (e.g., scales) or facilities (e.g., lighting too poor to read results by) making medical results inaccurate or invalid.

It often helps to direct such a protest to a Congressman or Senator, though one may send it directly to USAREC, Hampton, Virginia 23369. The letter should deal specifically with administration, procedures, and facilities at the AFEES, as outlined above; it may also be a complaint that the reevaluation dealt only with the medical papers and did not include a new examination.

Examination at Induction

The local board orders a man to report for induction in its area—either directly to the AFEES, or to a place from which the board provides transportation to the AFEES. The rules on postponement of induction are the same as for pre-induction exams, except that the local board will evidently retain the power to give two postponements of up to 60 days each. In addition, certain students can have induction orders postponed. In practice, many state directors routinely grant postponements of induction for a great variety of reasons, including: allowing an employer to find a replacement, finishing up business affairs, marriage, birth of a child, temporary family hardship. However, a person who is temporarily ill is wisest to report to an AFEES (if he can, and if he has medical reports which clearly will disqualify him) rather than request postponement of induction. If he is rejected at induction, his induction order is canceled and a new one can be issued only after he receives and passes a later re-examination, though he will not necessarily be reclassified 4-F.

The local board sends medical records and other forms from its file to the AFEES to which it normally sends its registrants. It marks the location of this AFEES and the man's AFQT (mental test) score on the upper left-hand corner of the induction order. When a man reports at a transfer AFEES, any other medical evidence in his file is usually not available to the examiners, though normally they will contact the local board's AFEES by telephone for a summary of previous examinations. Therefore, a man should be sure to bring with him copies of all the medical evidence he wants considered, both new and old.

A man who reports for induction is normally not given a complete medical examination, if the examiners have evidence that he has passed a pre-induction physical within one year. Instead he gets a "physical inspection." A doctor reviews any available medical reports from the pre-induction exam and asks the man if he has any new medical problems. The man is supposed to be "closely observed" for "communicable diseases and apparent defects not previously recorded." If he has brought new medical reports from civilian doctors, he should get a more complete check of the conditions claimed. He is asked about any pending court dates or new convictions. If he passed the pre-induction physical more than a year earlier, however, or never took a pre-induction physical, he gets a complete medical examination at induction.

If he passes examination or inspection, he is processed for induction. If he fails, he is sent home, a new DD Form 62 is issued, and the induction order is canceled.

Court Review

A man who refuses induction risks being convicted in federal court for violation of the draft law, punishable by up to five years in prison and a fine of up to $10,000. His lawyer can try to convince the U.S. Attorney to get him a new examination at the AFEES, and not to indict him, or to drop the indictment; sometimes this is successful. Otherwise the lawyer presents a defense in court that the man was improperly found acceptable. If successful, the man is acquitted and should be reclassified 4-F. If unsuccessful, he is convicted and may be sentenced to probation or prison.

A man who accepts induction can, with careful advance planning, have his attorney bring suit immediately in federal court to get a writ of habeas corpus releasing him from the military. The same kinds of arguments can be made as in a criminal case; if successful, the man should be released and reclassified 4-F. Habeas corpus is appropriate for the man who would rather remain in the military than risk prison if he loses in court.

A man who is faced with induction when he believes he should be classified 4-F can consider contacting an attorney to discuss court action. Local draft counselors can help find an experienced lawyer. CCCO tries to assist lawyers seeking its aid.

Medical Discharge from the Military

A man who had a medical condition before induction which should have led to a 4-F deferment, but who was inducted anyway, can sometimes get a medical discharge from the military. His Selective Service medical records become a part of his military papers. He must apply soon after induction, within four months. For advice, CCCO can make referrals to counselors who know military procedure. However, a man facing induction should not count on medical discharge, but should consider using all the steps listed above first, possibly including court action.

V. Summary of State Abortion Laws

This information is compiled by the authors from a variety of sources, and is up-to-date as of March 31, 1971

I. *Abortion on request* in the following states:

	Residency Requirement	Time Limit	By M.D.	In Hospital	Other Restrictions
ALASKA	30 days	"nonviable fetus" (no more than 20 to 24 weeks)	yes	yes	Unmarried woman less than 18 years needs permission of parent or guardian
DISTRICT OF COLUMBIA					No restrictions
HAWAII	90 days	same as Alaska	yes	yes	
NEW YORK		24 weeks	yes	yes (In New York City may be done in clinic)	After 24 weeks pregnancy may be terminated to preserve maternal life
WASHINGTON	90 days	16 weeks	yes	yes (or other places may be designated)	Need consent of husband if married, or parent/legal guardian if unmarried and under 18
WISCONSIN					No restrictions

II. *Abortions permitted under limited circumstances*, as specified below in the following states:

	To Preserve Maternal Life	To Preserve Maternal Health	To Preserve Maternal Mental Health	Fetal Deformity	Forcible Rape	Statutory Rape	Incest
ARKANSAS	X	X			X		X
CALIFORNIA	X	X	X		X	15 years	X
COLORADO	X	X	X	X	X	16 years	X
DELAWARE	X	X	X	X	X		X
GEORGIA	X	X		X	X	14 years	
KANSAS	X	X	X	X	X	16 years	X
MARYLAND	X	X	X	X	X		
NEW MEXICO	X	X	X	X	X	16 years	
NORTH CAROLINA	X	X		X	X		X
OREGON	X	X	X	X	X	16 years	X
SOUTH CAROLINA	X	X	X	X	X		X
VIRGINIA	X	X	X	X	X		X

	Time Limit	By M.D.	In Hospital	Residency Requirement	M.D. Approval	Other Qualifications
ARKANSAS		X	X	120 days	3 consultants	
CALIFORNIA	20 wks	X	X		yes	2-member Abortion Board to 12th week; 3-member after 12th week
COLORADO		X	X		3 member Abortion Board	16-week limit for rape and incest only
DELAWARE	20 wks	X	X	120 days	1 consultant & hospital review authority	After 20 weeks permitted to save maternal life or if fetus is dead. Residency not required if woman or husband works in Delaware, if woman has previously been patient of Delaware physician, or if life is in danger.
GEORGIA		X	X	yes	3 consultants & 3 member Therapeutic Abortion Board	
KANSAS		X	X		3 consultants	
MARYLAND	26 wks	X	X		Hospital Review Comm.	After 26 weeks abortion permitted to save maternal life or if fetus is dead.
NEW MEXICO		X	X		2 member Therapeutic Abortion Board	
NORTH CAROLINA	150 days	X	X	120 days	3 consultants	
OREGON		X	X	yes	1 consultant	
SOUTH CAROLINA		X	X	90 days	3 consultants	
VIRGINIA		X	X	120 days	Hospital Board	

III. To preserve the life or health of the mother, abortion is permitted in the following states: Alabama, Massachusetts.
IV. Abortion is permitted in the following states *only* to preserve the life of the mother: Arizona, Connecticut, Idaho, Illinois, Indiana, Iowa, Kentucky, Louisiana, Maine, Michigan, Minnesota, Missouri, Montana, Nebraska, Nevada, New Hampshire, New Jersey, North Dakota, Ohio, Oklahoma, Puerto Rico, Rhode Island, South Dakota, Tennessee, Texas, Utah, Vermont, West Virginia, Wyoming.
V. Abortion is permitted to save the life of the mother or in the event of rape with the approval of two consultants in the state of Mississippi.
VI. Unlawful abortion is prohibited but not defined in the state of Pennsylvania.
VII. Abortion is permitted in the state of Florida if there is substantial risk that pregnancy would result in defective birth, or if the pregnancy resulted from rape or incest.

Index

Abdominal injuries, 128–32
   non-penetrating, 131–32
   symptoms, meaning of, 129–31
Abdominal pain, 92–93, 129–31
   See also Stomach
Abortion, 324–26
   after rape, 328
   state laws, summarized, 471–74
Abscesses, 250
   of mouth, 215–16
Acetyl salicylic acid
   defined, 40
   See also Aspirin
Acid, see Hallucinogens
Acne, 217–22
   antibiotics and, 220, 222
   causes of, 217–18
   commonness of, 217
   diet and, 218, 220
   effects of, 217
   hormones and, 220–21
   menstruation and, 220–21
   squeezing of pimples, 221
   stress and, 220
   treatment of, 218–22
Addiction, see Drugs, mind-altering
Alcoholic beverages
   as cough treatment, 49
   epilepsy and, 66
   fever and, 46
   hepatitis and, 184
   during pregnancy, 320
   snakebite and, 238
   tests for presence of, 24
Alcoholism, 340–42

Allergies
   to bee stings, 240
   to detergents, 101
   to milk, 93–94
   to poison ivy, 100, 101
American Board of Internal Medicine, 5
American College of Surgeons, 5
American Medical Association (AMA), 9, 10
Amphetamines, 248, 257–58
   in weight reduction, 368–69
   See also Drugs, mind-altering
Analgesics, nature of, 39
Anemia, 357–58
   nature, causes, and treatment of, 57–58
Angina, 76–77
   See also Heart attacks
Animal bites, 234–37
Anorexia, 86
Anorexia nervosa, 86
Antibiotics, 130–31
   diarrhea and, 198–99
   in treatment of body odor, 99
Antihistamines
   for coughing and colds, 49, 178
   side effects, 68
Antiperspirants, 100
Ant stings, 240
Anus
   defined, 83
   functioning of, 84
   sensitivity of, 95
   See also Hemorrhoids

Anxiety, 59–60
  nervousness, 59
  See also Psychiatric problems
APC tablets, 40, 41
Appendicitis, 92–93, 130
Aphrodisiacs, 241
Appetite, loss of, 86
Army, *see* Draft deferral
Arrhythmia, 78
Arteries, 71–72
  cut, treatment of, 146–47, 150
  hardening of, 79–80, 82
Arteriosclerosis, 79
Artificial respiration, *see* Cardiac resuscitation
Aspiration, defined, 89
Aspirin, 40–41
  abdominal pain and, 130
  brands, differences between, 40
  buffered, 41
  codeine compared with, 42
  for colds, 177
  dosage, 40
    for children, 46
    for fever, 46
  kidney problems and, 40–41
  for menstrual discomfort, 204
  stomach irritation and, 41
Asthma
  cardiac arrest from, 162
  nature, causes, and treatment of, 53–54
  tear gas and, 50, 54
Atherosclerosis, 79
  heart failure and, 82

Backbone, broken, 112–13
  treatment of, 138
Bacterial endocarditis, 251
Bad breath, 222–24
Bad taste in mouth, 222–24
Bad Trips, 252, 264–66
Balance, loss of, *see* Dizziness
Baldness, 103–4
Barbiturates, 68, 254–57
  defined, 248
  duration of action, 255
  long-term effects, 256–57
  short-term effects, 255–56
  speed and, 258
Bat bites, 234–37
Bedbugs, 233
Bee stings, 240
Belching, 94–95
Bilirubin, 182
Birth control methods, 303–12
  abstinence, 308
  comparison of, 309–11
  condoms, 307–8, 309–11
  convenience, comparative, 309, 310
  cost, comparative, 311
  dangers, comparative, 310, 311
  diaphragm, 306–7, 309–11
  effectiveness, comparative, 309, 310
  esthetic aspects, comparative, 309–10
  future developments, 311–12
  intrauterine device (IUD), 305–6, 309–11
  jellies, creams, and foams, 308, 309–11
  list of, 303–4
  pills, 304–5, 309–11
    side effects, 225–27, 305
  rhythm, 304, 308
  selection of, factors to consider, 303
  side benefits, comparative, 310–11
  side effects, comparative, 310
  undesirable, 304, 308
  withdrawal, 304, 308
Bites
  animal, 234–36
  centipede, 241
  insect, 230–34, 239–41
  lizard, 239
  rabies, 234–37
  scorpion, 240

Bites (*cont.*)
  snake, 237–39
  spider, 239–40
Black eye, 118–19, 142
  treatment of, 40, 142
Bladder, *see* Urinary tract
Bleeding, 56–57
  from cuts, 146–47, 149
  from mouth, 216
  from nose, 207–10
  during pregnancy, 316
  from rectum, 193
Blister beetle, 241
Blood
  anemia, 57–58
  clots, 224–27, 250–51
  coughing up, 50–51
  nature and purpose of, 55–56
  pressure
    high (hypertension), 37, 75–76
    normal, 75
  spitting up, 50–51
  vomiting up, 50–51, 89–90, 91
Blueness of skin, 51–52, 163–64
Board certification, significance of, 5
Body odor, elimination of, 99–100
Body temperature, *see* Temperature, body
Bones, broken, *see* Fractures
Bonine, 230
Borborygmi, 96
Brain injury, *see* Head injury
Breastbone (sternum) injury, 120–23
Breathing
  detection of, 164
  difficulty (dyspnea), 50
  heavy, 50
  at high altitudes, 50, 52
  hyperventilation, 54–55, 73
  irregular, 112
  shortness of breath, 123–25
  slow, 112
  See also Asthma
Broken bones, *see* Fractures
Bronchitis
  from marihuana or hashish, 254
  See also Colds
Bruises, *see* Cuts
Bugs, *see* Insects
Buffered aspirin, 41
  See also Aspirin
Bullet wounds, *see* Gunshot wounds
Burns, 151–56
  classifications of, 98
  depth of, 151–52
  extent of, 152–53
  first degree, 151
    treatment of, 153–54
  second degree, 152
    treatment of, 154–55
  seriousness of, criteria for determining, 151
  shock from, 153
  smoke poisoning, 153
  sunburn, 151–52
    treatment of, 153–54
  tetanus from, 155
  third degree, 152
    treatment of, 155–56
  treatment of, 153–56

Calories, 349, 365
Cantharidin, 241
Capillaries, 71–72
Cardiac arrest
  causes of, 160–62
  recognition of, 163–64
  symptoms of, 163–64
  See also Heart attack
Cardiac massage, method for, 168–69
Cardiac resuscitation
  artificial respiration distinguished from, 159–60
  cardiac massage, 168–69
  how long to continue, 169–70

Cardiac resuscitation (*cont.*)
  mouth-to-mouth breathing, 166–68
  procedure, 166–70
  preparation for, 164–65
  when to employ, 160–62
Carsickness, 227–30
Casts, 138–41
Cat bites, 234–37
Centipede bites, 241
Central Committee for Conscientious Objectors, 449
Certification, board, significance of, 5
Chemical warfare agents, 278–91
  circumstances when most dangerous, 279
  incapacitating gases, 288–89
    BZ gas, 288–89
  mace, 290–91
  precautionary measures, 279–81
  tear gas, 281–88
  vomiting gases, 289–91
    DA, 290
    DC, 290
    DM, 290
  See also Tear gas
Chest injuries, 120–28
  breastbone (sternum), 120–23
  bullet wounds, 125–28
  cardiac arrest from, 162
  contusion and compression, 123
  lung collapse, 123–25
  ribs, 120–23
  stab wounds, 125–28
Chest pain, 76–77
  See also Heart attacks
Chiggers, 233
Childbirth, *see* Pregnancy
Children, *see* Minors
Chloral hydrate, 68
Cholera, 196–97
Circulatory system, *see* Blood; Heart entries

Clinics
  community (people's), 14, 17, 387
  directory of, 399–409
  medical costs in, 16
  quality of medical care in, 15–16
  student health, 14, 16
    confidentiality of medical records in, 16
  See also Emergency rooms; Hospitals
Cocaine, 259–60
Codeine, 42
  See also Opiates
Coitus, *see* Sex
Colds, 174–79
  antibiotics for, 174–77
  antihistamines for, 178
  aspirin for, 177
  causes of, 176
    misconceptions about, 174
  cough drops, 178–79
  cures, misconceptions about, 174, 176
  flu distinguished from, 175–76
  gargling, 177
  lozenges, 177
  non-prescription medications, 178–79
  nose sprays, 178
  pills, 177–78
  sores, 45
  strep throat distinguished from, 175–76
  treatment of, 176–79
  viruses, variety of, 174–75
  Vitamin C and, 174, 176
  See also Coughing
Cold temperatures, injuries from, 243–45
Colic, from CNS gas, 287
Colon, functioning of, 84
Coma, 69–70
Commitment of mental patients, *see* Mental patients

Community (people's) clinics, 14, 17, 387
  directory of, 399–409
Community mental health centers, 346
Compazine, 230
Concussions, *see* Head injuries
Condoms, *see* Birth control methods
Confidentiality of medical information, 16, 28–30
  privileged information, defined, 28
  reportable diseases, 29–30
Consciousness, alterations in, 69–70
  from brain injury, 110
  See also Drugs, mind-altering
Constipation, 96–97
  abdominal pain and, 130
  hemorrhoids and, 192, 194
  during pregnancy, 320–31
Contraception, *see* Birth control
Contusions, *see* Bruises
Convulsions, from fever, 45, 46
Cornea
  defined, 117
  See also Eye
Coronaries, *see* Heart attacks
Costs, *see* Medical costs
Coughing, 47–49
  antihistamines and, 49
  of blood, 50–51
  causes of, 47–48
  cough drops, 48–49
  cough medicines, 49
  cough suppressants, 49
  danger signals, 47
  expectorants, 49
  irritants and, 48
  marihuana and, 48, 254
  nervous, 48
  smoking and, 47, 48
  sneezing, 52
  See also Colds
Counseling, 17

Cramps, muscle, 242
Crotch, pain in, 191
Cuts, 141–50
  abrasions
    defined, 142
    treatment of, 143
  of arteries, 146–47, 150
  bleeding, 149
  cleaning, 146, 147–48
  closing up, 143–44
  of eyelids, 144–45
  of face and scalp, 145–46
  of hand, 144
  infections, 148–49
  lacerations
    defined, 142
    treatment of, 143–49
  police, dealing with, 150
  puncture wounds, 150
    defined, 142
  tetanus, 143, 150
  tourniquets, 146–47, 150
  treatment of, 143–50
  types of, 142
  See also Stab wounds
Cyanosis, 51–52, 163–64
Cystitis, 189, 302

Dandruff, 104–5
Darvon, 41, 42
DDT, 232, 233, 240
Dehydration, from vomiting, 189
Delirium, 64
  See also Fever
Delusions, 62
Demerol, 42
Democratic National Convention, 29
Demonstrators, medical care for
  in hospital clinics and emergency rooms, 14, 15–16
  in mass-arrest situations, 31–32
  See also Medical supplies and equipment; Tear gas
Deodorants, 99

Depilatories, 103
Depression, 60, 331-33
Dermis
  defined, 98
  See also Skin
Deviation, sexual, 336-40
Diabetes
  heart attacks and, 79
  urinary tract infections and, 190
  vaginal discharge and, 202
Diaphragm, *see* Birth control methods
Diarrhea, 94, 97, 132
  dysentery and, 195
  traveler's, 195-99
    avoidance of, 195, 197-99
    causes of, 195-96
    severe symptoms, 196-97
    treatment of, 198-99
Diet, *see* Nutrition
Dieting, *see* Obesity
Digestive process, 83-84
  See also specific entries
Dislocation, defined, 133
Dizziness, 62-63
  with headache, 37-38
  on standing up, 61
DMT, *see* Hallucinogens
Doctors, 4-6
  age of, quality and, 13
  board certification, significance of, 5
  competence of, 4
  confidentiality of patient information, 28-30
  criteria for selecting, 14-15
  general practitioners, 5-6
  group practice, 6
  hospital affiliations, 6
  hostile, dealing with, 24
  house calls, 18-19
  internships, 4-5
  keeping pace with expansion of knowledge, 6
  legal obligations to patients, 20-21, 27-28
  malpractice, 27-28
  medical society membership, significance of, 14
  referrals, 6
  refusal to provide treatment, 20-21
  residencies, 5
  role of, 4
  selection of, 14-15
  solo practitioners, 15
  specialization, 5
  training of, 4-5
  withdrawal from case, 27
  See also Hospitals; Medical care; Medical costs; Medicine
Dog bites, 234-37
DOM, *see* Hallucinogens
Douching, 200
  during pregnancy, 321
Doyle, Arthur Conan, 259
Draft deferment, 272-78
  alcoholism, 277
  appeals, 451-52, 464-68
  classification categories, 464
  confidentiality of records, 451
  counseling, where to find, 273
  doctor's examination, 273-76
  draft boards, 273
  drug addiction, 277
  enlistment exams, 462
  4-F classification, 449-70
  homosexuality, 277, 438-39
  induction
    court review, 470
    exam, 469
    refusal, 469-70
  informing draft board, 450-51
  medical discharge, 470
  medical interviews, 452-54
  official requirements for, 273, 410-48
    abdomen and gastrointestinal system, 411-12
    applicability of, 410
    arms, legs, etc., 416-21

Draft deferment (*cont.*)
   blood and blood-forming tissue diseases, 413
   body build, 432–33
   bone and joint problems, 416–21
   cancer, 445
   cellular tissues, 439–41
   chest, 433–35
   clavicles, 442
   dental conditions, 413–14
   ears and hearing, 414–15
   endocrine and metabolic disorders, 415–16
   eyes and vision, 421–25
   extremities, 416–21
   genitalia, 425–26
   head and neck, 428–29
   heart and vascular system, 429–31
   height, 432
   lungs, 433–35
   miscellaneous conditions and defects, 443–44
   mouth, 435, 436
   neurological disorders, 437–38
   nose, 435–36
   personality disorders, 438–39
   physical profile functional capacity guide, 446–47
   psychoneuroses, 438
   psychoses, 438
   ribs, 442
   scapulae, 442
   skin, 439–41
   spine and sacroiliac joints, 441–42
   systemic diseases, 442–43
   throat, 436
   tuberculosis, 434
   tumors
      benign, 444–45
      malignant, 444
   urinary system, 426–27
   venereal disease, 445
   vocational waivers, 448
   weight, 432
   1-Y classification, 449–50
   pre-induction exam, 456–61
      additional documentation, 460
      doubtful cases, 460
      exam records, 461–62
      holdovers and hospitalizations, 459–60
      medical exam
         described, 458
         form for, 457–58
      medical history form, 457
      mental testing, 457
      mistreatment, dealing with, 456–57
      profiling, 459
      psychological problems, 458–59
      uncooperativeness, 460–61
      waivers, 460
   reporting for pre-induction exam, 454–56
   postponements, 555
      records processing prior to, 455–56
      special instructions, 456
      transfer, 455
      voluntary, 454–55
   psychiatric, 277–78, 438–39
   for troublemakers, 278
   without examination, 452–54
Dramamine, 230
Dreaming, 67
Dropsy (edema), 82
Drug clinics, 17
   See also Drugs, mind-altering
Drugs, medicinal
   cardiac arrests from, 162
   cough suppressants, 49
   non-prescription, 40–41
   painkillers, 39, 40–41
      side effects, 40, 41
   during pregnancy, 264, 319–20
   prescription, 41–42

Drugs, medicinal (*cont.*)
  sedatives, 68
  for weight reducing, 368–69
Drugs, mind-altering, 246–72
  addiction, 277, 342–43
    defined, 246–47
  bad trips, 252, 264–66
  barbiturates, 254–57
  categories of, 248
  cocaine, 259–60
  contamination of, 250–52
  doctors' attitudes toward users, 249
  habituation, defined, 246–47
  hallucinogens, 260–66
  "hard-core," defined, 248
  hashish, 252–54
    defined, 248
  injections, medical problems from, 249–51
  marihuana, 252–54
    defined, 248
  misinformation about, 246–48
  opiates, 266–72
  during pregnancy, 264, 319–20
  purity of, 250–52
  safest ways to take, 251
  sedatives, 248
  stimulants, 257–58
  tests for presence of, 24, 248–49
  tolerance, defined, 247
  See also Hallucinogens; Opiates; other specific drug names
Dysentery, 97, 195
Dysmenorrhea, *see* Menstrual discomfort
Dysphagia, 85
Dyspnea, 50

Embolus, 225–27
Ear, 210–14
  discharge from, 112
  parts of, 210
  pinna, defined, 2
  wax, 211–12

Earache
  external canal, infection of, 211–12
  from foreign bodies, 212–13
  middle ear, infection of, 213–14
  outer ear, infection of, 211
  from toothache, 214
  from wax, 211–12
Edema (dropsy), 82
Electrocution, resuscitation of victim, 161–62
Electrolysis, 103
Emergencies
  defining, 17–18
  house calls, 18–19
  suggested procedure for, 17–19
Emergency rooms
  alcohol tests, right to administer, 24
  demonstrators, care of, in, 14, 15–16
  discriminatory treatment, dealing with, 24–25
  drug tests, right to administer, 24
  information required from patient, 22–23
  legal obligations to patient, 22–24
  medical costs, 16
  police
    presence of, 23–24
    reports to, 23
  quality of medical care in, 15–16
  refusal of services, 22
  See also Hospitals
Epidermis
  defined, 98
  See also Skin
Epilepsy, 64–66
  causes of, 65, 66
  treatment of, 65
Ergot, 64

Esophagus, defined, 83
Estrogens, 205
Excretion, process described, 84
Excrement, *see* Stool
Exercise
　as obesity treatment, 369
　during pregnancy, 321
Expenses, *see* Medical costs
Eye
　black, 40, 118–19, 142
　blunt injury to, 119
　cornea, defined, 117
　eyelid, lacerations of, 119–20, 144–45
　foreign bodies in, 115–18
　injuries, 115–20
　pupils
　　in brain injury, 111–12
　　described, 111
　sclera, defined, 116

Facial injuries, 114–15
　features, drooping of, 111
　lacerations, 145–46
Fainting, 60–62
　causes of, 61
　emotional, 60–61
　on standing up, 61
　treatment of, 62
Fatigue, anemia and, 57–58
Fatness, *see* Obesity
Feces, *see* Stool
"Fee for service" system, 9
Fees, *see* Medical costs
Fever, 42–46
　accompanying symptoms, 44–45
　alcoholic beverages and, 46
　aspirin for, 46
　causes of, 45
　with confusion, 45
　convulsions from, 45, 46
　delirium, 64
　as diagnostic tool, 42, 45
　fluctuation of, 44

fluid loss, combating, 46
　with headache, 38
　lowering, methods for, 46
　sores, 45
　treatment of, 45–46
　See also Temperature
First aid, 26–27
　for cuts, 149–50
　for fractures, 135–38
　kits, *see* Medical supplies and equipment
　liability for administering, 26–27
　psychiatric, 343–45
　splints, 135–37
　tourniquets, 146–47, 150
　for gunshot wounds, 158
　See also Cardiac resuscitation
Flagyl, 201
Flatulence, 94–96
Fleas, 233
Flu
　colds distinguished from, 175–76
　recovery, length of time for, 179
　shots, 176
　symptoms of, 175–76
Food, *see* Nutrition
Food poisoning, 87–88
Fractured skull, *see* Head injuries
Fractures, 132–41
　bleeding, 136, 138
　casts, dealing with, 138–41
　defined, 133
　detection of, 134, 136
　first aid for, 135–38
　from gunshot wounds, 158
　setting of, 134–35
　splints, 135–37
　types of, 133–34
Free clinics, 14, 17, 387
　directory of, 399–409
Freud, Sigmund, 259–60
Frigidity, 330, 339–40
Frostbite, 244–45

Gall bladder, functioning of, 84
Gas, 94–96
Gastritis, 90
Gastrointestinal tract
   functioning of, 83–84
   See also Abdominal entries; Stomach entries; related entries
General practitioners, 5–6
   See also Doctors
Genitals, *see* Urinary tract infections; Vaginitis; Venereal disease
Globus hystericus, 85
Gonorrhea, 291–97
   current epidemic of, 292–93, 300
   growing resistance to antibiotics, 293
   in infants, 294
   non-specific urethritis (NSU) distinguished from, 191
   preventive measures, 296–97
   symptoms, 293, 294–95
   treatment, 299–300
      need for, 292–93, 295
Grass, *see* Marihuana
Group practice, 6
Gunshot wounds, 156–59
   of chest, 125–28
   emotional effects, 159
   fatal, 158
   legal considerations, 159
   location of, 158
   from military weapons, 157
   resuscitation of victim, 161
   from shotguns, 157
   tetanus from, 159
   tourniquets for, 158

Hair, 102–4
   dandruff, 104–5
   depilatories, 103
   electrolysis, 103
   growth, factors influencing, 104
   shaving, 103
   transplants, 104
Hallucinations, 62
Hallucinogenic drugs, 164, 260–66
   bad trips, 264–66
   duration of action, 261–62
   long-term effects, 263–64
   short-term effects, 262–63
   types of, 260–61
Halitosis, 222–24
Hand, lacerations of, 144
Hard drugs, *see* Opiates
Hashish, 252–54
   defined, 248
   duration of action, 253
   long-term effects, 254
   short-term effects, 253
   See also Marihuana; Drugs, mind-altering
Headaches, 37–38
   with alterations in consciousness, 37–38
   in brain injury, 111
   with confusion, 37–38
   with dizziness, 37–38
   with fever, 38
   migraine, 64
   during pregnancy, 316
   present upon awakening, 37
   sleep-disturbing, 37
   with stiff neck, 38
   sudden, 37
Head injuries, 63, 108–15
   brain damage, 138
      in cardiac arrest, 164
      symptoms, 110–12
   delayed effects, 113–14
   facial injuries, 114–15
   fractured skull, 113
   hematoma, 114
   jaw, fractured, 114
   lacerations, 145–46
   seriousness of, 109–10
   treatment of, 37–38, 112–14
   types of damage, 109

Health departments, 385–86
Health insurance, see Medical insurance
Heart
  beat
    arrhythmia, 78
    irregular, 72–74
    Paroxysmal Atrial Tachycardia (P.A.T.), 74
    pounding, 73–74
    rapid, 73–74
    rate of (pulse), 72–73
  functioning described, 70–71
  rhythm, 72–74
Heart arrest, see Cardiac arrest
Heart attacks
  angina, 76–77
  cardiac arrest caused by, 162
  causes of
    arteriosclerosis, 79
    atherosclerosis, 79
    cholesterol, 80–82
    predisposing factors, 79–80, 81
  chest pain, 76–77
  nature of, 78
  obesity and, 81–82
  prevention, 80–82
  seriousness of, 78
  shock from, 77
Heartburn, 85
  during pregnancy, 317
Heart failure, see Cardiac arrest
Heart murmurs, 82–83
Heart massage, see Cardiac massage
Heart stoppage, see Cardiac arrest
Heat cramps, 242
Heat exhaustion, 242–43
Heat stroke, 243
Hematoma, 114
Hemoglobin, 56
Hemophilia, 56–57
Hemophilus vaginitis, 202
Hemoptysis, 50–51
Hemorrhoids, 192–94
  causes of, 192–93, 194
  nature of, 192
  during pregnancy, 317–18
  removal of, 194
  treatment of, 193–94
Hepatitis, 129–30, 179–85
  and alcoholic beverages, 184
  causes of, 179–81
  from injections, 180–81, 249–50
  jaundice from, 182–83
  mononucleosis distinguished from, 186
  protection from, 184–85
  serum, transmission of, 180–81
  symptoms, 182–83
    severity of, 181–82
  treatment of, 183–85
  types of, 180–81
Heroin, see Opiates
Hiccups, 52–53, 205–7
High altitudes, breathing at, 50, 52
High blood pressure, 37, 75–76
Hives, 101
Homosexuality, 277, 337–39
Honeymoon cystitis, 189–90, 302
Hormones, in weight reduction, 369
Hospitals
  alcohol tests, right to administer, 24
  bed, cost of, 9
  criteria for selecting, 13–16
  drug tests, right to administer, 24
  house staff, 5, 13
  legal obligations to patients, 22–24
  medical school affiliations, 7–8, 13
  non-profit, 8
  policy, setting of, 14
  private, 7, 12
  public, 7–8
  refusal of service, 22

Hospitals (*cont.*)
  trustees of, 14
  types of, 6
  voluntary, 8, 12
  See also Clinics; Emergency rooms
House calls, 18–19
House staff, 5, 13
Hypertension, 37, 75–76
Hyperventilation, 73
  as hiccups cure, 206
  nature, causes, and treatment of, 54–55

Illusions, 62
Immersion foot, 244
Impotence, 330, 339–40
Indigestion, 86–87
  heartburn, 85
  during pregnancy, 317
Induction into military services, *see* Draft deferral
Infections, 148–49
  See also Tetanus
Infectious hepatitis, *see* Hepatitis
Infectious mononucleosis, *see* Mononucleosis
Injections, 121
  dirty needles, 180–81, 249–50
Insects, 230–34, 239–41
  bedbugs, 233
  bees, 240
  centipedes, 241
  chiggers, 233
  fleas, 233
  lice, 231–32
  maggots, 234
  mange, 232–33
  mites, 232–33
  redbugs, 233
  scabies, 232–33
  spiders, 239–40
  ticks, 233–34
Insomnia, 66–68
Internship, 4–5

Intestinal tract, functioning of, 83
Intestines, 84
Itching, 100–1
  beneath plaster casts, 139–40
  rashes, 101–2
  treatment of, 40
IUD (intrauterine device), *see* Birth control methods

Jails, medical care in, 31–33
Jaundice, 182–83
Jaw, fractured, 114

Kidney
  infection, symptoms of, 130
  phenacetin (aspirin) and, 40–41
  stones, 131
  See also Urinary tract infections
Knife wounds, *see* Stab wounds

Lacerations, *see* Cuts
Lactase, 94
Laxatives, 96
  when not to use, 130
Lesbianism, 277, 337–39
Liability
  of doctor, 27–28
  of layman who performs first aid, 26–27
Lice, 231–32
Liniments, 40
Lips, cuts on, 144–45
Liver
  functioning described, 84
  See also Hepatitis
Lizard bites, 239
Lockjaw, *see* Tetanus
Lomotil, 198–99
LSD, *see* Hallucinogenic drugs
Lungs
  collapse of, 123–25
  See also Breathing; Chest injuries; Colds; coughing; Tear gas

Mace, 290-91
  See also Tear gas
Macrobiotic diets, 360-61
Maggots, 234
Malaria, transmission of, 249
Malcolm X, 342-43
Malnutrition
  in drug addicts, 251
  See also Nutrition
Malpractice, 27-28
Mange, 232-33
Marezine, 230
Marihuana, 252-54
  coughing and, 48, 254
  duration of action, 252-54
  long-term effects, 254
  during pregnancy, 320
  short-term effects, 253
  See also Hashish; Drugs, mind-altering
Mass arrests, medical care during, 31-32
MCHR, *see* Medical Committee for Human Rights
Meclezine (Bonine), 230
Medicaid, 11-12
Medical care
  good, general rules for finding, 13-17
  quality of
    for middle class, 10-11
    for poor people, 11-12
    for rich people, 9-10
    in rural areas, 12
  See also Doctors; Hospitals
Medical Committee for Human Rights, 29, 33, 387-88
  chapters, listing of, 393-98
  nature of, 13
Medical costs
  blanket fees, 9
  for clinic treatment, 16
  for emergency room treatment, 16
  "fee for service" system, 9
  for hospital beds, 9
  inflated, avoidance of, 10-11
  legal obligations for payment of, 27
  Medicaid, 11-12
  Medicare, 10
  for middle class, 10-11
  for poor people, 11-12
  prepayment plans, 9, 10-11
  prohibitive nature of, 9
  and quality of care, relationship between, 9-12
  for rich people, 9-10
  and selection of hospital or doctor, 14
  for welfare recipients, 11-12
Medical insurance, 10-11
  Medicaid, 11-12
  Medicare, 10
  system described, 10-11
Medical supplies and equipment, 371-87
  buying, 389
  determination of needs, 371-75
  free, 385-88
  kits, 374-84
    personal supply (simple) kits, 375-78
    portable (intermediate) kits, 378-81
    stationary (sophisticated) kits, 381-84
  types of, 374
  where to obtain, 384-89
Medicare, 10
Medicine
  average person's attitude toward, 3
  as a business, 3
  mystique of, 3
  self-policing activities, 4
  See also Doctors, related entries
Meningitis, 38
Menopause, 204-5
  nature of, 204
  symptoms of, 204-5
  treatment of, 205

Menstruation
  acne and, 220–21
  anemia from, 58, 357–58
  discomfort
    causes of, 203
    symptoms of, 203
    treatment of, 203–4
Mental illness, 30–31
  See also Psychiatric problems
Mental patients
  commitment proceedings, 30–31
    involuntary, 30–31
    voluntary, 30
  rights of, 31
Mescaline, *see* Hallucinogenic drugs
Methadone, 267, 271–72
Micturition syncope, 61
Migraine, 64
  See also Headaches
Military service, *see* Draft deferment
Milk, 351
  allergy to, 93–94
  need for, 197–98
Minors
  "emancipated," defined, 25–26
  obtaining treatment for, 25–26
Mites, 232–33
Monilia, 201–2
Mononucleosis, 186–87
  epidemics of, 186
  hepatitis distinguished from, 186
  symptoms of, 186–87
  treatment of, 187
Morphine, 39, 41, 42
  cocaine compared with, 259
  See also Opiates
Motion sickness, 227–30
Mouth
  abscesses, 215–16
  teeth injuries, 216
  See also Cuts

Mouth-to-mouth resuscitation, 166–68
  See also Cardiac resuscitation
Muscle
  cramps, 242
  ruptured tendons, 137
  strains, 134, 137
  weakness, 111
Mushrooms, poisonous, 88
Myocardial infarction
  defined, 78
  See also Heart attacks

Nasal decongestants, 208–9
Nausea, 88
  See also Vomiting
Neck
  broken, 112–13
    treatment of, 138
  stiff, 38
Nervous breakdown, 59
  See also Psychiatric problems
Nervousness, 59
  anxiety, 59–60
  See also Psychiatric problems
Nose
  bleeding, 207–10
  nasal decongestants, 208–9
NSU (non-specific urethritis), 191
Numbness, 111
Nutrition
  acne and, 218, 220
  beans, 353
  breads, 352–53
  calories, 349
  cereals, 352–53
  confusion about, 347–48
  general recommendations, 362–64
  on low budget, 351–54
  macrobiotic diets, 360–61
  milk and milk products, 351
  organic foods, 359–60
  planning for emergency situations, 354–55

Nutrition (*cont.*)
    during pregnancy, 322–23
    requirements for, 348–51
    vitamins, 355–58
    See also Milk

Obesity, 364–70
    age and, 367
    amphetamines for, 368–69
    diets, 365–67
        group support for, 367–68
    drugs for, 368–69
    health effects of, 364
    heart attacks and, 81–82
    hereditary causes of, 367
    hormone treatment of, 369
    medications for, 368–69
    physical causes of, 364, 367
    pills for, 368–69
    psychological help for, 369
    weight-reducing pills, 368–69
Opiates
    long-term effects, 268
    methadone, 267, 271–72
    morphine and heroin, differences between, 269–70
    nature of, 266–67
    overdoses, 270–71
    short-term effects, 266–68
    withdrawal from, 268–69
    See also Codeine; Morphine
Organic foods, 359–60
Otitis, *see* Earache
Overbreathing, *see* Hyperventilation
Overweight, *see* Obesity

Pain, 34–42
    abdominal, 92–93, 129–31
    characteristics of, 35
    chest, 76–77
    crotch, 191
    emotional vs. physical, 35
    headaches, 37–38
    individual variability in reaction to, 35
    intensity of, 35
    perception of, threshold levels in, 35
    physical vs. emotional, 35
    treatment of, 38–42
        aspirin, 40–41
        codeine, 42
        cold, 39–40
        counter-irritants, 40
        Darvon, 41, 42
        Demerol, 42
        heat, 39
        liniments, 40
        morphine, 41–42
        non-drug, 39–40
        non-prescription drug, 40–41
        prescription drug, 41–42
    when to worry about it, 35–37
    See also specific medical problems
Pancreas, functioning of, 84
Paranoia, 64
Parasitic infestation, 196
Paroxysmal atrial tachycardia (P.A.T.), 74
People's clinics, *see* Community (people's) clinics
Perversion, sexual, 336–40
Peyote, *see* Hallucinogenic drugs
Phenacetin
    defined, 40
    and kidney problems, 40–41
    See also Aspirin
Phlebitis, *see* Thrombophlebitis
Phlegm, *see* Coughing
Physicians, *see* Doctors
Piles, *see* Hemorrhoids
Pill, the, *see* Birth control methods
Pimples, *see* Acne
Planned Parenthood Agency, 326
Plasma, 56
Platelets, 56
Pneumothorax, 123–25

Poisoning
  food, 87–88
  mushroom, 88
Poison ivy, 100–1
Police, dealing with, 23–24, 150, 159
Political demonstrators, *see* Demonstrators
Pot, *see* Marihuana
Pregnancy
  abortion, 324–26, 328
  alcoholic beverages during, 320
  bleeding during, 316
  blood clots caused by, 225
  blurred vision caused by, 316
  breast-feeding, 324
  constipation during, 320–31
  deciding whether to have baby, 313
  delivery
    date, calculation of, 319
    home, 314–15
    natural childbirth, 315
  detection of, 312–13
  douching during, 321
  drug-taking during, 264, 319–20
  exercise during, 321
  headaches during, 316
  heartburn during, 317
  hemorrhoids caused by, 192, 317–18
  infant mortality, 314–15
  labor, 323–24
  maternal mortality, 314–15
  medical care, need for, 313–15
  medical problems of, 315–23
  morning sickness, 316–17
  nutrition during, 322–23
  sexual relations during, 320
  smoking during, 320
  swelling of feet and ankles caused by, 316
  travel during, 321–22
  urinary frequency during, 318
  urinary tract infections during, 189
  vaginal discharge during, 317
  varicose veins caused by, 318
Prepayment system, 10–11
Prisons, medical care in, 31–33
Privacy of treatment, right to, 28
Privileged medical information
  defined, 28
  See also Confidentiality of medical information
Prostrate gland, swelling of, 191
Psilocybin, *see* Hallucinogenic drugs
Psychiatric problems, 329–46
  alcoholism, 340–42
  amateur help for, 343–45
  anxiety, 59–60
  depression, 60, 331–33
  drug addiction, 246–47, 277, 342–43
  frigidity, 330, 339–40
  impotence, 330, 339–40
  obesity, 369
  professional help
    how to find, 345–46
    need for, 344–45
  sexual deviation and perversion, 336–40
  suicide, 333–35
  triggering factors, 329–30
  See also Mental illness; Mental patients
Psychotropic drugs, *see* Drugs, mind-altering
Ptomaine poisoning, 87–88
Public assistance recipients, medical assistance plans for, 11–12
Pulse, 72–73
  in brain injury, 112
Puncture wounds, 150
  See also Tetanus

Rabies, 234–37
Rape, 326–38

Rashes, 101–2
Rectum, *see* Anus; Hemorrhoids
Redbugs, 233
Red Cross, American, 386–87
Red blood cells, 56
Referrals, 6
Reportable diseases, 29–30
Residency, 5
Rib injuries, 120–23
Rural areas, medical care in, 12

Scabies, 232–33
Schistosomiasis, 196
Sclera, defined, 116
Scopolamine, 68
Scorpion bites, 240
Scratches, *see* Cuts
Seasickness, 227–30
Sedatives
　nature of, 39
　See also Barbiturates; Drugs
Selective Service, *see* Draft deferment
Serum, blood, 56
Serum hepatitis, *see* Hepatitis
Sexual relations
　counselors, 300–1
　deviation and perversion, 336–40
　among elderly people, 302–3
　frigidity, 330, 339–40
　honeymoon cystitis, 189–90, 302
　hymen, 302
　impotence, 330, 339–40
　manuals, 301–2
　during pregnancy, 320
　premarital experimentation, 302
　rape, 326–28
　See also Birth control methods
Shaving, 103
Shock, 106–8
　causes of, 106–7
　diagnosing, 107–8
　in heart attacks, 77
　nature of, 106
　treatment of, 108
Sinuses, congested, 37
Skin, 97–102
　bacteria, 99
　bluish color of, 51–52, 163–64
　burns, classification of, 98
　characteristics of, 97–98
　dermis, 98
　epidermis, 98
　itching, 40, 100–1, 139–40
　rashes, 101–2
　See also Sweating
Skull injuries, *see* Head injuries
Sleep
　dreaming, 67
　insomnia, 66–68
　requirements, individual variations in, 66–67
　sleepiness, in brain injury, 110
　sleeping pills, 68
Smoke poisoning, 153
Smoking
　asthma and, 53
　coughing and, 47, 48, 254
　heart attacks and, 79
　during pregnancy, 320
Snakebites, 237–39
Sneezing, 52
　See also Colds; Coughing
Sodium salicylate
　defined, 40
　See also Aspirin
Sore throat, *see* Colds; Strep throat
Spanish fly, 241
Specialists, 5
Speed, 248, 257–58
　and cardiac arrest, 162
Spider bites, 239–40
Spine, broken, 112–13
　treatment of, 138
Spit, bloody, 50–51
Splints, 135–37
Spock, Benjamin, 324

Sprains, 134, 137
  ankle, 39–40
Sputum, defined, 47
Stab wounds, 156–59
  of chest, 125–28
  emotional effects of, 159
  fatal, 158
  legal considerations, 150, 159
  resuscitation of victim, 161
  tetanus from, 159
  See also Cuts
Sternum
  defined, 85
  injury, 120–23
Stiff neck, 38
Stimulants
  defined, 248
  See also Drugs, mind-altering
Stitches, 143
Stomach
  belching, 94–95
  defined, 83
  gas, 94–96
  hiccups, 52–53
  indigestion, 86–87, 317
  inflammation of, 90
  irritation of, aspirin as cause, 41
  noises, 96
  See also Abdominal entries; Vomiting
Stool
  bloody, 91, 97, 129, 132, 193, *See also* Constipation; Diarrhea
STP, *see* Hallucinogenic drugs
Strains, 134
  treatment of, 137
Strep throat
  colds distinguished from, 175–76
  symptoms of, 175
  treatment of, 176–79
Student health clinics, 14, 16
  confidentiality of medical records in, 16
Stupor, 69

Suicide, 333–35
  See also Depression
Sunburn, 151–52
  treatment of, 153–54
Sunstroke, 241–43
Supplies and equipment, *see* Medical supplies and equipment
Swallowing
  of air, 95
  difficulty in, 85
Sweating, 98–100, 242
  drug control of, 99
  odor, elimination of, 99–100
  purpose of, 98
  types of sweat, 98–99
Swelling
  of feet and ankles, 316
  of legs, 82
  treatment of, 39–40
Syphilis, 291–94, 297–98
  current epidemic of, 298–99
  diagnosis of, 298–99
  growing resistance to antibiotics, 293, 295
  symptoms of, 293–94, 297–98
  transmission of, 249, 291, 294, 299
  treatment of, 299–300
    need for, 292–93

Tear gas, 278–91
  asthma and, 50, 54
  BBC, 283
  cardiac arrest from, 162
  CN, 282
  CNC, 282
  CNS, 283
  coughing of blood caused by, 51
  CS (pepper), 282–83
  mace, 290–91
  nature of, 281–82
  treatment for, 283–88
    CNS, 287–88
    CS, 287

Tear gas (*cont.*)
  decontamination of rooms, 286
  eyes, 284–85
  lungs, 286
  skin, 285–86
  See also Chemical warfare agents
Teeth
  broken or knocked out, 216
  toothache, 214–16
Temperature, body
  air temperature compared with, 42
  body's regulation of, 42–43
  normal, individual variations in, 43, 44
  oral, 43, 44
  range, normal, 42
  rectal, 43
  taking of, 43–44
  See also Fever
Tendon
  ruptured, 137
  See also Muscle
Tetanus, 140, 150, 170–73
  from burns, 155
  causes of, 171
  from gunshot and stab wounds, 159
  immunization, 171–73
  from injections, 250
  lethality of, 170–71
Thermometer
  use of, 44
  See also Temperature, body
Thrombophlebitis, 224–27
  from injections, 250–51
Ticks, 233–34
Title XIX, *see* Medicaid
Tingling, 111
Tiredness, anemia and, 57–58
Toothache, 214–16
Tourniquets, 146–47, 150
  for gunshot wounds, 158
Toxins, 171

Tranquilizers
  nature of, 39
  See also Barbiturates; Drugs
Trench foot, 344
Trichomonas, 201

Ulcers, 90–92
  antacid treatment for, 91–92
  bleeding, 57
  causes of, 90–91
  duodenal, 90
  gastric, 90
  peptic, 90
  symptoms of, 91
Ultraviolet lamps, 219
Urethritis, non-specific (NSU), 191
Urinary tract, functioning described, 188
Urinary tract infections, 188–91
  causes of, 189–90
  health significance of, 189
  location of, 188
  symptoms of, 188–89, 190
  treatment of, 190
  urine, characteristics of, 189
  See also Kidneys, Vaginitis
Urination
  fainting during (micturation syncope), 61
  frequent, 318
Urine, color of, 189

Vaginal discharge, during pregnancy, 317
Vaginitis, 199–202
  causes of, 199–201
  hemophilus, 202
  monilia, 201–2
  non-specific, 202
  trichomonas, 201
Varicose veins, 318
Veins, 71–72
  inflamed, *see* Thrombophlebitis
Venereal disease, 291–98
  current epidemic of, 292–93

Venereal disease (*cont.*)
    future of, 300
    from rape, 328
    transmission of, 291, 294
    treatment of, 299–300
        need for, 292–93
    See also Gonorrhea; Syphilis
Vertigo, *see* Dizziness
Virus
    symptoms of, 45
    See also Colds; Flu; Strep throat
Vision
    blurred or double, 111, 316
    See also Eye
Vitamins, 355–58
    A, 221
    B, 233, 357
    C, 353–54, 357
    E, 356
    See also Nutrition
Vomiting
    of blood, 50–51, 89–90, 91, 129
    and brain injury, 110–11
    bursting of blood vessels, esophagus, or stomach from, 89
    breathing down vomit (aspiration), 89
    dehydration from, 89
    of greenish material, 90
    and internal injury, 132
    process described, 88
    types of vomit, 129

Water, impurities in, 197–98
Weight reduction, *see* Obesity
Welfare recipients, medical assistance plans for, 11–12
White blood cells, 56
Wounds, *see* Bites; Burns; Cuts; Gunshot wounds; Stab wounds; Tear gas

X-ray treatment, 222

Yellow jaundice, *see* Hepatitis

ABOUT THE AUTHORS

STUART FRANK attended public school in New York, where he was born in 1934. He received his B.S. from MIT, and his M.D. in 1960 from New York University. He took his postgraduate training at Yale–New Haven Hospital, the Institute of Cardiology in London, and the National Heart Institute in Bethesda, Maryland. He practices medicine and cardiology in San Francisco, where he is also a Clinical Assistant Professor of Medicine at the University of California, San Francisco Medical Center. His community health involvements include working with the Haight-Ashbury Medical Clinic and helping to organize the Medical Committee for Human Rights.

ARTHUR FRANK is a physician specializing in internal medicine and public health in Washington, D.C. Like his twin brother Stuart, he was born in New York and attended MIT, where he received his B.S. He also secured an M.S. from the University of Pennsylvania before taking his M.D. at New York University in 1962. His postgraduate work included study at Stanford Medical Center and the National Heart Institute. He is currently a member of the faculty at Georgetown University School of Medicine and the Medical Director of the Georgetown University Community Health Plan. His past medical experience includes being Deputy Director of the Comprehensive Health Services Program OEO, and chairman of the Washington, D.C., chapter of the Medical Committee for Human Rights, and coordinating and planning medical care in demonstrations in Washington, D.C.